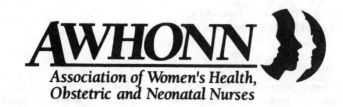

AWHONN

Association of Women's Health, Obstetric and Neonatal Nurses

Liability Issues in Perinatal Nursing

Donna Miller Rostant, RN, MSN, JD
Associate Attorney
Hall and Sickels, P.C.
Reston, Virginia

Rebecca F. Cady, RNC, BSN, JD
Associate Attorney
Grace, Brandon, Hollis, and Ramirez, L.L.P.
San Diego, California

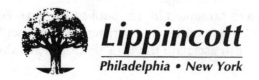
Lippincott
Philadelphia • New York

Acquisitions Editor: Jennifer E. Brogan
Coordinating Editorial Assistant: Susan V. Barta
Production Manager: Helen Ewan
Production Service: Diane Ratto, Michael Bass & Associates
Compositor: Andrea Reider, Michael Bass & Associates
Printer/Binder: Victor Graphics, Inc.
Second edition

9 8 7 6 5 4 3 2

Library of Congress Cataloging-in-Publication Data

Rostant, Donna Miller.
    Liability Issues in perinatal nursing / Donna Miller Rostant, Rebecca F. Cady.
      p. cm.
    At head of title: AWHONN, Association of Women's Health, Obstetric, and Neonatal Nurses.
    Includes bibliographical references and index.
    ISBN 0-397-55276-9
    1. Nurses—Malpractice—United States. 2. Maternity nursing—Law and legislation—United States.
I. Cady, Rebecca F. II. Association of Women's Health, Obstetric, and Neonatal Nurses. III. Title.
      [DNLM. 1. Malpractice—United States nurses' instruction. 2. Neonatal Nursing—United States
legislation. 3. Liability, Legal—United States nurses' instruction. WY 44 AA1R838L 1999]
KF2915.N83R67 1999
344.73'0414—dc21
DNLM/DLC
for Library of Congress
                                          98-27994
                                            CIP

CONTRIBUTORS

Suzanne McMurtry Baird, RN, MSN
Instructor in the Practice of Nursing
Clinical Placement Coordinator
Vanderbilt University School of Nursing
Nashville, Tennessee
Senior Consultant, Critical Care Obstetrics
Harvey, Troiano, and Associates, Inc.
Houston, Texas

Diana C. Ballard, RN, MBA, JD
Susman, Duffy and Segaloff, P.C.
Attorneys at Law
55 New Whitney Avenue
New Haven, Connecticut
President, Ballard Management Group
Health Care Consultants
175 East Mitchell Avenue
Cheshire, Connecticut

Cathy Beffa, JD, BSN, RN
Risk Management Consultant
FSM Health Care
St. Louis, Missouri

Paula Lashenske Burgess, BSN, MHA, ARM
Risk Manager
Duke University Medical Center
Durham, North Carolina

Kimberly E. Carr, RN, MSN
Supervisor, Children's Transport Team
Wake Med
Raleigh, North Carolina

Pamela Copeland, BSN, JD, ARM
Director, Risk Management/Associate General
    Counsel
Greater Southeast Community Hospital
Washington, D. C.

Carolyn A. B. Curtis, RN, BSN, MSN, CNM,
    FACNM
Acting Director
Nurse Midwifery Services
District of Columbia Health and Hospitals
Public Benefit Corporation
Washington, D.C.
Instructor
Howard University College of Nursing
Graduate Program
Washington, D.C.

Susan B. Drummond, RN, MSN
Clinical Nurse Specialist
Department of Obstetrics and Gynecology
Vanderbilt University Medical Center
Nashville, Tennessee

Patricia Fedorka, RNC, PhD
Assistant Professor
School of Nursing
Duquesne University
Pittsburgh, Pennsylvania
Staff Nurse
Allegheny General Hospital
Pittsburgh, Pennsylvania

Paula DiMeo Grant, RN, BSN, MA, JD
Court Mediator of Counsel
Ross and Hardies
Washington, D.C.
Adjunct Assistant Professor Nursing
Sacred Heart University
Fairfield, Connecticut

Carolyn J. Harris, RN, MSN, JD
Assistant Professor/Assistant Dean
Student Affairs
Howard University
Washington, D.C.

Teresa Dossey James, RN, CNM, MSN
Research Coordinator, OB/GYN Department
Wilford Hall USAF Medical Center
Lackland Air Force Base, Texas

Beverly Butler Karasick, RN, BSN, MSN
Vice President
Medical Management
University of South Florida
Tampa, Florida

Debi Law, RNC, BSN
Clinical Nurse
Duke Birthing Center
Duke University Medical Center
Durham, North Carolina

Michelle Murray, PhD, RNC
CEO
Learning Resources International, Inc.
Albuquerque, New Mexico
Perinatal Clinical Nurse Specialist
Lovelace Medical Center
Albuquerque, New Mexico
Adjunct Faculty
University of New Mexico
Albuquerque, New Mexico
and
University of Missouri, Kansas City
Kansas City, Missouri

Jan Nick, PhD, RNC
Assistant Professor
Loma Linda School of Nursing
Loma Linda, California

Pamela J. Reidy, Col. USAF, NC, BSN, MS
Clinical Quality Manager
Office of the Command Surgeon
Headquarters, Air Combat Command
United States Air Force
Langley Air Force Base, Virginia

Mary Catherine Rubert, RN, BA, BS, JD
Connelly and Connelly, P.C.
Attorneys at Law
North Babylon, New York
Clinical Assistant Professor
Community and Preventive Medicine
    Department
New York Medical College
Valhalla, New York

Lois L. Salmeron, EdD, RNC, BSN, MAT, MSN
Professor, Division Head, Health Services
Department Head, Nurse Science
Oklahoma State University
Oklahoma City, Oklahoma

Barbara Peterson Sinclair, MN, RNC, OGNP,
    FAAN
Professor of Nursing and Director, Institute of
    Nursing
California State University, Los Angeles
Los Angeles, California

Davia Solomon, BSN, JD
Associate
Joseph G. Hurley Law Corporation
North Hollywood, California

Mabel Smith-Pittman, RN, JD, PhD
Associate Professor, School of Nursing
College of Health Science
Old Dominion University
Norfolk, Virginia

Christine A. Sullivan, PhD, MSN, CNM, CNAA
Nurse-Midwife/Nurse-Administrator
Women's Health
Bixby Medical Center
Adrian, Michigan
Clinical Faculty
University of Michigan
Ann Arbor, Michigan

Trish King-Urbanski, MSN, RNC, CCE, SNM
Nurse Educator/Licensed Clinical Specialist
University Hospital
Albuquerque, New Mexico

In Chinese calligraphy the symbol used for *Chaos* means "crisis and opportunity." Because we live in a highly litigious society, it often seems we live in chaos. No where is it more evident than in the specialty areas that AWHONN represents, because perinatal malpractice cases are among the highest in number and monetary awards. Awareness of these facts may cause an uneasiness and, in fact, look like a crisis. However, a crisis can be an opportunity.

Knowledge of the law and its effect on the health care system, and ultimately the individual nurse, is essential for today's practicing perinatal nurse. It is through this knowledge that we are provided with many opportunities. Nurses can pro-actively identify legal risks and develop strategies to reduce them. This process of critical examination of legal risks can then improve our patient care. Informed consent is one example. Providing informed consent may protect health care professionals from the crisis of malpractice suits and also provides an opportunity for education. As informed consent is provided, we form partnerships with our patients and provide them the opportunity to increase control of their own health.

Career opportunities may also spring from increasing our knowledge of the law. Nurses provide their professional services to malpractice lawyers by reviewing charts of potential cases and advising the lawyer whether or not there is merit to the claim. For those cases that move forward, knowledgeable nurses may provide their professional services as expert witnesses for the plaintiff or the defendant. And some nurses may take the opportunity to further their education as a lawyer and work full time in this field.

The editors of *AWHONN's Liability Issues in Perinatal Nursing*, Donna Miller Rostant and Rebecca F. Cady, have provided us with an excellent resource. With the knowledge we glean from this book we can face what seems like chaos and crisis and provide ourselves with many opportunities.

Patsy Kennedy, RNC, WHNP
1998 AWHONN President

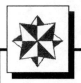

The Association of Women's Health, Obstetric and Neonatal Nurses

The Association of Women's Health, Obstetric and Neonatal Nurses (AWHONN), an organization comprised of 22,000 health care professionals, promotes excellence in nursing practice to improve the health of women and newborns. Through dynamic programs, services and community outreach, AWHONN strives to enrich not only the health and well-being, but the

ACKNOWLEDGMENTS

Undertaking a project of this magnitude was not an easy task and in the late night hours of editing, I frequently questioned the wisdom of agreeing to do so. However, knowing that nurses needed the information, that it was available, and that it could potentially prevent an untoward outcome was a driving motivation. Other motivating forces included the encouragement and support from many family members and friends. I could never have finished it without the support of either. Special thanks and much love go to my sons, Joey and Andy, for understanding and accepting my responsibility to the project as I worked late into the night. My husband provided me with the love and the encouragement to continue moving forward as deadlines loomed ahead. Special thanks to Rebecca Cady for her enthusiasm and drive which was like a breath of fresh air as we headed to the finish line. Fay Rycyna of AWHONN and Jennifer Brogan and Susan Barta of Lippincott-Raven were instrumental in pulling the final product together and getting over many last minute hurdles.

Finally, many thanks and much love to my mother and father, Barbara and the memory of Gordon Miller, to whom this book is dedicated. Thank you for teaching me to believe in myself and to know that I could accomplish anything if I tried hard enough. That belief carried me through my nursing education as well as law school and continues to drive me today. My father's unexpected death will prevent him from seeing the book in print, but I know he knows.

PREFACE

I became aware of the tremendous fear nurses had of being sued when I worked as a clinical educator in a large tertiary health care setting. With a full complement of attending obstetricians, midwives, residents, student midwives, perinatalogists, nurses, and student nurses, on a background of a largely indigent population with more than 10,000 deliveries per year, errors in patient care seemed inevitable. Part of my responsibilities included reviewing potential and actual lawsuits to determine if a meritorious defense could be mounted against a wily plaintiff's lawyer. I recall being frustrated in my many unsuccessful attempts to convince the risk manager that the alleged negligent action of the nurse could easily be understood when all of the circumstances were taken into consideration. Inadequate fetal heart rate monitoring could have resulted from antiquated or unavailable equipment. Patient assessment errors could easily be attributed to short staffing or mistakes made from fatigue. Each time the risk manager and defense counsel would sadly shake their heads, explaining that the law required a nurse's duty to be fulfilled and in spite of my many attempts to justify the act or omission, the law would likely determine that the plaintiff would be successful in their allegations. Huge verdicts or settlements often followed as the nurses involved would shake their heads in disbelief. No wonder nurses panicked every time the "perfect newborn" did not appear.

There is no question that an adverse outcome during the perinatal period has a devastating effect on the family unit. Expectations are great at the time of delivery and technological advances have led us to believe that a perfect infant will be born every time. When an infant is born with an injury, hopes are dashed, disappointment and despair move in, and despondency and anger follow. Often, a lawsuit results. A good plaintiff's attorney and an injured child, in front of a jury, can and often do yield multi-million dollar verdicts. For the defendant health care provider, devastation, depression, and feelings of decreased self worth quickly set in, for not only does the nurse grieve for the family's poor outcome, he or she must now face the reality of knowing that one or more of his or her actions led to the outcome. Such a tragic outcome for all involved and yet, in many instances, so preventable.

The writing of *Liability Issues in Perinatal Nursing* was undertaken to fulfill a void in the perinatal nursing arena—that is, a synopsis of the specific legal issues directly affecting the practice of perinatal nursing. It is no secret that nurses are increasingly being named as defendants in lawsuits. Substantial damage awards for obstetrical and neonatal malpractice make nurses in these areas attractive targets. Often, a simple lack of knowledge of legal responsibilities places a nurse at risk for being a defendant in a lawsuit. The editors hope that an awareness of legal issues in the perinatal setting will allow nurses to understand what the law requires of them while providing patient care and preventing nursing negligence and malpractice.

Although the twenty-four chapters encompass a wide variety of topics related to perinatal nursing liability, the book does not pretend to be an all-inclusive exploration of potential liability of health care providers. Nor should the book be used as a substitute for legal counsel and the editors caution the reader that no legal advice has been provided. Instead, the book is intended to provide an overview of the current legal issues within the perinatal setting. Each chapter has been written by an author with noted expertise in the area. Where appropriate, actual legal cases are used to illustrate key points and to demonstrate application of legal principles in the health care setting.

Unit I provides chapters illustrating an overview of the sources and classifications of law as well as an exploration of various theories of liability in which a nurse or institution can be held responsible for negligent acts or omissions. The standard of care for nurses is defined and analyzed, as is professional negligence and malpractice. The unit concludes with a chapter providing a well-defined look at the trial process.

Unit II begins with a general look at the scope of perinatal liability followed by critical care obstetrics which illustrates specific liability issues for nurses working with critically ill obstetric patients. Other chapters provide insight into responsibilities of the nurse assessing the patient in labor as well as fetal heart rate monitoring roles and responsibilities. The unit concludes with a summary of the responsibilities of the nurse when using pitocin during labor.

Unit III begins with a focus on the neonate, including resuscitation, transfer, and nursery responsibilities. Telephone triage and office nurse responsibilities are included as are home health and ambulatory nursing roles and duties.

Unit IV includes chapters on patient rights, informed consent, the HIV-positive patient, staffing, documentation, and liability of the nurse educator. Nurse-physician communication is included as is the nurse as an expert witness. The unit concludes with chapters that focus on professional liability insurance, advanced nursing practice, and computer technologies.

Many medical malpractice and professional negligence lawsuits can be prevented. Education and knowledge of legal principles and their application to the clinical setting provide better insight into the prevention of negligent actions. This book is intended to provide an overview of the law as it is applied in a perinatal setting. The book is not intended to provide legal advice and does not do so. Instead, it offers the reader an opportunity to gain insight into the often confusing world of malpractice litigation and proposes strategies to decrease liability exposure. Hopefully, the reader will find that *Liability Issues in Perinatal Nursing* fulfills its purpose.

CONTENTS

The Law in General

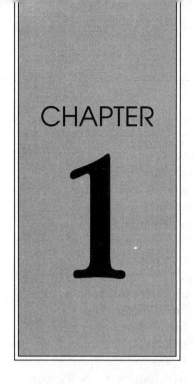

CHAPTER

1

Sources and Classification of Law

Donna Miller Rostant

Various laws and regulations affect the delivery of perinatal nursing care. To thoroughly understand the legal forces that impact nursing practice, one must understand the sources and classifications of law. This chapter provides a general overview of the definition and scope of law, forms of government, and sources and classifications of laws that affect the delivery of health care and the regulation of nursing.

DEFINITION AND SCOPE OF THE TERM "LAW"

Law is defined as that which is laid down, ordained, or established (Black, 1990). In a very generic sense, the word law means a body of rules of action or conduct prescribed by controlling authority, and having binding legal force (*United States Fidelity and Guaranty Co. v. Guenther,* 1930). The term law is very broad and quite correctly refers to many things, including reference to a body of principles, rules, or standards; commands that cause a person to act or not act in a certain manner; administrative agency rules and regulations; state legislative actions and judicial decisions; and long-established local custom that has the force of law (*United States Fidelity and Guaranty Co. v. Guenther*). Laws are essential to an orderly and civilized society.

ORIGINS OF LAW

Law is usually derived from one of three sources: legislation, judicial precedents or case law, or custom. Governmental bodies enact legislation or statutes, court decisions result in judicial precedents or case law, and long-standing patterns of custom result in customary law. Administrative agencies also set forth various rules and regulations that may affect health care providers. Regardless of the source, the nurse should be aware of the most pertinent laws that affect health care. Ignorance of the law is not a reasonable excuse in any liability setting.

GOVERNMENTAL BODIES AND LIMITATIONS ON LEGISLATION

Three levels of government exist in the United States: federal, state, and local. At the federal level, the United States Congress is comprised of senators and representatives from each state who have the overall goal of preserving and improving the welfare of the nation as a whole. Among the many functions of Congress is the enactment of federal legislation that applies to all states. In addition to the federal government, each state has its own state government with state-based congressional senators and/or representatives to enact state legislation. State governments enact laws that, in theory, only apply to the individual state. Finally, local municipalities within a state have representatives who may enact various ordinances for the efficient running of that particular community. No matter what the level, these forms of government are created by law and thus are obligated to conduct themselves and legislate within the powers bestowed upon them. Before a legislative body acts, it must have legal authority to do so. Thus no legislature can enact a law that is unauthorized by a higher level of authority.

The Supremacy Clause of the United States Constitution identifies the Constitution as the supreme law of the land, which obligates all forms of government to make laws consistent with its provisions (Article VI, Constitution of the United States of America). A specific power for the federal government to act must be found within the United States Constitution. That is, if the particular governmental power is not found, explicitly or impliedly, within the Constitution, it cannot exist. No legislative body, federal or state, can enact legislation that is contrary to the provisions of the Constitution.

The United States Constitution mandates that each state has its own legislative body. The makeup of the state legislature, its court system, and its government is set forth in the state constitution. The state constitution provides for state-controlled actions, consistent with those of the United States Constitution. Unlike the United States Constitution, state constitutions provide for plenary power, which allows a state to have unlimited powers restrained only by the limitations set forth in the United States Constitution. Generally, the ability to regulate health care in a particular state is within the state's police powers. The police powers of a state allow a state to place restraints on individual freedom as well as property rights of persons for the overall protection of the public safety, health, and morals. Thus a state can regulate licensing of health care providers subsequent to its role to protect the public safety and health. The state can enact legislation to protect these same principles. However, the police power of a state is always subject to the limitations found within the federal and state constitutions. That is, unless a law can survive a constitutional challenge, it is not valid.

Laws are presumed to be constitutionally valid. In most cases, the standard of review for whether a law is constitutional or not is the rational basis test. The rational basis test simply requires that the law have a rational basis to the goal the legislature intended to accomplish. The burden is on the person challenging the law to show there is not a rational relationship between the law and the goal it is intended to accomplish. This is the lowest level of scrutiny applied to a law and as a practical matter, most laws can readily withstand a rational relationship test.

A law must meet a higher level of scrutiny if the class of persons it affects is a "protected class." Some classes of persons are "protected" because of the special characteristics of the group. Laws that affect persons of a particular alienage or race are subject to strict scrutiny. If a law affects only a "protected" class of persons, the state must show more than a rational relationship between the law and the goal it hoped to achieve. Illegitimate children and gender provoke an intermediate level of scrutiny in which the person challenging the law must show he or she is a member of the protected class. Once the person is proved to be a member of the protected class, the state must show it had a substantial interest in achieving the goal. If the law affects a protected class (usually a particular race or aliens) or if a fundamental right is involved, the standard of review for the law is elevated substantially. Some examples of fundamental rights include the right to vote, the right to privacy, and the right to travel freely between the states. When a protected class or a fundamental right is involved, the state must have a compelling interest in achieving the goal intended.

Statutes

Statutes are formal written enactments (laws) of a legislative body. To alert all to their presence, statutes are published in various sources for persons to review.

Federal Statutes

Federal statutes are those laws enacted by the United States Congress that apply to each state. One example is the "anti-dumping" legislation of 42 U.S.C. Section 1395dd, which is contained within the Consolidated Omnibus Budget Reconciliation Act of 1986 (COBRA). This legislation prohibits a hospital from transferring patients solely as a result of financial status. COBRA was enacted in response to a national epidemic of "dumping," that is, the practice by hospitals of refusing emergency care to indigent patients outright or of transferring such patients without regard to the necessity for stabilizing their condition, to other (typically public) hospitals. All hospitals receiving Medicare funds are obliged to follow the provisions of anti-dumping legislation or be subject to civil penalties (*Owens v. Nacogdoches County Hospital District,* 1990).

Federal statutes are commonly referred to as codes and may be published in one of three ways. Individual slip opinions are laws that have been recently enacted. Federal laws are also compiled within a certain time period, such as a session of Congress, and published. Finally, all federal laws are published in a complete unified code book. The unified codes are published in a series of hardcover books that contain all of the public laws currently in effect. The United States Code (U.S.C.) is the official publication of federal statutes and is printed by the U.S. Government Printing Office. The Codes may also be found in two unofficial publications, the United States Code Annotated (U.S.C.A.) and the United States Code Service (U.S.C.S.). The Codes are organized by subject matter (Cournoyer, 1989). The Codes and other legal resources are also available on the Internet at www.counselquest.com.

State Statutes

States also enact legislation. Although the federal government is concerned with the safety and welfare of the nation as a whole, regulation of occupational groups, including health care providers, is left to the individual states. State statutes are also published. The name of the statutes differs from state to state. For example, in North Carolina state laws are referred to as the North Carolina General Statutes; in Virginia, they are commonly known as the Code of Virginia. Most public libraries as well as state courthouse libraries have the complete publication of statutes for the particular state.

In a medical malpractice or nursing negligence case, relevant statutes are reviewed to determine whether the individual health care provider complied with the statutory restrictions or requirements. An example of state legislation that affects nursing practice is mandatory state licensure. Each state has a requirement that all persons functioning in the role of a registered nurse be licensed by the state before nursing care can be delivered to state citizens. Such licensure is granted by the state, usually through the State Board of Nursing, once the nurse completes an appropriate course of academic and clinical study and successfully completes a competency examination. Performing functions of a registered nurse without a license is a violation of most state statutes and will expose a nonregistered nurse to harsh penalties including possible criminal penalty. Some exceptions apply; for example, persons in an office-based setting may be delegated duties by a physician that ordinarily fall within the scope and purview of professional nurses. The physician retains ultimate responsibility for the office personnel. This is an example of how "custom" and "tradition" provide accepted, although not ideal, practice.

NURSE PRACTICE ACTS. The definition of nursing may vary from state to state. Each state has a Nurse Practice Act, which sets forth the legal definition of nursing, as well as provisions that govern the practice of nursing in the individual state. Display 1-1 illustrates Section 90-171.20(7) of the North Carolina General Statutes, which defines the functions of a registered nurse. Display 1-2 illustrates Section 90-171.20(8) of the North Carolina General Statutes, which defines the functions of a licensed practical nurse. The nurse should review the provisions of the statute carefully. Note that in the North Carolina example, the registered nurse is responsible for assessing the patient. The licensed practical nurse can *participate in the assessment,* but the scope of practice does not include performing the actual nursing assessment.

Nurse Practice Acts define the practice of nursing and allow an administrative body, usually the State Board of Nursing, to impose various disciplinary actions if the conduct of a licensed nurse violates a provision of the act that threatens the health and safety of a citizen.

Thus, the State Board of Nursing is not only authorized to determine an applicant's eligibility for nursing licensure, but also has the power to deny, revoke, or suspend the licensure of a nurse.

STATE STATUTES THAT DEFINE HEALTH CARE. Often a state will enact legislation intended to identify the scope of practice as well as deviations therefrom. For example, each state sets forth the definition of nursing and medical practice. Most states also have statutes that identify when malpractice has occurred as well as the burden of proof required in a medical malpractice case. North Carolina General Statute Section 90-21.12, set forth next, identifies the standard of health care and the proof necessary to prove medical negligence has occurred.

Section 90-21.2. Standard of Health Care

In any action for personal injury or death arising out of the furnishing or the failure to furnish professional services in the performance or medical, dental or other health care, the defendant shall not be liable for payment of damages unless the trier of the facts is satisfied by the greater weight of the evidence that the care of such health care provider was not in accordance with the standards of practice among members of the same health care profession with similar training and experience situated in the same or similar communities at the time of the alleged act giving rise to the cause of action.

Note that the language in this statute applies to health care providers including physicians and nurses. Most states have similar statutes.

DISPLAY 1-1

Practice of Professional Nurses

Chapter 90. Medicine and Allied Occupations

Article 9A. Nursing Practice Act

Sec. 90-171.20. Definitions

As used in this Article, unless the context requires otherwise:

(7) The practice of nursing by a registered nurse consists of the following nine components:

a. Assessing the patient's physical and mental health, including the patient's reaction to illnesses and treatment regimes;

b. Recording and reporting the results of the nursing assessment;

c. Planning, initiating, delivering, and evaluating appropriate nursing acts;

d. Teaching, delegating to, or supervising other personnel in implementing the treatment regime;

e. Collaborating with other health care providers in determining the appropriate health care for a patient, but, subject to the provisions of G.S.90-18.2, not prescribing a medical treatment regimen or making a medical diagnosis, except under supervision of a licensed physician;

f. Implementing the treatment and pharmaceutical regimen prescribed by any person authorized by State law to prescribe such a regimen;

g. Providing teaching and counseling about the patient's health care;

h. Reporting and recording the plan for care, nursing care given, and the patient's response to that care; and

i. Supervising, teaching, and evaluating those who perform or are preparing to perform nursing functions and administering nursing programs and nursing services.

Most states also have statutes dealing with informed consent and the components of the informed consent discussion. Some statutes provide a rebuttable presumption that informed consent has been given if the patient signs the informed consent form, whereas others offer no such presumption (North Carolina General Statute Sec. 90-21.13). Generally, because of their age, minors cannot give informed consent. Many states offer an exception to the general rule where the minor is pregnant or emancipated.

Other state health care-related statutes might include reporting of communicable diseases, disposition of a stillborn fetus, and living will and natural death legislation. The perinatal nurse should be familiar with statutes that impact on nursing care delivery.

Ordinances

In its most common meaning, ordinance is a term used to designate the enactments of a legislative body of a municipal corporation.

Because state law is a higher authority than local ordinances, they rarely play a significant role in perinatal liability.

Case Law

Case law is often referred to as the "common law" or "judge-made law." Case law is made when there is no particular law or point that applies to the fact situation at hand. It is impossible to include, within a statute, all the potential factual situations that can occur. As a result, judges and juries are often called upon to interpret a particular statute as it applies to a specific factual situation. To return to an illustration in our example set forth in Display 1-1, the definition of registered nursing includes the "assessment of patients." That is, the nurse must assess each patient. However, consider the following scenario:

> A labor and delivery nurse was called by a physician and informed that a patient was coming in to the labor and delivery suite. The

DISPLAY 1-2

Practice of Professional Nurses

Chapter 90. Medicine and Allied Occupations

Article 9A. Nursing Practice Act

Sec. 90-171.20. Definitions

(8) The practice of nursing by a licensed practical nurse consists of the following five components:

a. Participating in assessing the patient's physical and mental health including the patient's reaction to illnesses and treatment regimes;

b. Recording and reporting the results of the nursing assessments;

c. Participate in implementing the health care plan developed by the registered nurse and/or prescribed by any person authorized by State law to prescribe such a plan, by performing tasks delegated by and performed under the supervision or under orders or directions of a registered nurse, physician licensed to practice medicine, dentist, or other person authorized by State law to provide such supervision;

d. Reinforcing the teaching and counseling of a registered nurse, physician licensed to practice medicine in North Carolina, or dentist; and

e. Reporting and recording the nursing care rendered and the patient's response to that care.

physician added that the fetus was in a breech position and a cesarean delivery was likely to be performed. The physician arrived at the hospital before the patient. When the patient arrived, the nurse ushered her into the labor room. The physician examined the patient, confirmed that the fetus was in a breech position, and told the nurse that a cesarean delivery was necessary because of the fetal presentation. Because the physician was in the room with the patient, conversing in a nonurgent manner, the nurse left the room and began preparing for the cesarean delivery. When the nurse returned to the room and listened to the fetal heart rate for the first time, she discovered that the fetus was in severe distress. An emergency cesarean delivery was performed but the child was born with severe physical and cognitive deficits.

Could the nurse be excused from completing an initial assessment of the patient until an hour after her arrival in the labor suite because the physician told her the patient was fine? In a similar case, a jury found that the nurse was not excused from assessing the patient and awarded $3 million to the patient. Expert witness testimony by the patient's nursing expert convinced the jury that the duty to assess was an independent nursing function that could not be delegated, even to the physician (*Duncan A. McMillan, Darlene S. Philips, and Ray A. Phillips v. Frye Regional Medical Center and American Medical International, Inc.,* 1992).

When a judge from a lower court evaluates a particular dispute between parties where there is no statute, administrative rule, or ordinance directly on point, he or she looks to previous decisions of judges who were faced with a similar situation. This precedent is often referred to as common law or judge-made law. Because there is no national common law, each state has its own body of common law. Judges come to a decision by considering the factual situation in light of the local customs and beliefs of the community. The judge tries to decide what a similar person in the community would do if placed in similar circumstances. After making a decision as to who is right, the judge writes an opinion

that sets forth the rationale for ruling the way he or she did. Thus the judge has set a precedent. If followed by many other judges, the precedent becomes common law (Cournoyer, 1989). Precedent is usually protected by the doctrine of *stare decisis.* Stare decisis simply means "the previous decision stands" (Black, 1990). The doctrine provides subsequent judges and parties with a sense of predictability over the outcome of a specific factual situation. Lower court judges must abide by former decisions. If they do not, the aggrieved party will appeal the case. Unless there are compelling reasons to deviate from a prior decision, the earlier decision holds great weight for similar factual situations and judges will look to those decisions for guidance. Stare decisis permits stability and allows judges to conserve resources and avoid reinventing the wheel for each case, thus relieving an already overloaded judicial system.

An attorney will research previous cases with similar factual patterns to predict what the outcome will be in a particular situation. A case with a substantially similar fact pattern is said to be "on point." If the prior decision is favorable in the cases on point, the attorney will argue that the earlier law applies to the case at issue. If the prior decisions are unfavorable to the attorney's position, he or she will try to distinguish the earlier case by arguing that the facts are not the same. If the facts are the same, the attorney must try to convince the judge that the law is no longer applicable and that a new law must be made.

Reporting Judicial Decisions

Judicial opinions are often printed in books known as reporters. Most states have a state reporter where decisions can be found. A case is most easily found by the full case citation, although various indexes are available that list the cases by the names of the parties involved. A full case citation includes the name of the parties involved, the volume number of the reporter in which the case is found, the abbreviated name of the reporter, the page number on which the case is found, and the year in which the case was decided. Interpretation of a federal court case citation and a state case citation are set forth in Table 1-1.

Administrative Agency Rules

Administrative agencies are creatures of statutes. That is, administrative agencies are created by statutes to assist the legislature in carrying out functions that require expertise in other disciplines. The State Board of Nursing and the State Board of Medicine are examples of state-based administrative agencies. These agencies are created to assist legislators in the regulation of health care and health care providers. An administrative agency must act within the limits set forth in the statute that created it. No agency can take an action that exceeds the scope of authority provided to it. If it does, the action is void. Administrative agencies function in a quasi-legislative and quasi-judicial role. That is, they can enact rules and regulations, conduct hearings, and write opinions. An administrative agency decision is, if challenged, usually appealed to the state court for a review of its decisions. The state court can uphold or overturn a decision by an administrative agency. State courts can also review agency rules and regulations for reasonableness and legality. Like a state, an agency cannot pass a regulation that is unconstitutional.

CLASSIFICATION OF LAWS— CIVIL AND CRIMINAL LAW

There are federal and state laws dealing with criminal and civil issues. Criminal laws are laws enacted to protect the health and welfare of society as a whole. A violation of a criminal law is a violation committed against the state. The Constitution of the United States indicates that all men possess freedom of life, liberty, and the pursuit of happiness. Liberty has been interpreted to include the ability to walk freely without unreasonable restraint. Because the Constitution protects the liberty of individual citizens, the burden of proof required to convict a defendant of a crime, and thus deny him his liberty, is high. The parties involved in a criminal action are the state and the defendant. The state, through its district attorneys, must prove that the defendant is guilty beyond a reasonable doubt. If the prosecution can successfully prove a defendant's guilt, penalties are rendered against him. Penalties for a violation of a criminal statute include fines, imprisonment, or both. The fines are paid to the state, and not the victim of the criminal action.

Nurses are rarely involved in criminal actions relating to the delivery of nursing care. Criminal actions require the intent (known as *mens rea*) to commit a crime as well as the act of committing

Table 1-1. Legal Case Reporters

	Citation	Parties	Vol. no.	Reporter	Page no.	Year case decided
State Court Case	*Boyd v. Bulala,* 239 Va.218 (1990) 389 S.E. 2d 670	R.A. Bulala, M.D., Helen C. Boyd	389 or 239	Southeastern 2nd or Virginia	670 or 218	1990 1990
Federal Court Case	*American Hospital Association v. Elmore,* 801 F.2d 983 (1st Cir. 1987)*	American Hospital Association, Elmore	801	Federal Reporter 2nd	983	1987

*The parenthetical provides the name of the circuit court that decided the case. In this instance, the case was decided in the 1st circuit.

the crime (known as *actus res*). Absence of one or the other will not support a criminal action. In some jurisdictions gross recklessness may rise to the level of criminal homicide. Gross recklessness is more than mere negligence. A person who practices nursing without a license may incur criminal penalties.

Conversely, civil laws are those laws that serve to protect the interests of private citizens or corporations. A civil violation is a violation committed against a private individual or corporation. The parties involved in a civil action are the plaintiff or aggrieved party and the defendant. The burden of proof in a civil action is not as great as that required of a criminal action because there is no threat to a defendant's liberty. Thus, the plaintiff must merely show that the greater weight of the evidence is in his or her favor to successfully win a civil action. If successful, damages are awarded directly to the plaintiff to compensate the plaintiff for his or her losses. In a negligence action, economic and noneconomic damages are often awarded to an injured plaintiff. Economic damages include the out-of-pocket expenses that can be easily valued, for example, medical bills, lost wages, and future health care needs. Noneconomic damages include pain, suffering, and mental anguish the plaintiff has undergone as a result of the defendant's negligence. Loss of consortium damages may also be awarded if the injuries to the plaintiff caused another party, such as a spouse, to suffer. See Table 1-2 for a comparison of criminal and civil actions.

During trial, the jury is provided with evidence of economic damages and testimony regarding noneconomic damages. The jury is then free to award the amounts they feel are appropriate to compensate the plaintiff for the negligence of the defendant. Damages are awarded to put the plaintiff in the position he or she would have been but for the negligence of the defendants. Some states restrict the amount a jury can award in a medical malpractice action. In Virginia, if a jury finds that a defendant physician negligently treated a prenatal patient who is not yet in labor, and the negligence proximately resulted in an injury to the newborn, even if the newborn's injury will require millions of dollars in health care treatment and supplies, a Virginia jury's verdict, if it is over one million dollars, will be reduced to the statutory cap of $1 million, by law (Va. Code Section 8.01-581.15). Without the restrictions on the amount a jury can award to an injured plaintiff, such as those found in Virginia, juries are free to award what they believe is fair compensation for the injured plaintiff. Other states have statutes that limit noneconomic damages in personal injury and wrongful death actions. For example, Maryland limits the recovery of noneconomic damages in a personal injury action to $500,000, with annual increases of $15,000. (Courts and judicial proceedings, Section 11-108).

Table 1-2. Comparison Between Criminal and Civil Actions		
	Criminal Law	Civil Law
Offense committed against	Society as a whole	Individual person or corporation
Parties	State v. Defendant	Plaintiff v. Defendant
Burden of proof	Beyond a reasonable doubt	By the greater weight of the evidence
Punishment	Fines, imprisonment, or both	Compensation directly to the injured party

Statutes, which limit or cap jury awards, have been subject to constitutional challenge on many grounds. Allegations that the caps interfere with a plaintiff's right to a jury trial have not been successful. In *Bulala v. Boyd* (1990), the defendant appealed a jury verdict that awarded $8.3 million to a child who was injured during the birth process and her parents.

Mrs. Boyd was approximately 36 weeks pregnant when she went into labor. She was admitted to Clinch Valley Community Hospital in Virginia in active labor. At 4:00 A.M., a nurse called Dr. Bulala to notify him of Mrs. Boyd's arrival and status. Dr. Bulala's standing order at the hospital mandated that unless the patient had complications, he was only to be called when the baby crowned. Mrs. Boyd reached complete dilation at 7:00 A.M. but because there were not complications and the baby was not yet crowning, Dr. Bulala was not called. Approximately 45 minutes later, a nurse found that the fetal heart rate had dropped dramatically below normal. The evidence revealed that fetal hypoxia had existed for approximately one hour but because of inadequate monitoring, was not discovered. At 8:00 A.M., the nurse called Dr. Bulala at his home and reported the complications. Mrs. Boyd was taken immediately to the delivery room where she gave birth to a severely neurologically injured baby girl, Veronica. At the time of Veronica's birth, Virginia had enacted a medical malpractice statute that limited recovery in a medical malpractice action to a total of $750,000. The jury awarded in excess of $8 million for the injuries to Veronica, her mother, and father. Punitive damages were also awarded.

The defendant appealed the verdict alleging that the verdict was subject to the $750,000 cap. The Supreme Court of Virginia agreed that the cap's limitation applied to the case and in spite of the enormous medical expenses, pain, suffering, and anguish experienced by Veronica and her family, reduced the jury's award.

The court looked to an earlier case for analysis, *Etheridge v. Medical Center Hospitals, et al.* (1989). In *Etheridge,* the court reduced a jury verdict of $2,750,000 awarded to the plaintiff for injuries she sustained as a result of medical negligence. The plaintiff was a normal, healthy 35-year-old mother of three young children who underwent surgery to repair a jawbone. A jury found that during the surgery, one or both of her physicians were negligent. The physician's negligence proximately resulted in severe, substantial, and permanent injuries including severe brain damage that left her with little memory and intelligence. She is confined to a wheelchair and unable to provide care to herself or her children. After the jury's verdict was rendered, the defendant appealed. The court turned to recent legislation enacted by the State of Virginia. The legislation, based on results from a study commissioned by the State Corporation Commission's Bureau of Insurance that revealed medical malpractice insurance rates had risen dramatically, determined that the cost and potential unavailability of malpractice insurance for health care providers caused a significant problem adversely affecting the public health, safety, and welfare, which necessitated the imposition of a limitation on the liability of health care providers in medical malpractice actions. Although the statute protects only a select group of persons—health care providers—and actually harms a select group of persons—those persons who are injured by health care providers—the court found that it nonetheless passed the rational basis test and was thus constitutional.

CONCLUSION

Many legal forces affect the delivery of nursing care. Nurses must be aware of federal and state statutes that impact nursing practice. Knowledge of relevant court decisions is also helpful for the nurse in the perinatal setting. The doctrine of stare decisis explains a court's predisposition to rule a certain way and allows the nurse to plan nursing care accordingly to prevent personal and professional liability. Finally, the nurse should be familiar with the role and functions of the State Board of Nursing in a state where he or she practices as well as the components of the Nurse Practice Act.

REFERENCES

Beckman, J. P. (1996). Nursing negligence, analyzing malpractice in the hospital setting. Thousand Oaks, CA: Sage Publications.

Beckman, J. P. (1995). Nursing malpractice. Seattle: University of Washington Press.

Black, H. C. (1990). Black's law dictionary (6th ed.). St. Paul, MN: West.

Cournoyer, C. (1989). The nurse manager and the law. Rockville, MD: Aspen.

Cushing, M. (1988). Nursing jurisprudence. Norwalk, CT: Appleton & Lange.

Furrow, B., Johnson, S., Jost, S., & Schwartz, R. (1992). Health law, cases, materials and problems (2nd ed.). St Paul, MN: West.

CASE CITATIONS

Bryan Joseph Phillips, by and through his guardian ad litem, Duncan A. McMillan, Darlene S. Phillips and Ray A. Phillips v. Frye Regional Medical Center and American Medical International, Inc., 89 CvS 2149 (Catawba County, November 17, 1992).

Bulala v. Boyd, 389 S.E.2d 670, 239 Va. 218 (1990).

Etheridge v. Medical Center Hospitals, et al., 376 S.E.2d 525, 237 Va. 87 (1989).

Owens v. Nacogdoches County Hospital District, 741 F. Supp. 1296 (E. Dist. Tex. 1990).

United States Fidelity and Guaranty Co. v. Guenther, 281 U.S. 34, 50 S.Ct. 165 (1930).

CHAPTER 2

Theories of Liability

Rebecca Cady

When a complaint is filed, as will be described in Chapter 5, usually the plaintiff asserts several different legal theories otherwise known as causes of action against the health care providers involved. This chapter explores the various causes of action that are likely to appear in a perinatal lawsuit as well as some of the common defenses. It is important for the perinatal nurse to realize that in addition to professional negligence, the lawsuit may also include allegations of intentional torts, which, significantly, would not be covered by any available malpractice insurance, and which could ultimately result in the forfeiture of the nurse's personal assets should the plaintiff win the suit. It is also important to note that, although generally the plaintiff in such a lawsuit is the patient, the spouse and/or the heirs of the patient may also be entitled to join in the lawsuit as plaintiffs in their own right, and under separate legal theories.

UNINTENTIONAL TORTS

Professional Negligence

This cause of action, which will be described in detail in Chapter 4, is the most common, and often the only cause of action present in most lawsuits against health care providers. In brief, this theory asserts that the health care provider did not act within the appropriate standard of care while caring for the patient. This theory of liability must be asserted by the patient, or if a minor, by the legal guardian. This theory also includes any emotional damage to the patient caused by the health care provider's negligence. In most states, any physician negligence that causes injury to the fetus and resultant emotional anguish to the mother therefore breaches a duty owed directly to the mother (*Burgess v. Superior Court,* 1992). A hospital also owes the mother such a duty of care, and the mother has a right to recover for emotional distress resulting from the negligently caused stillbirth of her fetus (*Johnson v. Superior Court,* 1981).

Lack of Informed Consent

This theory is often included in a perinatal lawsuit when certain procedures or tests result in less than optimal outcomes for the mother and/or baby. This theory asserts that had the patient been appropriately counseled by the physician regarding the risks and benefits of the procedure or test in question, the patient would not have consented to the procedure or test. The physician owes to the patient a duty of reasonable disclosure of the available choices with respect to proposed therapy and the dangers inherently and potentially involved in each (*Cobbs v. Grant,* 1972). In most states, the informed consent cause of action presents two issues: (1) what was the scope of disclosure, and (2) what would a reasonable, prudent patient have decided to do if given the proper informed consent (*Cobbs v. Grant,* 1972). Although the issue of the scope of disclosure (that is, what information a skilled practitioner of good standing would provide under similar circumstances) must be determined by expert testimony, the issue of what a prudent person in the patient's position would have decided if adequate informed consent had been given is *not* required to be proven by expert testimony.

The nurse's role in this theory is fairly limited, as the nurse does not obtain the patient's informed consent, but merely serves as a witness to the patient's signature on the informed consent document. The patient is the person who must assert this theory, and in the perinatal setting, it is only the mother who can assert this theory, as the fetus obviously cannot give its informed consent. In a recent case, the court held that a physician violated a patient's right to informed consent by failing to inform her of the risks of pitocin induction of labor prior to its use. The court held that even though the physician exercised his medical judgment and determined that a repeat c-section was not medically indicated, he nevertheless denied the patient the right to withdraw her consent to a trial of labor (*Bankert v. United States,* 1996). Lack of informed consent is often pled by plaintiffs in conjunction with a cause of action for battery, an intentional tort.

Negligent Infliction of Emotional Distress

This theory asserts that while negligently caring for the patient, the health care provider negligently caused emotional distress. In most states, negligent infliction of emotional distress as to the patient is not an independent cause of action, but is included in the general tort of professional negligence, and involves the same elements of duty, breech, causation, and harm (*Christensen v. Superior Court,* 1991). Thus any purported cause of action for negligent infliction of emotional distress brought by a patient of

alleged medical malpractice is superfluous, and is properly subsumed within the cause of action for negligence (California Civil Code Section 3333). This does not mean that the mother cannot recover damages for emotional distress when something happens to her fetus as a result of a health care provider's negligence; it does mean that there is only one cause of action, for professional negligence, that may include the emotional distress to the mother. In a recent case, the California Supreme Court held that a mother can recover monetary damages under a direct victim theory of liability for emotional distress she has suffered as a result of the in utero death of her fetus allegedly caused by the professional negligence of her physician (*Zavala v. Arce,* 1997). This emotional distress could include fright, nervousness, grief, anxiety, worry, mortification, shock, humiliation and indignity, physical pain, or other similar distress (*Zavala v. Arce,* 1997).

The patient is not the only one who can claim this theory. The patient's spouse or other close relative may be able to assert a separate cause of action for negligent infliction of emotional distress. There are two theories upon which a third party (a person who isn't the patient) may claim negligent infliction of emotional distress.

The first theory is the direct victim theory. The essential elements of this theory require that the nonpatient plaintiff have a preexisting consensual relationship with the offending health care provider, and that the health care provider's alleged conduct was so outrageous that liability should be imposed (*Bro v. Glaser,* 1994). This theory is difficult to establish in the perinatal setting, except as previously noted with respect to claims by the mother, as the spouse or family would be unlikely to have the required preexisting relationship with the health care provider.

The second theory is the bystander theory. In order to proceed under the bystander theory, the nonpatient plaintiff must show that he or she (1) is closely related to the injured party, (2) was present at the time of the injury-producing event and was contemporaneously aware that an injury was being caused to the injured party, and (3) as a result, suffered serious emotional distress (*Thing v. LaChusa,* 1989). In the perinatal setting, the spouse and/or family present at a delivery with poor maternal or fetal outcome may have a viable cause of action for negligent infliction of emotional distress under this bystander theory.

Wrongful Death

This theory of liability asserts that the health care provider wrongfully caused the death of the patient. This does not necessarily mean that the health care provider acted intentionally, but usually means that the health care provider's negligence caused the death. This theory is often asserted instead of a separate cause of action for professional negligence. A wrongful death cause of action can arise in the perinatal setting in two different ways. First, it obviously would be used if the mother died as a result of malpractice. Second, it could also be used if the fetus was born alive, but failed to survive. This cause of action could not be used in the case of a stillbirth (*Justus v. Atchison,* 1977). Who can bring this cause of action depends on who died. In cases where both the mother and liveborn fetus die, the plaintiffs would most likely be the spouse and any surviving children, and there would be two separate causes of action, one for the death of the mother and one for the death of the liveborn child. If the mother is the only one to die, the plaintiffs would be the spouse and all surviving children. If the liveborn fetus dies, the plaintiffs would be both parents.

Wrongful Birth/Wrongful Life

These theories are often seen in the perinatal area. The parents can claim wrongful birth, and the child can claim wrongful life when the following occur: (1) the health care provider negligently counseled, tested, and treated the mother of the child regarding genetic defects and disabilities; (2) the negligent counseling, testing, and treating caused the parents to be unaware of the possibility of the child's having a hereditary condition, thereby depriving them of the opportunity to choose not to conceive a child with a genetic defect or of the opportunity to make an informed decision regarding aborting the pregnancy; (3) the health care provider's

negligence was a cause of the child being born; (4) the child was born with a congenital or genetic ailment or defect; (5) the parents/child sustained special damages consisting of money expended to compensate for the extraordinary additional medical care and training necessitated by the child's ailment or defect (California BAJI 6.08). The damages in these cases can be staggering, often resulting in verdicts of tens of millions of dollars. Some states also allow parents to bring a cause of action for wrongful life when they bear a healthy but unwanted child as a result of a failed surgical sterilization procedure. However, the damages for a failed sterilization case can vary greatly depending on the law of the individual state. For example, a recent case held that although parents could claim actual medical expenses, they could not recover damages for emotional anguish (*Crawford v. Kirk,* 1996).

INTENTIONAL TORTS

These theories involve actions by the health care provider that are intentional in nature. Attorneys for plaintiffs often add these theories to a complaint for several strategic reasons. First, these causes of action are not generally covered by professional liability insurance, and thus may expose the individual health care provider to personal financial liability for damages awarded on these causes of action. Second, intentional torts are frequently subject to punitive damages, which can reach staggering amounts and which are not generally subject to any monetary caps on damages awards that may apply to the negligence causes of action. Third, some states provide that the plaintiff can be awarded costs and attorneys' fees if he or she prevails on certain intentional tort claims. It has been the author's experience that most of the time, plaintiffs' attorneys attempt to include these causes of action for their "shock value" to gain a psychological advantage over the health care providers during the discovery process. It would be wise for the perinatal nurse confronted by allegations of intentional torts to consider demanding separate counsel in order to ensure that his or her defense is not subject to a conflict of interest with the hospital. If the allegations could possibly subject the nurse to criminal liability, then it would be prudent to obtain an attorney experienced in criminal defense. Many times, however, defense counsel can persuade the court to in effect remove some intentional tort causes of action from the complaint by the process of filing a demurrer, which will be discussed in Chapter 6.

Spoliation of Evidence

Spoliation of evidence is probably the most commonly pled intentional tort against non-physician health care providers. This theory asserts that the health care provider intentionally acted in such a way that records pertaining to the patient were destroyed, damaged, lost, or concealed (California BAJI 7.95). This theory also requires that the health care provider knew of the existence of a claim by the patient, and that the patient's opportunity to prove her claim was substantially interfered with (California BAJI 7.95). The patient is usually the person who can assert this cause of action, although if the patient has died, the spouse and/or surviving children may assert it as well. This theory usually arises any time corrections are made to the medical records in an improper fashion, or when parts of the record are missing. The problem with defending this cause of action is that even if the corrections were made at the time of the care and thus before the health care provider could be aware of the existence of a claim, the nature of improper corrections (that is, those not dated, timed, or signed) leaves open the inference that the changes were made after the lawsuit was filed.

In the perinatal setting, this cause of action is most often applied when portions of the fetal monitor strips are unable to be located. Obviously, the strips can be critically important evidence of what transpired during a delivery, including not only the fetal heart pattern and contraction pattern, but usually also handwritten notations regarding personnel present, and nursing and medical actions taken. Perinatal nurses should therefore take care that all strips are removed from the fetal monitor and placed in the patient's chart after a delivery or when the patient is discharged or transferred to another room prior to delivery.

The perinatal nurse should also take care that any corrections to the medical record be made in the proper fashion, by putting a single line through the erroneous entry, noting "error" above it, and dating, timing, and initialing the cross-out. One must also take care that any late entries be properly charted by writing the actual time of charting, "late entry for," and the time when the events to be documented actually occurred.

Even if a plaintiff does not prevail on this cause of action, introduction of evidence that the chart was not properly kept and that improper corrections were made can lead the jury to infer that the health care providers' actions, which seem to amount to tampering with the chart, are evidence of their culpability with respect to the negligence cause of action. Therefore, it is critical from a loss-prevention standpoint that each perinatal nurse be scrupulous regarding his or her charting.

Battery

Patients often assert the claim of battery along with one for lack of informed consent. In many jurisdictions, performing medical care without informed consent, and not in an emergency situation, is equivalent to committing battery. A battery is defined as an intentional, unprivileged, and unconsented-to offensive contact (California BAJI 7.50). However, patient complaints arising out of disputes over informed consent do not always amount to battery. Some courts believe that as a matter of public policy, the patient who disputes informed consent should be limited to bringing that complaint as a cause of action for negligence when the essential character of the treatment contemplated by both patient and physician was therapeutic in nature (*Freedman v. Superior Court,* 1989). Likewise, courts have held that a patient whose consent has been exceeded by a well-meaning physician attempting therapeutic treatment should be relegated to a negligence cause of action (*Cobbs v. Grant,* 1972).

A surgical procedure performed without consent *may* be considered a technical battery (*Berky v. Anderson,* 1969). However, a cause of action for battery based on lack of informed consent is usually very narrowly drawn, and the courts tend to prefer the majority trend to catagorize actions for failure to obtain informed consent as negligence (*Cobbs v. Grant,* 1972). If the doctor failed to meet his or her duty to disclose pertinent information to obtain informed consent, the action should be pled in negligence (*Cobbs v. Grant,* 1972). Typically, causes of action for battery based on lack of informed consent are reserved for cases involving extreme circumstances such as performing a different procedure than the one that was consented to (*Cobbs v. Grant,* 1972).

Fraud

This cause of action is asserted by the patient when the health care provider allegedly has misrepresented certain important facts to the patient, which caused the patient to act in a way she wouldn't have acted except for the misrepresentation. This claim is usually seen in conjunction with a claim for lack of informed consent. Fraud can be asserted as either intentional/affirmative misrepresentation or concealment or both. A cause of action for affirmative misrepresentation requires the following elements:

1. Defendant must have made a representation as to a past or existing material fact.
2. The representation must have been false.
3. The defendant must have known that the representation was false when made or must have made the representation recklessly without knowing whether it was true or false.
4. The defendant must have made the representation with an intent to defraud the plaintiff, that is, he or she must have made the representation for the purpose of inducing the plaintiff to rely upon it and to act or refrain from acting in reliance thereon.
5. The plaintiff must have been unaware of the falsity of the representation, must have acted in reliance upon the truth of the representation, and must have been justified in relying upon the representation.
6. Plaintiff must have sustained damage as a result of the reliance upon the truth of the representation. (California BAJI 12.31)

An action for fraud/concealment requires the following elements: (1) the defendant must have concealed or suppressed a material *fact;* (2) the defendant must have been under a duty to disclose the facts to the plaintiff; (3) the defendant must have intentionally concealed or suppressed the fact with the intent to defraud the plaintiff; (4) the plaintiff must have been unaware of the fact and would not have acted as she did if she had known of the concealed or suppressed fact; (5) the concealment or suppression of the fact caused the plaintiff to sustain damage (California BAJI 12.35).

In determining liability for fraud the courts distinguish between statements of *fact* and those of *opinion.* "A representation of opinion is ordinarily not actionable" (Witkin, 1988). In states that limit monetary awards in medical negligence cases, courts often look upon a fraud cause of action as an attempt to circumvent the monetary award limitations in medical negligence cases. In a landmark case, the court held as follows: "even though the plaintiff alleges false representations on the part of the physician or fraudulent concealment, our courts have always treated the action as one for malpractice" (*Tell v. Taylor,* 1961). The *Tell* case holding was further echoed in a recent case in which the court stated that worker compensation fraud by a doctor is unethical, illegal, and immoral. However, the court nevertheless stated that the physicians' actions were directly related to the professional services they were rendering in their capacity as health care providers and plaintiff was required to comply with the provisions of the law related to actions against health care providers (*Davis v. Superior Court,* 1994).

Intentional Infliction of Emotional Distress

This cause of action asserts that the health care provider intentionally caused emotional distress to the patient or family. The essential elements necessary for a claim of intentional infliction of emotional distress are (1) the defendant is engaged in outrageous conduct; (2) the defendant intends to cause the plaintiff to suffer emotional distress; (3) the plaintiff has suffered severe emotional distress; (4) such outrageous and unprivileged conduct of the defendant was the cause of the emotional distress suffered by the plaintiff (California BAJI 12.70). The plaintiff must allege specific facts showing outrageous conduct that is intentional or reckless and outside the bounds of decency, all of which are required for properly asserting a cause of action for intentional infliction of emotional distress (*Ochoa v. Superior Court,* 1985). Courts have held that *no* cause of action for intentional infliction of emotional distress is stated where allegations fall short of showing extreme or outrageous conduct (*Perati v. Atkinson,* 1963).

MISCELLANEOUS CAUSES OF ACTION

Loss of Consortium

This cause of action is always brought by the patient's spouse. When one spouse is injured in a way that substantially affects his or her capacity to participate in the marriage, then the other spouse has an independent cause of action for loss of consortium (*Rodriguez v. Bethlehem Steel Corp.,* 1974; *American Export Lines, Inc. v. Alvez,* 1980). This claim compensates the noninjured spouse for any lost love, companionship, or affection that may have resulted from his spouse's injuries. Loss of consortium means that the patient, because of the health care provider's negligent actions, was unable to perform her usual marital and household duties. This cause of action cannot be asserted in a wrongful death case, because the wrongful death cause of action encompasses the loss of consortium. This cause of action is dependent upon the negligence cause of action, so if the provider is found to not have been negligent, there will be no award for loss of consortium.

Breach of Fiduciary Duty

This cause of action is always brought by the patient. This theory asserts that the health care provider had a fiduciary duty to the patient, which was breached. There have been only a few situations in which courts have recognized a cause of action against a physician for breach of fiduciary duty (*Cole v. Wolfskill,* 1920; *Schurman v. Look,* 1923), involving financial dealings between physician and patient and fraudulent concealment of an injury to avoid discovery until after the statute of limitations has run. A cause of action has been recognized for a breach of fiduciary duty if a physician fails to disclose his or her research and economic interests prior to obtaining consent to perform the medical procedure at issue (*Moore v. Regents of University of California,* 1990). However, under *Cobbs v. Grant* (1972), failure to disclose adequate information should be pled as negligence. Other than these specific categories, no fiduciary duty is recognized in the physician/patient relationship giving rise to a cause of action other than medical negligence. The courts have not specifically addressed the issue of whether a nurse owes such a duty to his or her patients, but one can assume the nurse does owe such a duty because of the similarity between the doctor–patient and nurse–patient relationships.

Invasion of Privacy

This cause of action is most often brought by the patient, and occasionally by the spouse. This theory asserts that the health care provider violated the patient's right to privacy. Legally protected privacy interests are usually of two different types: informational and autonomical. In the medical setting, informational privacy would be the most frequently invoked, and would specifically deal with the patient's medical information. In some states such as California, the state constitution specifically gives everyone a right of privacy (California Constitution Article 1, Section 1). A cause of action for violation of the state right to privacy in California would require (1) the health care provider engaged in conduct that invaded plaintiff's privacy interests; (2) plaintiff had a reasonable expectation of privacy as to the interests invaded, that is, the patient did not consent to the invasion; (3) the invasion of privacy was serious; (4) the invasion of privacy caused damage or injury to plaintiff (California BAJI 7.25.1). In other states, the federally recognized right of privacy would apply. The Fourteenth Amendment of the United States Constitution establishes the right of individuals to make independent decisions about their medical care (*Roe v. Wade,* 1973). This theory arises most commonly in the perinatal setting when information about a patient or her medical condition is given to others without the patient's consent. An example of this would be talking to the press regarding a mother with multiple gestation without her consent to do so. Privacy issues are discussed in detail in Chapters 14 and 24.

EMTALA

The Emergency Medical Treatment and Active Labor Act (42 U.S.C., Section 1395 dd) addresses the problem of patient dumping. This law requires that for persons seeking treatment for an emergency medical condition, the hospital is required to screen and stabilize the patient prior to transferring that patient to another facility. With respect to pregnant patients, EMTALA defines an emergency medical condition as (a) the patient is having contractions, (b) there is inadequate time to safely transfer the patient, or (c) transfer poses a threat to the health or safety of the woman or the fetus. A physician can certify that a woman is in false labor following observation for a reasonable period of time. Screening must be done by a qualified medical professional, such as a nurse. However, under the law, only a physician can really determine if a woman is in active versus false labor. Therefore, the nurse must at least talk to the physician to make this determination, even if the nurse is a CRNM. However, the physician is not actually required to see the patient. If these rules are not followed, the patient can file a civil action against the health care providers, the federal government can fine the facility up to $50,000 per violation, revoke Medicare status, revoke tax exempt status, and can revoke the facility's license. Some states, such as California, have passed similar legislation that adds penalties on the state level, such as revocation of state licenses (California Health and Safety Code Sections 1317 et seq.)

DEFENSES

Various legal and factual defenses exist that can be asserted on behalf of health care provider defendants who are sued. In defending against causes of action for negligence, the health care provider would obviously introduce expert testimony related to the elements of the negligence cause of action, that is, that he or she did not have a duty, did not breach a duty, the breach of the duty did not cause the harm suffered, or there was no harm suffered. The health care provider defendant accused of battery would assert that consent had been given, or that consent was not needed due to the emergency exception.

When a health care provider is sued for failure to obtain informed consent, the emergency exception defense may also apply. This defense asserts that there existed an emergency situation such that the patient's consent could not practically be obtained, and the situation warranted, in the physician's best judgment, immediate action to safeguard the patient's life. This defense would be established through the testimony of a defense expert physician.

General defenses include the statute of limitations, contributory negligence, comparative negligence, and good samaritan acts.

The statute of limitations that applies to each particular cause of action can vary, and the statute of limitations can vary from state to state. Generally, with respect to causes of action for medical/nursing negligence, the plaintiff must file the lawsuit one year from the time he or she knew or should have known about the possibility of negligence having occurred, or three years from the date of the incident. Plaintiffs who suspect negligence can be required to take the burden of finding out more information about the occurrence of negligence. Statutes of limitations regarding actions brought by minors for injuries suffered at birth typically allow the child to file a lawsuit until at least eight years of age, and sometimes up to the age of 21. If the plaintiff has failed to file the lawsuit within the appropriate time frame indicated by the applicable statute of limitations, then the court must order the entire case dismissed.

Contributory and comparative negligence theories are used to show that even if the nurse was negligent, the patient and others involved in the patient's care were also negligent. These theories attempt to apportion the amount of damages awarded according to the level of fault of each party. As an example, if a labor and delivery nurse was negligent in failing to timely notify the physician of repeated severe late decelerations, and the physician was negligent for failing to perform an emergency c-section once she was notified, and the patient smoked crack cocaine while pregnant and while in labor, and the baby was born with severe developmental disabilities, then the nurse and doctor would assert the contributory negligence of the mother as a factor in the child's condition. The nurse and doctor would also assert that each of them individually should not be totally responsible for the child's condition, because each of them was also negligent. The jury would then attempt, with the assistance of expert testimony, to apportion the amount of responsibility to be borne by the mother, the nurse, and the doctor. In this example, the jury might find that the mother was 75% responsible for the child's condition due to her substance abuse, that the nurse was 10% responsible due to her failure to timely notify the doctor about the fetal heart rate problems, and that the doctor was 15% responsible due to her failure to perform an emergency c-section once she was notified. Or either of the defendants could assert, through expert testimony, that another health care provider who, for whatever reason is not a defendant in the case, was partially or totally responsible for the patient's poor outcome. This is known as the "empty chair" defense. After the jury makes its determination about proportional fault, then the proportions are applied to the amount of damages the jury determines the plaintiff has sus-

tained. These theories basically make sure that defendants are held responsible only for those amounts of the damages that they caused, and that the award is reduced by any amounts of damage that were caused by the plaintiff, as the plaintiff has a duty to avoid harming themselves.

When the health care provider while off duty has stopped to assist a person, such as when happening upon the scene of a car accident, most states have what are known as good samaritan laws, which prevent the person so assisted from suing the health care provider for professional negligence. The reasoning behind these laws is that we want to encourage health care providers who are off duty to stop and assist others; therefore we will protect these health care providers from being sued as a result of their voluntary assistance of persons in need. If the good samaritan law applies, the court must dismiss the entire case.

CONCLUSION

There are many different legal theories plaintiffs can assert against health care providers should a lawsuit be brought. There are various defenses that can be asserted by the health care providers to rebut the plaintiff's claims. The perinatal nurse should be aware of these theories and their consequences as part of a personal risk management plan. By being aware of the legal responsibilities owed to patients and their families, the perinatal nurse can conduct himself or herself in such a manner as to avoid incurring liability, and to avoid the potential of personal financial responsibility for failure to meet these responsibilities.

REFERENCES

Battaglia, F. C., & Meschia, G. (1986). An Introduction to Fetal Physiology. New York: Academic Press.

Bristow, J., Rudolph, A. M., Itskovitz, J., & Barnes, R. (1983). Hepatic oxygen and glucose metabolism in the fetal lamb. Journal of Clinical Investigation, 71(1), 96–102.

California Civil Jury Instructions (BAJI). (1994). The judges of the superior court of Los

Angeles county, California. (8th ed.). St. Paul, MN: West.

California Civil Code section 3333.

California Constitution, Article 1, Section 1.

Freeman, K. S., Carite, T., & Nagoette, K. (1991). Fetal heart rate monitoring (2nd ed.). Baltimore: Williams & Wilkins.

Friedman, W. F. (1972). The intrinsic physiologic properties of the developing heart. Progress in Cardiovascular Diseases, 15(1), 87–111.

Gilbert, R. D. (1980). Control of fetal cardiac output during changes in blood volume. American Journal of Physiology, 238(1), H80–86.

Lewis, A. B., Donovan, M., & Platzker, A. C. (1980). Cardiovascular responses to Autonomic blockade in hypoxemic fetal lambs. Biology of the Neonate, 37(5–6), 233–242.

Parer, J. T. (1994). Fetal cerebral metabolism: The influence of asphyxia and other factors. Journal of Perinatology, 14(5), 376–385.

Rankin, J. H., Meschia, G., Makowski, E. L., & Battaglia, F. C. (1971). Relationship between uterine and umbilical venous PO2 in sheep. American Journal of Physiology, 220(6), 1688–1692.

5 Witkin. (1988). Summary of California law, torts (9th ed.) section 678, page 779.

CASE CITATIONS

American Export Lines, Inc. v. Alvez, 446 U.S. 274 (1980).

Bankert v. United States, 937 F. Supp. 1169 (1996).

Berky v. Anderson, 1 Cal. App. 3d 790 (1969).

Bro v. Glaser, 22 Cal. App. 4th 1398 (1994).

Burgess v. Superior Court, 2 Cal. 4th 1064 (1992).

Christensen v. Superior Court, 53 Cal. 3d 868, 882 (1991).

Cobbs v. Grant, 8 Cal. 3d 229 (1972).

Cole v. Wolfskill, 49 Cal. App. 52 (1920).

Crawford v. Kirk (Tex. App.) 939 SW 2d 633 (1996).

Davis v. Superior Court, 27 Cal. App. 4th 623 (1994).

Freedman v. Superior Court, 214 Cal. App. 3d 734 (1989).

Johnson v. Superior Court, 123 Cal. App. 3d 1002 (1981).

Justus v. Atchison, 19 Cal. 3d 564 (1977).

Moore v. Regents of University of California, 51 Cal. 3d 120 (1990).

Ochoa v. Superior Court, 39 Cal. 3d 159 (1985).

Perati v. Atkinson, 213 Cal. App. 2d 472 (1963).

Rodriguez v. Bethlehem Steel Corp., 12 Cal. 3d 382 (1974).

Roe v. Wade, 410 U.S. 113 (1973).

Schurman v. Look, 63 Cal. App. 347 (1923).

Tell v. Taylor, 191 Cal. App. 2d 366 (1961).

Thing v. La Chusa, 48 Cal. 3d 644 (1989).

Zavala v. Arce, Daily Journal D.A.R. 13347 (1997).

CHAPTER

3

Defining the Standard of Care

Patricia Fedorka

Standards are the basis for nursing practice and are instrumental in determining whether or not a nurse is found negligent in a court of law. It is, therefore, vital that the nurse have a thorough understanding of what standards are, how they apply to nursing practice, their role in evaluating nursing care and patient outcomes, and how they are utilized to determine whether the nurse has "breached a duty" in the care provided to a patient.

This chapter reviews and discusses the various sources that may establish and prescribe standards in the perinatal setting. They include: (1) state statutes (nurse practice acts); (2) the American Nurses Association (ANA); (3) national professional nursing organizations; (4) documentary evidence; (5) the Joint Commission for the Accreditation of Healthcare Organizations; (6) hospital policies and procedures; and (7) expert witness testimony. Each of these sources is discussed in detail.

Nursing is a dynamic profession that has undergone many changes over the past years in response to technological advances in health care, consumer demands, and changes in the health care delivery system. Nowhere are these changes more evident than they are in the field of perinatal nursing. Regardless of their source, standards in nursing generally and in perinatal nursing specifically should be dynamic and vital in order to reflect the current state of knowledge in the nursing practice.

Consumers have demanded change and health care providers have responded with options in anesthesia, decrease in medical interventions, increased patient input in decision making, participation of patient and significant others in the birth experience, and nontraditional health care settings.

The complexity and advances in technology in the perinatal setting have also affected nursing practice. There is a constant demand for increased specialization and more complex skills. Nurses carry out procedures that historically were considered the exclusive purview of the physician, such as interpretation of electronic fetal monitoring strips and insertion of internal fetal monitors and intrauterine pressure catheters. If nurses are not actually implementing procedures, they are responsible for assessing and monitoring the patient for negative or untoward outcomes.

The climate of today's health care delivery system has placed nurses in settings in which they function in a more independent role, often without any immediate support available. This is very evident in the homecare setting. Home health nurses manage the care of women with antepartal complications ranging from hyperemesis with IV therapy for hydration to preterm labor with terbutaline pumps.

Despite the various changes that the health care system has undergone and the impact on practicing nurses, assurance of quality of care has always been of prime importance to the nursing profession. The development, acceptance, and implementation of standards is one way to ensure optimal patient outcomes.

Standards are considered the "minimal" requirements that determine the acceptable level of care (see Display 3-1 for standard definitions). In theory there should be no difference in the level of care provided a patient in a teaching hospital compared to the care in a community hospital, or a rural hospital compared to a suburban one. National standards protect the patient population from receiving varying and differing levels of care depending on the institution in which they receive treatment (Guido, 1997). In *Shilkret v. The Annapolis Emergency Hospital Association, et al.* (1975), a claim of negligence was brought against several physicians and the Annapolis Emergency Association hospital. The physicians named in the suit included the two obstetricians who treated the mother throughout her pregnancy and delivery, an anesthesiologist in attendance at the birth, and a pediatrician. The infant was born with brain damage and had to be permanently institutionalized due to alleged negligence at birth, which resulted in an intracranial bleed complicated by subsequent treatment rendered by the pediatrician. Originally the court applied the strict locality rule, which localized the standard of care to the specific community, and directed a verdict for the defendants. However, the court of appeals that later heard the case found for the plaintiffs. Expert witnesses for the plaintiff testified that the physicians did not meet national standards when providing care for the mother and the infant. The court of appeals held that physicians and hospitals are required to meet national standards and to use the degree of care and skill that is expected of a reasonably competent physician or hospital in the same or similar circumstances. In rendering its decision the court held that:

DISPLAY 3-1

Definitions

Standards—"Authoritative statements by which the nursing profession describes the responsibilities for which its practitioners are accountable. Consequently, standards reflect the priorities of the profession. Standards provide direction for professional nursing practice and a framework for the evaluation of practice. Written in measurable terms, standards also define the nursing profession's accountability to the public and the client outcomes for which nurses are responsible." (ANA, 1991, p. 1)

Standards of Care—"Authoritative statements that describe a competent level of clinical nursing practice demonstrated through assessment, diagnosis, outcome identification, planning, implementation, and evaluation." (ANA, 1991, p. 21)

Standards of Nursing Practice—"Authoritative statements that describe a level of care or performance common to the profession of nursing by which the quality of nursing practice can be judged. Standards of clinical nursing practice include both standards of care and standards of professional performance." (ANA, 1991, p. 21)

Standards of Professional Performance—"Authoritative statements that describe a competent level of behavior in the professional role, including activities related to quality of care, performance appraisal, education, collegiality, ethics, collaboration, research, and resource utilization." (ANA, 1991, p. 21)

Recognizing the significant developments which have marked the increased urbanization of our society, a majority of American courts have now abandoned the strict locality rule as being too narrow. We, too, conclude that it can be sustained no longer given the current state of medical science. . . . The dynamic impact of modern communications and transportation, the proliferation of medical literature, frequent seminars and conferences on a variety of professional subjects, and the growing availability of modern clinical facilities are but some of the developments in the medical profession which combine to produce contemporary standards that are not only much higher than they were just a few short years ago, but also are national in scope. Whatever may have justified the strict locality rule fifty or a hundred years ago, it cannot be reconciled with the realities of medical practice today.

The ease and opportunity for rapid sharing of information and new technology makes "lack of current knowledge" an unacceptable rationale for regional or local variances in the care that patients receive. Ignorance of applicable nursing standards or lack of knowledge of current nursing practice is never a defense for substandard nursing care. The ANA speaks to the nurse's professional responsibility to keep current and competent (ANA, 1991).

STATE STATUTES

Nurse Practice Acts

"Nursing, like other professions, is responsible for ensuring that its members act in the public interest in the course of providing the unique service society has entrusted to them" (ANA, 1995, p.17). "Legal contracts between society and the professions are defined by statutes and associated regulations. State nurse practice acts and related legislative and regulatory initiatives serve as the codification to act in the best interest of society. Nurse practice acts grant nurses the authority to sanction nurses who violate the norms of the profession and act in a manner that threatens public safety" (ANA, 1995, p. 19).

All 50 states and the District of Columbia have their own nurse practice acts that define "nursing" for that particular state. Normally, nurse practice acts discuss the scope of nursing in general, broad concepts, which do not provide specific guidelines for nursing practice. Although the definitions may be similar, differences exist from state to state. Therefore, each nurse is responsible for knowing the scope of practice in the state in which he or she practices. This applies to a variety of nursing roles, for example, licensed practical nurses, registered nurses, nurses in advanced nursing roles such as nurse midwives, and nurse practitioners who function under an expanded scope of practice. Nursing actions that are within the scope of practice for a registered nurse may be illegal for a licensed practical nurse to assume. The same situation can occur comparing scope of practice for a nurse practitioner and a registered nurse. Although it is quite acceptable for a nurse practitioner to make a medical diagnosis, it is outside the scope of practice for a registered nurse to do so.

Neither physician orders nor institutional policy may take precedence over the state's nurse practice act. A nurse who acts outside of the nurse practice act, or whose actions exceed those allowed under the act, may actually be violating a state's medical practice act, which ultimately determines the scope of physician practice. The nurse may be infringing on activities that only a physician may legally perform. If this is the case, the nurse could be found in violation of both the nurse practice act and the state's medical act, which is clearly a deviation from the standard of care.

State boards of nursing are usually given the authority to (1) prescribe regulations setting forth educational requirements and admission standards for licensure of nurses, and in some states, advanced practice nurses; (2) delineate the tasks that nurses and advanced practice nurses are permitted to carry out either independently or in collaboration with physicians; and (3) establish criteria and administrative processes for disciplining nurses usually with authority to impose appropriate penalties (Bernzweig, 1996, p. 81). The most common reasons for revoking a license are abuse of drugs and failure to meet applicable nursing standards.

There have been many changes in state legislation in recent years in regard to disciplining nurses. The state bears the responsibility of safeguarding the health and safety of the general population and one aspect of the safeguard consists of ensuring competent care from properly licensed nurses. As our society becomes more and more mobile, the abuse of practicing nursing without a license continues to be a problem. Areas addressed by the nurse practice acts include, but are not limited to, fraud and deceit, criminal activity, negligence, risk to clients and physical or mental incapacity, violation of the nursing practice act or rules, disciplinary action by another jurisdiction, incompetence, and unethical conduct (ANA, 1986). State laws vary in their authority to impose sanctions on nurses. However, the ANA recommends that State Boards of Nursing have the ability to protect the public from incompetent practitioners by having the power to enforce recommended disciplinary acts ranging from public or private reprimand; denying application for a license; suspending, restricting, or revoking a license; requiring a nurse to submit to care/counseling or participate in a program of education; or requiring a nurse to practice under supervision (ANA, 1990).

In *Commonwealth of Pennsylvania, State Board of Nurse Examiners v. Rafferty* (1984), a registered nurse was assigned to a patient who had developed serious complications that left him comatose and on a ventilator. During a bath, the registered nurse tested the patient for spontaneous respirations by disconnecting the respirator. Subsequently the patient's vital signs deteriorated and he began to have premature ventricular contractions (PVCs). The defendant nurse asked the opinion of a second registered nurse, who instructed the defendant nurse to call a code while the second nurse began ventilating the patient. Instead of calling the code, the defendant nurse left the patient's bedside and asked the opinion of yet a third nurse and a medical resident. Only then did the defendant nurse call the code. The resuscitation attempt was unsuccessful, and the patient was pronounced dead. The plaintiff's nurse expert witness, qualified as an expert in the field of critical care, testified that the defendant nurse's actions of (1) taking the comatose patient off the ventilator; (2) failure to call a code in a timely manner; and (3) leaving a patient who was experiencing PVCs were deviations from acceptable nursing standards. The State Board of Nursing revoked the license of the defendant nurse for violations of the nursing regulation requiring a nurse to carry out nursing care actions that promote, maintain, and restore the well-being of individuals.

As nurses' roles expand and change with the health care environment the Nurse Practice Acts (NPA) must reflect these expanding roles. Nurses must not only be knowledgeable of their current Nurse Practice Act but must also be instrumental in working with the legislature to revise and update the NPAs as necessary.

THE AMERICAN NURSES ASSOCIATION (ANA)

The American Nurses Association is the "official" organization of professional nurses. Since its inception in 1896, its main areas of focus have been economic interests, education, entry into practice, ethics, clinical standards for nursing practice, professional status, and research (ANA, 1987).

The American Nurses Association has been instrumental in the development of standards for the nursing profession since the 1960s with revisions to reflect the current state of nursing. The ANA's first practice standards were published in 1973, titled *Standards of Nursing Practice*. These standards were broad in scope, applied to all professional nurses regardless of specialty, and focused primarily on the nursing process. They were revised in 1991 and replaced with the *Standards of Clinical Nursing Practice*. These standards "describe a competent level of professional nursing care and professional performance common to all nurses engaged in clinical practice" (p. 3). The *Standards of Clinical Nursing Practice* consists of two components: (1) standards of care and (2) standards of professional performance. (See Displays 3-2 and 3-3.)

The *Code for Nurses with Interpretive Statements* was first published by the ANA in 1950 and a revised edition was published in 1976. This document addresses ethics and nursing standards. The *Code for Nurses with Interpretive Statements* (Display 3-4) provides a basis for ethical decision making (ANA, 1985).

In 1974, in recognition of increasing specialization and the subsequent need for applicable standards, the ANA published the first specialty standards. The clinical specialties included (1) Community Health Nursing, (2) Geriatric Nursing, (3) Maternal and Child Nursing, (4) Mental Health Nursing, and (5) Medical Surgical Nursing. At present the ANA publishes standards that address over 24 specialty areas (American Nurses Association, 1997).

NATIONAL PROFESSIONAL NURSING ORGANIZATIONS

Although the ANA has published generic standards applicable to all nurses, as well as 24 sets of broad standards addressing clinical specialties, many nurses felt a need for more specific standards and guidelines to supplement the general standards already in existence, hence the development of specialty professional nursing organizations. These organizations serve several purposes. They play a vital role in developing standards and guidelines that establish minimum safe standards specific to the specialty. They are also instrumental in disseminating information of relevance to the specialty area often through their own journals, newsletters, and reports. They often develop and/or sponsor educational programs to enable nurses to keep their knowledge and technical skills up to date. This can offer the

DISPLAY 3-2

Standards of Clinical Nursing Practice

Standards of Care

Standard	Statement
I. Assessment	The nurse collects client health data.
II. Diagnosis	The nurse analyzes the assessment data in determining diagnoses.
III. Outcome Identification	The nurse identifies expected outcomes individualized to the client.
IV. Planning	The nurse develops a plan of care that prescribes interventions to attain expected outcomes.
V. Implementation	The nurse implements the interventions identified in the plan of care.
VI. Evaluation	The nurse evaluates the client's progress toward attainment of outcomes.

American Nurses Association. (1991). *Standards of clinical nursing practice* (pp. 9–11). Washington, DC: Author. Reprinted with permission.

DISPLAY 3-3

Standards of Clinical Nursing Practice

Standards of Professional Performance

Standard	Statement
I. Quality of Care	The nurse systematically evaluates the quality and effectiveness of nursing practice.
II. Performance Appraisal	The nurse evaluates his/her own nursing practice in relation to professional practice standards and relevant statutes and regulations.
III. Education	The nurse acquires and maintains current knowledge in nursing practice.
IV. Collegiality	The nurse contributes to the professional development of peers, colleagues, and others.
V. Ethics	The nurse's decisions and actions on behalf of clients are determined in an ethical manner.
VI. Collaboration	The nurse collaborates with the client, significant others, and health care providers in providing client care.
VII. Research	The nurse uses research findings in practice.
VIII. Resource Utilization	The nurse considers factors related to safety, effectiveness, and cost in planning and delivering client care.

American Nurses Association. (1991). *Standards of clinical nursing practice* (pp. 13–17). Washington, DC: Author. Reprinted with permission.

additional benefit of permitting nurses to accrue continuing education credits. The organizations often sponsor research grants to encourage nurses to add to the current body of nursing knowledge. And last, these organizations often play an important part in the development and implementation of the certification process for its members.

In the area of perinatal nursing there are several specialty organizations, which develop standards and guidelines that serve as a basis for nursing care (see Display 3-5). The perinatal nurse should be familiar with the applicable organizations and their standards and guidelines. The professional standards should also be used as a basis for the development of hospital policies, for although hospital policies may

exceed national expectations, they should never be less stringent.

In *Bolduan v. Highland Park Hospital* (1997), Mrs. Bolduan was pregnant with her fourth child when she entered Highland Park Hospital on August 6, 1993, in labor. Her labor was augmented with Pitocin. During labor the fetal monitor strip began to show variable decelerations. The nurse continued to increase the pitocin and failed to implement any interventions appropriate for prolonged variable decelerations such as position change, oxygen administration, increasing nonadditive intravenous fluids, and physician notification. The fetal heart rate continued to deteriorate. Shortly after the physician arrived, the infant was delivered by caesarean section. However, the infant

DISPLAY 3-4

Code for Nurses with Interpretive Statements

1. The nurse provides services with respect for human dignity and the uniqueness of the client, unrestricted by considerations of social or economic status, personal attributes, or the nature of health problems.

2. The nurse safeguards the client's right to privacy by judiciously protecting information of a confidential nature.

3. The nurse acts to safeguard the client and the public when health care and safety are affected by the incompetent, unethical, or illegal practice of any person.

4. The nurse assumes responsibility and accountability for individual nursing judgements and actions.

5. The nurse maintains competence in nursing.

6. The nurse exercises informed judgement and uses individual competence and qualifications as criteria in seeking consultation, accepting responsibilities, and delegating nursing activities to others.

7. The nurse participates in activities that contribute to the ongoing development of the profession's body of knowledge.

8. The nurse participates in the profession's efforts to implement and improve standards of nursing.

9. The nurse participates in the profession's efforts to establish and maintain conditions of employment conducive to high quality nursing care.

10. The nurse participates in the profession's effort to protect the public from misinformation and misrepresentation and to maintain the integrity of nursing.

11. The nurse collaborates with members of the health professions and other citizens in promoting community and national efforts to meet the health needs of the public.

American Nurses Association. (1985). *Code for nurses with interpretive statements* (p. 1). Washington, DC: Author. Copyright 1985 by American Nurses Association. Reprinted with permission.

suffered brain damage and was permanently impaired. Ms. Bolduan sued the hospital and physician on behalf of her child, alleging that injudicious use of pitocin resulted in the permanent brain damage of her infant. The nurse testified that she increased the pitocin because the physician instructed her to. However, the physician denied ordering the increase and there was no written order or any notation in the chart of a verbal order. The jury verdict found the hospital liable for the negligent action of the nurse, who did not follow national standards in the administration of pitocin. The hospital was ordered to pay the plaintiffs $11 million. The physician was found not liable.

DOCUMENTARY EVIDENCE

There is a variety of documentation methods utilized by health care institutions, and each of the systems has advantages and disadvantages. Inherently, the type of documentation system is not as important as the nurse's ability to properly and consistently implement it according to

DISPLAY 3-5

Specialty Nursing Organizations in the Areas of Perinatal Nursing

American Nurses Association (ANA)
600 Maryland Avenue SW
Suite 100 West
Washington, DC 20024-2571
(202) 651-7000

American College of Nurse Midwives (ACNM)
818 Connecticut Avenue NW
Suite 900
Washington, DC 20006
(202) 728-9860

Association of Women's Health, Obstetric and Neonatal Nursing (AWHONN)
2000 L Street NW
Suite 740
Washington, DC 20036
(800) 673-8499 (U.S.)
(800) 245-0231 (Canada)
(800) 395-7373 (Fax on demand)
(202) 261-2400
(202) 728-0575 (Fax)
http://www.awhonn.org

National Association of Neonatal Nurses (NANN)
1304 Southpoint Boulevard
Suite 280
Petaluma, CA 94954-6859
(800) 451-3795

National Association of Pediatric Nurse Associates and Practitioners (NAPNAP)
1101 Kings Highway North
Suite 206
Cherry Hill, NJ 08034
(609) 667-1773

institutional guidelines. Also, the documentation system should reflect the national and institutional standards under which the unit functions. For example, for a perinatal nurse working in labor and delivery, the charting system should allow for fetal heart rate assessments at time intervals consistent with American College of Obstetrician and Gynecologists (ACOG) and AWHONN standards. For the low-risk patient, evaluation of the fetal heart rate is carried out every 60 minutes in the latent phase, every 30 minutes in the active phase, and every 15 minutes in the second stage of labor. For the high-risk patient, evaluation of the fetal heart rate is carried out every 30 minutes in the latent phase, every 15 minutes in the active phase, and every 5 minutes in the second stage of labor. Also, according to national standards the evaluation of the fetal heart rate should consist of baseline FHR, accelerations, decelerations, long-term variability, and short-term variability when appropriate. The charting system should also encourage the evaluation of contractions including frequency, duration, intensity, and resting tone. Nurses must be instrumental in developing and refining documentation systems that reflect their unit's individual needs based on applicable national and institutional standards.

Regardless of the system employed, the nurse's documentation is the only evidence that nursing assessments were carried out, physician orders were implemented, the nursing process was utilized, patient's responses were evaluated, communication took place with the physician and other health care providers, and standards were maintained. In many obstetrical malpractice cases that are litigated, the statute of limitations may be 18 years or more. By that time, most nurses would have little recollection of the particulars of the case. Often, the only proof of what transpired is the written documentation. The old adage "if it's not charted, it wasn't done" is widely quoted by nurse expert witnesses and is often still accepted in court.

Thorough documentation will be of the utmost benefit to the nurse as he or she tries to reconstruct events when questioned as to the nurse's actions and their rationale. The most proficient nurse will not appear competent if pertinent activities or events have not been charted. Many judges and juries interpret inadequate charting as an indication that substandard care was given to the patient.

Standards can be adhered to and yet a bad outcome may still occur. Accurate, thorough documentation of appropriate interventions serves to insulate the health care provider from liability. In *Cangelosi v. Our Lady of the Lake Regional Medical Center, et al.* (1989), the plaintiffs alleged that between the intubation and extubation for gallbladder surgery, negligence caused a fracture of two tracheal rings leading to a permanent tracheotomy and subsequent medical procedures. However, the evidence established that the physicians, nurses, and hospital did not deviate from the standard of care during intubation and extubation of an endotracheal tube during surgery despite the untoward results. All the physicians' and nurses' documentation was indicative of a normal insertion and removal with no unusual or abnormal symptoms during the 53 hours of intubation. Also, testimony and hospital records showed that the cuff pressure was routinely checked and the endotracheal tube routinely suctioned. The certified nurse anesthetist testified that she never used a stylet during intubations. The plaintiff's expert opinion was that the damage to the trachea occurred sometime during the intubation process. However, he did admit that tracheal stenosis can occur in the absence of substandard care. He also admitted that if a fracture had occurred during intubation, blood would have been seen when the patient was suctioned. Documentation indicated that blood was not present. An additional expert for the plaintiff, although he thought the injury was caused by the intubation, also admitted that he found no cases in the medical literature of fractured trachea rings for intubation when a stylet was not used. The jury found for the defense.

Defensive charting is a necessary component of today's litigious society. If documentation is done in a factual, accurate, and timely manner, consistent with policies and standards, it is an invaluable asset that can protect the nurse from liability. The following are some of the "Dos and Don'ts" of charting:

- Follow institutional guidelines for charting.
- Chart legibly, spell correctly, and use only institutionally approved abbreviations.
- Use clear, objective language.
- Correct any errors according to institutional policy; never erase or use correction fluid.
- Chart only your own observations and actions.
- Make an entry for every observation.
- Every entry should be dated, timed, and signed.
- Make use of late entries when appropriate.
- Chart all physician visits, examinations, results, review of fetal monitoring strips, and so on.
- Chart all communication with physicians and other health care providers, what information was relayed, and what the response was.
- If the physician's response is not timely or appropriate, document the use of the chain of command.
- Chart all changes in patient status that are indicative of deterioration, and actions taken in response to the changes.
- Chart all assessments, interventions, treatments, responses, and evaluations.
- Document all teaching, including discharge teaching, and evaluate patient understanding.
- Chart medication administration, amount, route, time, site, and response.
- Document all safety precautions, such as side rails up, and so on.
- Identify yourself after every entry.
- *Never* document in advance.
- *Never* replace or falsify any information.

Drug reference books such as the *Physicians' Desk Reference* and medication insert enclosures are other sources of information that the nurse is responsible for knowing and utilizing. Medication errors are cited as a common cause of nursing liability (Gobis, 1995). At a minimum, the responsibilities of the nurse administering medication include the correct patient, the correct medication, the correct dose, the correct route, the correct time, the correct injection techniques, knowledge of potential side effects, contraindications, and antidotes.

A physician's order will not protect a nurse from liability if a medication error occurs that results in damage. The nurse is responsible for questioning any physician order for a medication that is not within the normal range for dosage or administration route, or is contraindicated due to allergies or concurrent medical problems. The nurse is also responsible for questioning any order that is not clearly written. A drug reference book should always be easily accessible and the extra time taken to verify pertinent information. The majority of medication errors are easily preventable

ESTABLISHED REFERENCES

Nurses are also responsible for knowing information disseminated by professional organizations including standards, committee opinions, and technical reports. For nurses working in a perinatal setting the majority of standards and guidelines are developed by the professional organization AWHONN, formerly known as NAACOG (Nurses' Association of the American College of Obstetricians and Gynecologists). NAACOG published the first edition of standards in 1974, revising and updating them over the years, and has recently published the fifth edition. In addition to standards, AWHONN has published a variety of nursing practice resources such as *Fetal Heart Rate Auscultation 1990,* which gives specific guidelines for auscultation of the fetal heart rate and addresses correct techniques, evaluation, and documentation. AWHONN also has published position statements and committee opinions on issues such as *The Role of the Registered Nurse in the Management of the Patient Receiving Analgesia by Catheter Techniques* (1996) and the *Nurse's Role in Administration of Prostaglandin* (1995). AWHONN has also been instrumental in developing nursing practice competencies and educational guidelines for a variety of issues including fetal monitoring and ultrasound examinations. NAACOG published other valuable information in their practice resource guides, which include staffing recommendations for perinatal units. When involved in a lawsuit, nurses will be held to the published standards of their professional organization. Other important sources of information for the nurse include instructions from the Food and Drug Administration (FDA) or the manufacturer's instructions for correct use of equipment such as internal fetal heart rate monitors and intrauterine pressure catheters.

Textbooks

Textbooks, procedure books, and other authoritative publications are important sources of information that are utilized by nurse experts to form their opinion. A nurse may appear incompetent when he or she is not aware of information related to his or her specialty that is published in an undergraduate textbook.

In-Service Training Manuals and Information

Information presented during the initial orientation to the employing institution or any subsequent inservices can be considered information that the nurse is responsible for knowing and implementing.

In *Santa Rosa Medical Center v. Robinson* (1977), a patient fell and struck his head. The patient complained of pain in his head and vomited during the night. He was lethargic, his speech was slurred, and he was not very responsive to verbal stimuli. No physician was notified for over 8 hours, during which the patient's condition deteriorated. When medical attention was obtained the patient was diagnosed with an extradural hematoma, which resulted in a craniotomy and permanent, irreversible brain damage. The nurse expert testified that the nurses breached numerous standards and had been negligent in their duty to (1) assess the patient's condition, (2) recognize the importance of the symptoms, and (3) notify the physician in a timely manner. The court allowed the admission of a head injury film and tape that was used in in-service training of the nursing staff at the hospital. The information presented in the film and tape verified that the nurses had been trained in identifying the signs and symptoms of a head injury. The fact that the nurses did not recognize the significance of the patient's symptoms did not excuse the staff from notifying the physician in a timely manner. The delay in physician notification and the lack of subsequent treatment was held to be directly related to the poor outcome that the patient experienced. Not only does a nurse have an ethical and legal responsibility to notify the physician of any change in a patient's condition that could indicate deterioration in status, but the nurse also has a duty to use the chain of command if the physician does not respond in a timely manner. The jury found for the plaintiff, who was awarded over $450,000 in 1977.

The Joint Commission for the Accreditation of Healthcare Organizations

The Joint Commission for the Accreditation of Healthcare Organizations (JCAHO) is an example of a federal organization that sets standards for health care institutions: hospitals, long-term care facilities, ambulatory care, psychiatric and mental health care, and hospice care. Health care institutions are responsible for adhering to the standards proposed by the Joint Commission for the Accreditation of Healthcare Organizations. Noncompliance with standards may serve as sufficient cause for an organization to lose its accreditation and therefore become ineligible for third-party reimbursement payments.

JCAHO also sets national standards for hospitals. In *Shilkret v. The Annapolis Emergency Hospital Association et al.* (1975), the court stated that a hospital that has been accredited by the JCAHO is required to provide the care and skill expected of other JCAHO accredited hospitals and that there existed a national standard of care for accredited hospitals in caring for obstetrical patients. These standards included the availability of special facilities and specialists consistent with advances in the profession. The *Comprehensive Accreditation Manual for Hospitals: The Official Handbook, 1996,* states that "Standards establish a set of expectations against which current and future performance can be measured. . . . Standards are based on the idea that if you carry out important functions well, outcomes generally will be positive. Joint Commission standards define the functions and processes that must be carried out effectively in order to achieve good patient outcomes" (p. USI-1).

The JCAHO handbook is divided into several sections with individualized standards and indica-

tors used for evaluation. Although one section is devoted entirely to nursing, other sections include (1) care of patients, (2) management of information, (3) education, and (4) assessment of patients. These areas have standards that either directly address nursing interventions or have implications for nursing care and documentation. For example, one of the standards under the "Assessment of Patients" section mandates that a patient history and physical, including the nursing assessment, must be completed within 24 hours of a patient's admission as an inpatient. Another standard addresses medical records and record keeping and requires that every patient must have a nursing assessment at least once a shift, or more often if there is a change in patient status. These standards are applicable to all nurses working in perinatal settings and should be incorporated into the unit's institutional policies and procedures.

The following is an overview of the responsibilities of the nurse executive as listed by the JCAHO, 1996.

- To insure that nursing standards of patient care and standards of nursing practice are consistent with current nursing research standards and nationally recognized professional standards
- To implement the finding of current research from nursing and other literature into the policies and procedures governing the provision of nursing care
- To promote quality patient care, nursing services, including nursing care, on a continuous basis, 24 hours a day, 7 days a week, to those patients requiring such care and service. To accomplish this goal, the hospital provides a sufficient number of qualified nursing staff members to
  - assess the patient's nursing care needs;
  - plan and provide nursing care interventions;
  - prevent complications and promote improvement in the patient's comfort and wellness; and
  - alert other care professionals to the patient's condition, as appropriate.

JCAHO standards are fairly general and are normally incorporated into institutional policies and procedures for implementation. Many nurses are unaware of the source and rationale of these standards and the necessity of compliance for future hospital accreditation.

Hospitals that do not meet accreditation standards can be denied federal reimbursement for patient care.

Hospital Policies, Procedures, and Protocols

Hospital policies should be based on national guidelines if applicable. Although hospital policies may be more stringent than national policies, caution should be used. Holding nurses to standards that are difficult if not impossible to achieve does a disservice to the nursing staff. Policies and procedures should reflect achievable goals that result in good patient outcomes.

Hospital policies and procedures are scrutinized during a malpractice lawsuit as one basis for determining if the nurse has met or breached a duty. The American Nurses Association, in the publication *Liability Prevention & You, 1990,* states that failure to follow hospital procedure is one of the most frequent allegations against nurses.

JCAHO mandates that hospital policies be dated, reviewed periodically, and updated to reflect changing national standards, nurse practice acts, and changes within the health care setting. The hospital's policies and procedures must be accessible to the staff. Nurses should take an active part in ensuring that the policies and procedures reflect the current practice of their specialty. Also, when policies are updated, the old policies should not be destroyed until the statute of limitations has passed. Plaintiff's lawyers can demand the policies that were in effect at the time of an alleged incident that led to a malpractice case.

Hospital policies need not necessarily be written to be considered valid. In *Hartman v. Riverside Methodist Hospital et al.* (1989), an unwritten policy was still considered binding. This case focused on a case of emergency surgery. The surgery was uneventful, but due to the emergency status of the procedure, the patient had food in her stomach. The recovery room nurse was advised of this. The nurse was also aware that the anesthesiologist never wanted narcotics given to his postoperative patients without his approval. Nevertheless, when the patient awoke in pain, without consulting the anesthesiologist, the nurse administered Dilaudid, which along with the earlier medications relaxed the trachea and esophagus, resulting in regurgitation and aspiration and ending in death 43 days later. The jury found the nurse negligent by her act of administering a narcotic without the approval of the anesthesiologist, an unwritten policy, and found in favor of the family of the deceased patient.

THE EXPERT WITNESS

The expert witness plays an important role in presenting nursing standards for the jury to consider. The expert nurse's duty is (1) to present to the jury what the nursing standards were at the time the incident took place, and (2) to give an opinion as to whether the nurse adhered to the standards and acted as a reasonable and prudent nurse would have in the same or similar circumstances. If a nurse failed to meet the standards of care and breached his or her duty, the nurse was, by definition, negligent. Courts have spoken to the necessity of only a qualified "expert" being allowed to address standards and the adherence to those standards in the following malpractice cases. In *Northern Trust Company v. The Upjohn Company* (1991), the plaintiff, Ms. Moran, entered the hospital in 1978 to have her pregnancy aborted. Although Ms. Moran had a history of hypertension and was taking medication to control it, her blood pressure was normal upon entering the hospital. The nurse documented at the initial interview that Ms. Moran was in generally good health. After the initial assessment an IV was started, and the physician began the abortion procedure. The method chosen to terminate the second trimester pregnancy was the administration of Prostaglandin F2 Alpha (Prostin), which was manufactured and distributed by Upjohn. Instillation of the Prostin began about 4:20 P.M. and was completed about 4:25 P.M. The physician then left the room to write in the patient's chart. Initially, Ms. Moran suffered some of the typical side effects associated with the drug, including nausea, vomiting, cough, and irregular pulse rate. However, by 4:30 P.M. her blood pressure had elevated to 230 over 75. The physician was notified of the change and was called back to the patient's room where he diagnosed a mild reaction to the Prostin and instructed the nurse to keep monitoring her closely. About 4:40 P.M Moran's blood pressure improved, but her pulse was thready, she became cyanotic, and she experienced shortness of breath. The nurse started oxygen administration and attempted to notify the physician. As a resident entered the room to assist while waiting for the physician to respond to his page, Ms. Moran went into cardiac arrest. Cardio-pulmonary resuscitation began immediately and the patient was eventually resuscitated. However, she sustained brain damage, which involved permanent memory loss, disorientation, and difficulty in performing normal daily activities. Ms. Moran required residential care in a nursing home environment after her release from the hospital. In January 1980, a suit was filed against Upjohn, the physician, and the hospital due to the alleged negligence of the nurses. The trial went before a jury in 1989 and lasted 8 weeks. The jury returned a general verdict in the plaintiff's favor against all defendants in the amount of over $9 million. The expert witness for the plaintiff testified that the hospital was negligent because (1) its nursing personnel failed to obtain the presence of a physician, and (2) its nursing personnel failed to "appreciate the existence of an emergency represented by the events described up to and including Ms. Moran's failure to improve with oxygen." On appeal, the court held, based on expert testimony, that the nurse was not negligent and reversed the judgment entered against the hospital.

In *Hiatt v. Groce and Bethany Hospital* (1974), an action was brought by a maternity patient against a hospital and nurse for personal injuries sustained as a result of alleged failure of a nurse to notify the plaintiff's physician that delivery of the patient's child was imminent, resulting in an unattended birth with consequent injuries. On the evening of January 23, 1970, the plaintiff, Mrs. Hiatt, who was 24 years old, entered the hospital for the birth of her second child. She was in early labor and labored all night. The next morning the husband reported that he told the nurse, who was reading a magazine in the nurses' station, that his wife's contractions were getting stronger. His testimony was that the nurse continued to read the magazine and then said she would check Mrs. Hiatt. After performing a vaginal exam, the nurse stated that Mrs. Hiatt was only 7 cm dilated and that it would be quite a while before she had the baby. The husband reportedly told the nurse that his wife delivered their first child shortly after she reached 8 cm dilation, to which the nurse responded that she was in charge and would take care of calling the doctor when she thought it was necessary. Approximately an hour later, the husband again approached the nurse at the nurses' station, where she was again reading a magazine, and reported that the contractions were getting stronger. The nurse came to the room and examined Mrs. Hiatt and reported she was now 8 cm dilated. Mr. Hiatt asked the nurse to please call the physician as their first child came almost immediately when his wife reached 8 cm. The nurse stated she was in charge and would call when she thought it was necessary. The nurse then left the room and went to the nurses' station where she continued to read her magazine. Within a few minutes, Mrs. Hiatt screamed she was going to have the baby. The husband ran to the nurses' station, to get the nurse. After determining that Mrs. Hiatt was indeed crowning with the infant, she paged the physician. The physician did not arrive in time and the infant was delivered by the nurse. The nurse later testified under oath that although the hospital records state the baby was delivered by the physician, she in fact had delivered the baby but was under orders from the nursing supervisor not to document it. The birth resulted in lacerations to the perineum that caused Mrs. Hiatt permanent damage to nerves in the area resulting in pain and sexual dysfunction. The case was submitted to the jury solely upon the issue of negligence of the defendant nurse. The court held that: "In determining whether a registered nurse used the learning, skill and conduct required of her, the jury is not permitted to arbitrarily set a standard of its own or determine the question from its personal knowledge. On questions of nursing expertise concerning the standard of care of a nurse, only those qualified as experts are permitted to testify. The standard of care is established by members of the same profession in the same or similar communities under like circumstances."

Experts are also instrumental in explaining and interpreting the standards in terms that the lay members of a jury can understand. At the deliberation portion of the trial the jury will consider the "facts" of the case, which include expert testimony. The jury must decide whether the nurse did or did not adhere to said standards. The causation factor must also be proven, for a nurse is not considered negligent if the breached duty did not cause the particular injury or if no damage occurred, even if she or he did not meet applicable nursing standards. A bad patient outcome is not always an indication of malpractice (*Gibson and Sheppard v. Bossier City General Hospital, et al.,* 1991).

Most expert witnesses have a library of information in their specialty area, which may include a variety of national and state standards and guidelines, such as nurse practice acts, JCAHO manuals and standards, and guidelines published by the applicable professional organizations. In addition, the expert will usually request the pertinent hospital policies and procedures relevant to the case, such as pitocin administration guideline, fetal distress protocols, glucose monitoring procedures, and so on. Texts and other authoritative material from the period of time in which the incident took place may be reviewed and used as a basis for an opinion on whether the nurse met or breached standards.

Occasionally there are national guidelines published by professional organizations that are very specific in such areas as the intervals for monitoring and evaluating fetal heart rates for low-risk and high-risk patients, which makes determining the standards and evaluating whether a nurse adhered to standards relatively simple.

In *Alef v. Alta Bates Hospital et al.* (1992), the plaintiffs alleged that negligent Doppler monitoring of the fetal heart rate during labor and delivery by the nurse was the proximate cause of an infant's permanent brain damage. Physician experts testified that the baby's brain damage occurred during the second stage of labor. The plaintiffs alleged that inadequate monitoring by the labor and delivery nurse resulted in the decelerations going unnoticed. The labor and delivery nurse attending the patient testified that during the second stage of labor she listened to the fetal heart rate "after every contraction," for approximately 15 seconds. Based on the testimony of an expert in obstetrical nursing the jury found that the standard for monitoring the fetal heart rate with a Doppler during the second stage of labor was breached by the registered nurse. Evidence established by the expert nurse witness established that (1) the standard of care in 1981 for Doppler monitoring of the fetal heart rate was to assess throughout the complete contraction and for 30–40 seconds afterward in order to detect late decelerations that could be an indication of hypoxia; (2) the labor and delivery nurse caring for the patient, by her own admission, did not monitor as the standard required and therefore did not properly assess for late decelerations. The expert stated that the purpose of fetal heart rate monitoring is to detect changes in the fetal heart rate that are indicative of fetal distress, thus allowing prompt additional measures to prevent injury or limit further damage to the fetus. The plaintiff's expert physician testified that if the fetal distress had been detected and timely intervention had occurred, the infant's brain damage would probably have been prevented.

In the same case, it was established that the standard can be the same for physicians and nurses in specific areas such as fetal heart rate monitoring. Because this was the standard of care to which the patient was entitled, the hospital was required to provide that minimum level of care. It was irrelevant whether the monitoring was performed by a physician or a nurse as both are qualified to perform the function.

However, in many instances there is no specific standard or guideline that addresses the exact issues in the case. In these instances when guidelines are broad, the expert nurse witness gives an interpretation and opinion as to whether standards were met. In these instances, the expert witness for the defense will have an opinion that may differ drastically from that of the plaintiff's expert. In *Fraijo v. Hartland* (1979), the court upheld the notion that a nurse is not bound do to exactly what another nurse would do, but only to conduct herself or himself as a reasonable and prudent nurse. If there is more than one recognized method of diagnosis or treatment and not one of them is used exclusively by all practitioners, a physician or nurse is not negligent if in exercising best judgment, the person selects one of the approved methods that later turns out to be a wrong selection or one not favored by other practitioners. There might be a variety of options that would fulfill the nurse's duty to the patient.

In *Morella v. Bryn Mawr Hospital et al.* (1997), the patient was a 26-year-old gravida 5 para 5 who delivered her last child on October 5, 1992. During her immediate postpartum period, the registered nurse charted at 6:45 A.M. that the patient "verbalized reluctance to have tubal today—states she wants to think about it some more. Advised to discuss this with her M.D." The same information was documented on the clinical record sheet. The nurse went off duty at 7:00 A.M. and no further documentation was made. The patient underwent a tubal ligation later that afternoon with no complications. She later sued the physician and hospital stating she had not given informed consent, as she never had the opportunity to discuss her reservations about the procedure with the physician. In the physician's deposition, the physician stated she never read the chart, and was unaware of the patient's reluctance. The physician also stated that she would have expected the nurse to contact her directly if such a situation occurred. The expert nurse witness for the plaintiff testified that a standard of nursing care is to inform the physician that the patient was reconsidering the surgery, and that it is also a standard of nursing care for the nurse to reassess the patient at some point to ensure that the patient had an opportunity to discuss her reluctance with the physician. Because the standards were not met, the nurse did breach her duty to the patient.

The nurse expert for the defense gave the opinion that the nurse did meet the standard of care by instructing the patient to confer with the physician and that it was the patient's responsibility to follow through. The nurse expert also stated that the nurse had charted the information in the chart and that it was the responsibility of the physician to read it. The jury found for the defense.

There are some instances within the law where an expert is not needed to identify pertinent standards or to address whether standards were met. These exceptions include (1) legal duty established by law, (2) *res ipsa loquitur*, and (3) not helpful to a jury.

Legal Duty Established by Law

If the standard of care is statutorily established by the state nurse practice act, it is a matter of law and therefore a matter for the judge to decide, not the jury. The expert witnesses are only used if they can assist the jury in understanding the issues in the case. In a jury trial, questions of "fact" are left to the jury to decide and questions of "law" are decided by the court. In a nonjury trial, the court decides questions of both fact and law. The court can take the matter out of the jury's hands and "direct a verdict" for either the defense or plaintiff. For example, if a registered nurse artificially ruptures membranes and damage occurs to either the mother or fetus, the nurse will be found negligent due to the fact that she acted outside her scope of practice. (Most state nurse practice acts do not recognize artificial rupture of membranes as a registered nurse function; it is in the domain of the physician and nurse midwife.) A nurse expert would not be needed to testify as to standards and the breach that occurred because it is a matter of law that the nurse functioned outside the nurse's scope of practice. The court could direct the verdict in favor of the plaintiff.

Res Ipsa Loquitur—"The Thing Speaks for Itself"

The term *res ipsa loquitur* was first mentioned in the 1863 English case, *Byrne v. Boadle,* 1863, where a barrel of flour rolled out of a warehouse window onto a pedestrian. Because a barrel of flour should *not* roll out of a warehouse window in the absence of negligence even though it could not be proven who actually pushed the barrel out of the warehouse window, it was presented to the jury that without direct evidence, the conclusion could be drawn that the accident was the owner's fault (Restatement, supra, 328D, comment a; W. Prosser & W. Keeton, supra, 39, at 243; J. Lee & B. Lindahl, supra, 15:19).

This legal doctrine negates the need for an expert witness in that the defendant's liability is self-evident even to a lay person. The rule of *res ipsa loquitur* applies if three conditions are present: (1) the injury would not ordinarily have occurred unless there was negligence; (2) whatever caused the injury at the time was under the exclusive control of the defendant; (3) the injured person did not contribute to the negligence (contributory negligence) or voluntarily assume the risk. Some classic examples of *res ipsa loquitur* are cases where an operative sponge is left in a surgical patient, an infant is dropped in the nursery by a staff member, or burns and other injuries occur when the patient is unconscious from anesthesia.

In these cases the evidence is not in dispute and jurors would know from their own experience that negligence occurred. An expert witness would not be needed. The decision must be made by the court to invoke *res ipsa loquitur.*

Not Helpful to a Jury

Expert witnesses are only used if they can assist the jury in understanding the issues in the case. If the jury can understand the issues there is no need for expert witness testimony. However, in most medical negligence cases, standard of care testimony is required. As stated earlier there are often many ways to implement standards. The expert can address these issues and describe the situation, as well as how and why the nurse met the standard. The subjective evaluation is the basic rationale for differing opinions and testimony presented by "opposing" experts.

It cannot be stressed too strongly that nurses have both a professional and a legal responsibility to be competent in their area of practice.

This includes knowing applicable standards pertaining to the area of perinatal nursing in which the nurse functions. Lack of knowledge will never be an acceptable defense for negligent nursing care. This puts the responsibility on the practicing nurse to stay current, be involved in the appropriate professional nursing organizations, and be proactive in the development and refinement of institutional policies and procedures. Patients are becoming ever more discriminating in evaluating the health care provided to them and expect and deserve competent and compassionate care. Implementation of standards, regardless of the source, should not only insulate nurses from claims of negligence but also serve as the basis for high-quality nursing care to all patients regardless of where they receive care.

REFERENCES

American Academy of Nursing. (1987). The evolution of nursing professional organizations: Alternative models for the future. Kansas City, MO: American Nurses Association.

American Nurses Association. (1973). Standards of nursing practice. Washington, DC: Author.

American Nurses Association. (1975). A plan for implementation of the standard of nursing practice. Kansas City, MO: Author.

American Nurses Association. (1980). Nursing: A social policy statement. Washington, DC: Author.

American Nurses Association. (1983). Standards of maternal–child nursing practice. Washington, DC: Author.

American Nurses Association. (1984). Standards for professional nursing education. Washington, DC: Author.

American Nurses Association. (1985). Code for nurses with interpretive statements. Washington, DC: Author.

American Nurses Association. (1986). Enforcement of the nursing practice act. Kansas City, MO: Author.

American Nurses Association. (1990). Liability prevention & you: What nurses & employers need to know. Kansas City, MO: Author.

American Nurses Association. (1991). Standards of clinical nursing practice. Washington, DC: American Nurses Publishing.

American Nurses Association. (1995). Nursing's social policy statement. Washington, DC: American Nurses Publishing.

American Nurses Association. (1997). Catalog of publication. Washington, DC: Author.

Association of Women's Health, Obstetric and Neonatal Nurses (AWHONN). (1991). Nursing practice competencies and educational guidelines for antepartum fetal surveillance and intrapartum fetal heart monitoring. Washington, DC: Author.

Association of Women's Health, Obstetric and Neonatal Nurses (AWHONN). (1993). Nursing practice competencies and educational guidelines for limited ultrasound examination in obstetric and gynecologic/infertility settings. Washington, DC: Author.

Association of Women's Health, Obstetric and Neonatal Nurses (AWHONN). (1995). The nurse's role in administration of prostaglandin. Washington, DC: Author.

Association of Women's Health, Obstetric and Neonatal Nurses (AWHONN). (1998). Standards & guidelines (5th ed.). Washington, DC: Author.

Bernzweig, E. P. (1996). The nurse's liability for malpractice (6th ed.). St. Louis, MO: Mosby.

Gardner, S., & Hagedorn, M. (1997). Legal aspects of maternal-child nursing practice: Concepts and strategies in risk management. Menlo Park, CA: Addison Wesley Longman.

Gobis, L.A. (1995). Medication errors: Learn from your colleagues' mistakes. RN, 58(12), 59–63.

Guido, G. W. (1997). Legal issues in nursing, Norwalk, CT. Appleton and Lange.

Moniz, D. (1992). The legal danger of written protocols and standard of practice. Nurse Practice 17, 58–60.

Joint Commission for Accreditation of Healthcare Organizations. (1997). Comprehension accreditation for hospitals: The official handbook. Oakbrook Terrace, IL: Author.

Nurses' Association of the American College of Obstetricians and Gynecologists. (1990). Fetal heart rate auscultation. Washington., DC: Author.

Nurses' Association of the American College of Obstetricians and Gynecologists. (1991). Nursing practice, competencies and educational guidelines: Antepartum fetal surveillance and intrapartum heart monitoring. Washington, DC: Author.

Prosser, W. (1971). Handbook of the law of torts (4th ed.). St. Paul, MN: West.

CASE CITATIONS

Alef v. Alta Bates Hospital et al., 5 Cal. App. 4th 208, 6 Cal. Rptr. 2d 900 (Cal. 1992).

Bolduan v. Highland Park Hospital, 95 L 403 Cir. Ct., Lake Co., Ill. (1997).

Byrne v. Boadle, 2 H. & C. 722, 159 Eng. Rep. 299 (1863).

Cangelosi v. Our Lady of the Lake Regional Medical Center, et al., 564 S.2d 654 (La. 1989).

Commonwealth of Pennsylvania, State Board of Nurse Examiners v. Rafferty, 508 Pa. 566, 499 A.2d. 289 (Supreme Court of Pa. 1984).

Ewing v. Aubert, 532 S.2d 876 (La. App. 1988).

Fraijo v. Hartland Hospital, 99 Cal. Rptr. 3d 331, 160 Cal. Rptr. 246 (1979).

Gibson and Sheppard v. Bossier City General Hospital, et al., 594 S.2d 1332 (La., 1991).

Hartman v. Riverside Methodist Hospital et al., 62 Ohio App. 3d 599, 577 N.E.2d 112 (1989).

Hiatt v. Groce, 215 Kan. 14, 523 P.2d 320 (Kans. 1974).

Morella v. Bryn Mawr Hospital et al. (Delaware County, 1997).

The Northern Trust Company v. The Upjohn Company, 213 Ill. App. 3d 390, 572 N.E.2d 1030, 157 Ill. Dec. 566 (Ill. 1991).

Santa Rosa Medical Center v. Robinson, 560 S.W.2d 751 (Tex. 1977)

Shilkret v. The Annapolis Emergency Hospital Association, et al., 276 Md. 187, 349 A.2d 245 (1975).

Ybarra v. Spangard, 154 P.2d 687 (Cal. 1944).

CHAPTER 4

Professional Negligence and Nursing Malpractice

Davia Solomon and Rebecca Cady

When a lawsuit is brought against a health care provider by a patient or the patient's family, the most common claim is that the health care provider has been professionally negligent. Such claims are subject to certain rules and theories of law that have been created to provide some measure of protection against meritless claims. This chapter explores the rules and theories surrounding claims of professional negligence against health care providers.

SOURCES OF LEGAL RESPONSIBILITY

General liability springs from three sources: criminal, contractual, and tort. Contract and tort cases are both considered to be civil actions. In a civil action, the plaintiff is a private citizen or entity who believes they have been wronged in some fashion. The standard of proof by which the plaintiff is required to prove his or her case is called a *preponderance of the evidence*. This is a lower standard than that used in criminal cases, and requires only that the jury decide which evidence is more believable to support any fact than any other evidence (LaFave and Scott, 1986). As a review, ordinary negligence, or "a person doing something which the reasonably prudent person would not do; or failing to do something which the reasonably prudent person

would do under the circumstances" is a necessary ingredient for tort liability (Restatement [Second] of Torts, 1972).

In a contractual civil case, the rights of the parties are dependent upon the failure of one of the parties to live up to some agreement between the two of them. Penalties for civil liability consist of monetary compensation for injuries or damages sustained.

Acts that violate criminal laws are the basis for liability in the criminal arena. The plaintiff in criminal cases is always the state or federal government and its respective citizens, who ensure that the guilty party is punished in some way for violating the public safety or welfare (LaFave and Scott, 1986). The standard of proof needed to convict a person of a crime is "beyond a reasonable doubt." Penalties for criminal liability include fines and imprisonment.

Perinatal injuries can give rise to liability in either contracts, torts, or criminal law. An example of the application of contract law would be when the nurse contracts to perform nursing services for compensation to be paid by the patient or family. If the nurse promises to provide services and inexcusably does not perform the services, a suit could follow holding the nurse liable for damages resulting from his or her breach of this contract. Contract cases are rare in nursing due to the nature of today's nursing practice. In a contract case, the damages consist of what injuries result from the failure of a party to perform what they have agreed to do in exchange for consideration, that is, payment, and nurses could therefore have legal liability under a contracts theory (Prosser, 1941).

Criminal liability can result from the nurse failing to obey the laws of the state. Although criminal law is not generally used to regulate nurses and physicians, it is of some benefit that each state require that nurses become generally familiar with state and federal regulations, which call for criminal penalties for prohibited conduct. The most common criminal allegations against nurses are practicing without a license and refusing to provide emergency care in an emergency department (Brent, 1997). It should be clear that homicide is prohibited in every jurisdiction and that homicide is defined variously in different jurisdictions. For a nurse to take steps to ensure the death of a patient when the patient's spouse seemed to indicate that his wife would be better off dead would be considered a criminal act punishable by a term in jail (*State v. Shook,* 1990). This is because the public generally does not want medical care providers independently and unilaterally making such decisions. In this example, in addition to a criminal action, the aggrieved husband and family may also have the right to file a civil tort cause of action seeking damages for the death of the patient. If the head of the hospital contributed to the violation of a criminal statute or the head of the hospital or other hospital personnel aided the nurse, the hospital could similarly be exposed to criminal penalties as well as civil damages.

ORDINARY NEGLIGENCE

Ordinary negligence is a person doing something that the reasonably prudent person would not do; or failing to do something that the reasonably prudent person would do under the circumstances (Prosser, 1941). All negligence claims require proof of four elements: duty, breach, causation, and harm. An action for ordinary negligence requires first that the person being sued owed some duty to act or not act to the person bringing the lawsuit. In a famous

New York case, a woman named Kitty Genovese was being stabbed to death outside the windows of many apartment dwellers while she screamed and cried for help. Many people later admitted hearing her cries and doing nothing about it. If the family of this victim had brought a lawsuit against those who heard her cries and did not act, the law would not support this claim because no legal duty exists to respond to a stranger's cries for help. The law does not impose a duty to rescue a stranger (Restatement [Second] of Torts, 1972).

PROFESSIONAL NEGLIGENCE OR MALPRACTICE

As discussed in Chapter 3, special rules apply when one is trying to show that a medical professional was negligent. Professional negligence and malpractice really mean the same thing, that is, when a professional has acted in such a way so as to breach a duty owed to someone, usually the patient, which causes harm.

Res Ipsa Loquitur

This legal doctrine, which is Latin for "the thing speaks for itself," provides a circumscribed way to show professional negligence in certain narrow cases without testimony regarding the standard of care. This doctrine establishes that when the facts are easily understood by ordinary people and when such occurrences do not happen unless negligence of some kind occurred, then expert testimony is not required to establish that the defendant was negligent. For this doctrine to be used in the medical malpractice case, the plaintiff must establish that the event involved must (1) be of a kind that ordinarily does not occur in the absence of someone's negligence, (2) be caused by an instrumentality or agency within the exclusive control of the defendant, and (3) not have been due to any voluntary action or contribution on the part of the plaintiff (Prosser & Keeton, 1984). Part of the reason for the application of this doctrine in medical cases is that doctors and nurses have proved in the past to be reluctant to divulge information to a plaintiff, which makes it difficult, if not impossible, for the plaintiff to prove his or her case. In a classic California case, a patient awoke from an appendectomy operation with an injury to his right shoulder and neck. The team of doctors and nurses declined to state what had occurred during the surgery, leaving plaintiff with few options in explanation for his condition. The court, in applying the doctrine of *res ipsa loquitur,* stated: "Without the aid of the doctrine a patient who received permanent injuries of a serious character, obviously the result of someone's negligence, would be entirely unable to recover unless the doctors and nurses in attendance voluntarily chose to disclose the identity of the negligent person and the facts establishing liability" (*Ybarra v. Spangard,* 1944).

When this doctrine is applied, the plaintiff need not present expert testimony as to the standard of care that was breached. If the plaintiff can establish the preconditions for the use of this doctrine, courts reason that a jury can decide the facts without the use of expert testimony and the burden of proof may shift to the defendant, requiring the defendant to introduce evidence to rebut or explain the inference of negligence (Prosser & Keeton, 1984).

Professional negligence that cannot be proven by the doctrine of *res ipsa loquitur* requires the establishment of four elements: duty, breach, causation, and harm.

Duty/Breach

The question of duty was addressed in an early Alabama case. A woman went to the hospital to have a baby. She and her husband believed the baby was coming imminently. The wife asked the nurse to call the doctor but the nurse determined that the doctor was unnecessary at the time. The husband asked the nurse to remain with the wife when the nurse sent the husband from the room. Unfortunately, the nurse likewise left the patient and ignored the repeated call button requests for assistance. The baby was born on its own and strangled in the umbilical cord. The jury found that the nurse had failed in her duty to observe the laboring woman and to use such judgment as was required of a nurse to summon the physician to attend the birth. The

jury felt the duty extended to all things that should be obvious to a nurse if she were attending reasonably to the duties incumbent on her as a professional (*Birmingham Baptist Hospital v. Branton,* 1928).

Depending on the jurisdiction, the nurse's duty will be found in statutory codes, regulatory laws such as those governing the board of nursing, and/or case law. In professional negligence cases involving nurses, the duty can also be found in the customs and practices of nurses, which rise to the level of standards in the profession. Each element involved in the standard of care can be the subject of spirited argument, which is often the gist of a malpractice action when it reaches the trial court.

Once a duty on the part of the health care provider arises, the duty must then be breached in order to result in potential liability. Generally the breach is obvious and does not require elucidation and detail. In a 1988 Connecticut case, a baby was born who subsequently developed breathing problems. The delivery room nurse attempted to suction the baby and administer oxygen, but the baby did not respond. The physician inserted an endotracheal tube, but the nurse could not find the proper tube to fit the endotracheal tube for suctioning. Then the doctor asked for an ambu bag. The nurse handed it to him attached to a mask too large for the infant. The doctor and nurse could not remove the mask. The doctor performed CPR until proper equipment arrived, but the baby had suffered severe hypoxia and cerebral palsy. At the trial, the nurse testified that it was her responsibility to equip the delivery room and to know how to use the equipment; she failed to remove the mask but didn't know why she had failed; it was her responsibility to stock supplies in the delivery room but she didn't restock suction tubes because she assumed she wouldn't need them; prior to the incident she had not worked for 9 weeks; and she had never assisted in a delivery room where an ambu bag was used. The jury found the hospital negligent and based its decision on the expert testimony introduced at trial that the hospital breached its duty to the patient by not giving the nurse a refresher course, updating her knowledge of her working circumstances, or orienting the nurse to the equipment necessary for use in the delivery room (*Mather v. Griffin Hospital,* 1988).

Proximate or Legal Causation

The next element necessary to successfully prove a malpractice action is called proximate or legal cause. Proximate cause has been defined as a cause "which in natural and continuous sequence, unbroken by any controlling, intervening cause, produces injury, and without which it would not have occurred" (*Johnson v. Minneapolis, St. Paul & S. S. M. Ry. Co.,* 1926). In a medical negligence case, unlike most other negligence cases, the causal connection between the defendant's conduct and the plaintiff's injury is almost always in issue, and must also be proven by expert testimony. The plaintiff has the burden of proving the causal connection between the injuries and the defendant's malpractice. For example, plaintiff may be able to prove that a defendant's care fell below the standard of care in not properly monitoring the fetal heart tones in a hypoxic infant, but may not be able to prove that the infant's brain damage was the proximate result of inadequate monitoring. Furthermore, causation must be established to a reasonable medical probability, that is, it is not enough for the expert to say that the breach might have caused the injury, but instead he or she must say that the breach, to a reasonable medical probability, caused the injury.

By way of example, consider the following: You are a labor and delivery nurse and you do not recognize late decelerations on the fetal monitor nor do you inform the physician. If, in fact, the infant is born without complications, or if the complications arose prior to the delivery phase, that is, if the child had a genetic disorder, you would not be held liable despite your breach of the standard of care. The nurse who misses the sponge count on a patient who dies of a heart attack during the night cannot be held liable for the death of the patient if, in fact, the heart attack had nothing to do with the errant sponge still floating around in the peritoneal cavity. An erroneous prescription, which calls for a dosage that would be lethal, does not result in liability to anyone if an alert nurse does not administer it. The duty and breach of duty must, to a reasonable medical probability, be the cause of a claimed injury to be considered as one of the elements required to prove professional negligence.

Harm

The final element of a cause of action for professional negligence is injury and damages. Where there is a duty, and a breach of that duty, and that breach causes some effect, the effect must be injurious to be actionable (Prosser, 1941). For example, if a labor and delivery nurse failed to obtain a group B strep vaginal culture ordered by a patient's physician and the patient was in fact a group B strep carrier but the infant was born without group B strep sequelae, then, as no harm occurred, the nurse could not be found liable for a claim of professional negligence

DUTIES OF THE GENERALIST NURSE

Aside from the duty to do the right thing and to avoid the wrong thing, a practicing nurse has a general duty to possess the knowledge, skill, and judgment commensurate with his or her education, experience, and position. The adequacy of a nurse's performance is tested with respect to the performance of other nurses (*Fraijo v. Hartland Hospital,* 1979). A registered nurse's duty is identical to that owed by the hospital, that is, to exercise the care required by the patient's condition and to protect the patient from danger (*Daniel v. St. Francis Cabrini Hospital of Alexandria, Inc.,* 1982). A registered nurse who has worked in a highly specialized field exclusively for many years might be seriously at risk in suddenly accepting assignments in other highly specialized fields when the nurse knows or should know that he or she is no longer reasonably current. It would be the duty of the nurse, if so assigned, to call attention to the administration and the other medical professionals that the field upon which he or she has been asked to embark is not one in which he or she claims expertise. It would be incumbent upon this nurse to venture no further except in emergency situations where no other person with greater skill was available.

Many hospitals, doctors offices, military establishments, and government health departments have special procedures particular to the type of patients they treat, diseases they see, or superior orders they obey. For a nurse to depart from the protocols so established would be a serious dereliction except for compelling reasons otherwise. Any departure from such instructions would place the nurse in jeopardy unless the nurse is able to justify conduct inconsistent with such protocols. Evidence that the hospital has specific procedures from which the nurse deviated can be devastating to the defense of the nurse if injury follows such departures. The health care industry has recognized that it has a duty to deliver a minimum quality of nursing care throughout the country (JCAH, 1981; ANA, 1954, 1966). Each state enforces a code or set of standards that governs the delivery of health care in hospitals, through its health department, state board of nursing, or other agency. And, although each state is responsible for the requirements for the practice of nursing within its boundaries, national standards of nursing practice were developed in 1973 (ANA, 1973; Kelly, 1974).

Investigations into liability invariably include searching out the existence of manuals, general instruction materials, minutes of seminars, and similar communications. Information showing that the hospital has established a standard that in its own judgment is the standard to be observed is compelling evidence of liability if harm results from a deviation by an employed nurse. If, in a nurse's opinion, a standard called for by the hospital or the doctor differs from a standard that his or her nurse's training suggests is a community standard, it is a nurse's duty to reconcile this difference. If the community standard is stricter, the nurse is on notice that any standard that falls below the community standard may harm the patient and create liability for those who observe a lower standard. If the procedure proscribed is higher or safer or better than what the nurse believes to be the community standard, he or she would be well advised to abide by the higher standard because proof that injury occurred as a result of a departure from an employer's standard is very likely to result in a jury awarding money to the patient who has been injured.

To a professional whose job includes supervision of others, the duty to supervise and to call attention to problems is an affirmative duty. If a nurse observes conduct of other staff members that threatens the health and safety of the patients, it is the nurse's affirmative duty to call that conduct to the hospital's attention and to warn the patients. It is the nurse's duty to do all that is reasonably possible to prevent harm to the patient even if the hospital does not heed the warning.

A physician may make a request, prepare a prescription, give an instruction, or perform a procedure that is clearly inappropriate. It is the duty of a nurse to question any action by any person that, in the nurse's opinion, is counter to good medical practice; if the nurse is not satisfied with the response, the nurse has an affirmative duty to call it to the attention of others who have the power and responsibility to evaluate and allay the nurse's concern, that is, to use the hospital's chain of command. Although this is obviously an area where circumspection and tact are called for, it is never appropriate for a nurse to shirk his or her own responsibility for fear of ruffling the feathers of others. The health and protection of the patient are paramount.

The degree of duty can differ among nurses. The obstetrician/gynecologist who holds himself/herself out as a specialists' specialist, for example, the perinatologist, has the duty to have a higher degree of skill and to use that skill than does the ordinary general practitioner who is delivering babies. So too, a nurse practitioner who specializes in perinatal matters or the nurse who has attained specialty certification in her area of practice is held to a higher standard than the general duty nurse who does not.

ADVANCED PRACTICE NURSES

An advanced practice nurse is a registered nurse who has completed an additional course of study in a nursing specialty that provides specialized knowledge and skills to function in an expanded role (Inglis & Kjervik, 1993). Inherent in the expansion of the role are expanded legal responsibilities and liabilities. In 1983, the Missouri Supreme Court became the first court to address an interpretation of the nurse practice act for Missouri. The court acknowledged that the state had recognized the expanded role of nurses when the practice act was revised in 1975. By recognizing the expanded role of the advanced practice nurse, the state also articulated the legal premise that the nurse would also have the responsibility to act in a professional manner and know the limits of his or her professional knowledge. This would include the duty to act within the limits of standing orders and protocols and the duty to refer to a physician when a patient's needs exceeded the scope of the nurse's practice (*Sermchief v. Gonzales,* 1983). Other duties that the advanced practice nurse has are consistent with his or her area of practice. Advanced practice nurses have been accused of negligence for failure to inform of known risks and delay in proper treatment by the nurse practitioner (*Gugino v. Harvard Community Health Plan,* 1980), failure to consult a physician when there is a change in condition by the nurse midwife (*Lustig v. The Birthplace,* 1983), negligent administration of an anesthetic, failing to attempt corrective measures, and failure to seek help in a timely manner by the nurse-anesthetist (*Brown v. Dahl,* 1985). In most of these cases, the courts held that the standard of care was that of a nurse specialist with the same education, skill, and training. The expert testimony was that of a similar nurse specialist, not a medical expert.

In a landmark California case, *Fein v. Permanente Medical Group* (1985) the appellate court held that the trial court had erred when it sent an instruction to the jury to the effect that the standard of care required of a nurse practitioner when the nurse practitioner examines a patient or makes a diagnosis is the standard of care of a physician and surgeon duly licensed to practice medicine in California. Even though the reversal did not go so far as to relieve the nurse practitioner of her liability in that case, the courts now recognize that the professional standard that the advanced practice nurse will be measured against will be that of another advanced practice nurse.

In 1989 in the state of Indiana, the court of appeals officially stated that a nurse practitioner is a specialist under the Indiana statute and is held to the standard of care appropriate to persons of such superior knowledge and skill (*Planned Parenthood of Northwest Indiana v. Vines,* 1989). The court reiterated that the standard of care and how the nurse practitioner breached that standard must be established by expert testimony. This was a case where a nurse practitioner was claimed to have been negligent in inserting an IUD. Testimony was given that there is a universal minimum standard for the insertion of IUDs. Interestingly, the standard for a nurse practitioner in this particular case was declared by the court to be that of a physician doing the same work; however, in general, nurse practitioners are held to the standard of nurse practitioners, not doctors.

CASE EXAMPLE

A significant drama occurred in a hospital in San Jose, California, where a mother died from hemorrhage following an incision of the cervix made to relieve a constricted band of muscle during childbirth. The hospital, nurses, and doctor were sued. The pregnant woman was given pitocin to induce labor. The doctor made and left unsutured an incision in the cervix. The nurse informed the doctor three times within the next 2 hours that she felt that the patient was bleeding excessively. The doctor reassured her that was normal and told the nurse that the way to measure the blood loss was to figure out how long the perineal pads took to become soaked. The nurse kept changing the pads but never took vital signs. She didn't call the doctor because she felt he wouldn't come in any event. She was also still doing her timing tests and felt that they were not yet completed.

The doctor did state on his postpartum orders that he should be called if the postpartum flow was greater than normal. Three hours after surgery, the nurse thought an emergency existed; a half hour later the nurse was relieved by an incoming nurse who was "horrified" by the doctor's treatment of this patient. The incoming nurse felt the patient was going into shock and called the doctor, who arrived at the hospital 10 minutes later. Oxygen and adrenaline were administered, and an attempt at blood transfusion was unsuccessful because the doctor couldn't find a vein. The patient died. In reviewing the case, the appellate court said: "The measure of duty of a hospital toward a patient is to exercise that degree of care, skill, and diligence used by hospitals generally in that community and required by the express or implied contract of the undertaking, the hospital is liable for want of ordinary care, whether from incompetency of a nurse or failure in duty of a fully qualified nurse" (*Goff v. Doctors General Hospital of San Jose,* 1958).

The expert testimony blamed the treating physician for not suturing the incision and not continuing to observe it, and for failing to do a cut-down to find the vein for the critically needed transfusion. The nurse's performance regarding vital signs was below the standard for nurses. Had the minimum standards been observed, the mother's perilous condition would have been clearly revealed. The nurse should have called the doctor no matter what she considered his opinion or his attitude; above all, she should have notified her supervisor immediately. The hospital owed this woman a duty of protection and needed to exercise such reasonable care toward the patient as her condition required. The court indicated that any negligence on the part of the nurses in the San Jose case would be imputed to the hospital as they were employees of the hospital working within the scope of their duties.

It should be noted that although this is a classic tort case, the appellate court added that these duties are "required by the express or implied contract of the undertaking." Again the breakdown of liabilities into criminal, contract, and tort come into play. The court here included the observation that the conduct of the doctor and nurses on behalf of the hospital was a breach of the agreement between the patient and the hospital, which, if not actually written, is certainly implied when the patient comes through the door.

One may wonder why contract provisions are not invoked more often in cases such as this. The reason is that the principles involving contract cases are really founded on agreements between people who voluntarily deal with each other as opposed to tort matters where strangers interact with each other. The other, more profound difference relates to the measure of damages. The measure of damages in contract actions is far more constrained, that is, the court usually will grant only those damages actually suffered by the party. An interesting point arises here. Before the caps or limitations on damages that became fashionable in many states in the early 1980s, there were no limits to damage recoveries in tort actions. Damages in contract actions were and are more or less limited by what could naturally follow as a result of the breach.

CONCLUSION

Knowing the legalities that surround nursing functions is not as important as knowing, understanding, and observing good nursing techniques. It should be reassuring to know that fidelity to the rules and regulations promulgated by hospitals and good nursing schools will prevent most troublesome events in a nursing career. The most common allegations of nursing negligence are summarized in Display 4-1. However, causes of medical malpractice and suits where nurses are sought to be held responsible share common patterns.

Often, danger lurks when the responsibility for the care and attention to the patient is passed from one health care provider to another. Negligence and malpractice cases also have a pattern of occurrence involving days when professionals are distracted or preoccupied. Problems arise, not so much from lack of skill or lack of understanding by the nurse, but far more often by carelessness that would not occur in calmer times or when the nurse is not preoccupied with ancillary activities.

The law fairly well parallels common sense in what is required of nurses and hospitals and the protections afforded them by law. By maintaining common sense, the nurse can reduce his or her risk of having to defend against allegations of professional negligence.

DISPLAY 4-1

Most Common Allegations of Negligent Conduct Against Nurses

Negligent administration of medications—includes negligent preparation, incorrect dosages, route of administration, incorrect patient.

Failure to act (only when the nurse had the duty to act)—includes failure to take vital signs, failure to communicate patient condition to doctor, failure to report symptoms, failure to monitor or assess.

Error in use and/or supervision of equipment—causing burns on patients (use of hot packs, electrical equipment, and so on), use of obviously unsafe equipment, use of side rails.

Errors in surgical area—leaving a foreign object in patient, falls, burns, trauma to body parts from moving patient.

Failure to follow physician orders

Failure to follow hospital procedures, policies

Failure to provide proper patient care

Failure to exercise sound judgment

Aiding or allowing the negligent conduct of another—includes failure to supervise properly.

Failure to refer

REFERENCES

American Law Institute. (1972) Restatement (second) of torts. St. Paul: American Law Institute.

American Nurses Association. (1981). Standards of nursing practice, ANA statement of functions 54. American Journal of Nursing, 868–871, 992–996, 1130.

American Nurses Association. (November 1966). ANA revised standards for nursing services, News, 66. American Journal of Nursing, 2461–2462.

American Nurses Association. (1973). Standards of Nursing Practice, Washington, DC; American Nurses Association.

Brent, Nancy J. (1997). Nurses and the law: A guide to principles and applications. Philadelphia: W. B. Saunders.

Inglis, A., & Kjervik, D. (Summer, 1993). Empowerment of advanced practice nurses: Regulation reform needed to increase access to care. The Journal of Law, Medicine and Ethics, 21(2); 193–205.

Joint Commission of Accreditation of Hospitals. (1981). Accreditation manual for hospitals. Oakbrook Terrace, IL: Author.

Kelly, L. Y. (July 1974). Nursing practice acts. American Journal of Nursing, 74(7); 1310–1319.

LaFave, Wayne, & Scott, Austine. (1986). Criminal law (2nd ed.). St. Paul, MN: West.

Prosser, W. (1941). Handbook on the law of torts (2nd ed.). St. Paul, MN: West.

Prosser & Keeton, (1984). Law of torts, (5th ed.). St. Paul, MN: West.

CASE CITATIONS

Birmingham Baptist Hospital v. Branton, 218 Ala. 464, 118 So. 741 (1928).

Brown v. Dahl, 705 P.2d 781 (Wash. App. 1985).

Daniel v. St. Francis Cabrini Hospital of Alexandria, Inc., 415 So.2d 586 (La. App. 1982).

Fein v. Permanente Medical Group, 38 Cal. 3d 137, 695 P.2d 665 (1985).

Fraijo v. Hartland Hospital, 99 Cal. App. 3d 331 (1979).

Goff v. Doctors General Hospital of San Jose, 166 Cal. App. 2d 314, 333 P.2d 29 (1958).

Gugino v. Harvard Community Health Plan, 380 Mass. 464, 403 N.E.2d 1166 (1980).

Johnson v. Minneapolis, St. Paul & S.S.M. Ry. Co., 54 N.D. 351, 209 N.W. 786 (1926).

Lustig v. The Birthplace, No. 83-2-07528-9 (Washington, King's County Superior Court, dec. Sept. 9, 1983).

Mather v. Griffin Hospital, 540 A.2d 666 (Conn. 1988).

Planned Parenthood of Northwest Indiana v. Vines, 543 N.E.2d 654 (1989).

Sermcheif v. Gonzales, 660 S.W.2d 683 (Mo. Banc. 1983).

State v. Shook, 393 S.E.2d 819 (N.C. 1990).

Ybarra v. Spangard, 25 Cal. 2d 486, 154 P.2d 687 (1944).

CHAPTER 5

Trial Process

Mable Smith-Pittman

Many patients initiate lawsuits out of anger, revenge, and dissatisfaction with the medical outcome. A study by Imershein and Brents (1992) revealed that significant factors in the participant's decision to sue were "some form of retribution and/or deterrence, a desire to punish, to make the incident public, or to prevent future mistakes" (p. 41). The patient seeks an advocate who will promote the patient's cause. This person is usually an attorney. The involvement of an attorney may create a further deterioration in the relation between the patient and health care provider. Heckman (1989) stated that what starts as a communication problem between the physician and the patient becomes a battle between the attorney and the insurance company. What starts out as a means of emotional vindication turns into a battle called "malpractice litigation"; this approach fails to meet either party's objectives.

EVALUATION OF THE CASE

Once contacted, the attorney interviews the client to gain information about the possible cause of action. With the client's permission, the attorney requests the medical records to determine whether the documented information supports the client's allegations. The attorney who has limited medical knowledge will usually hire a medical or nursing expert to evaluate the merits of the case, based on the documentation and the information obtained from the interview.

Before a lawsuit is initiated, the attorney must evaluate the merits of the case. All lawsuits must be grounded in fact and filed in good faith. An attorney who files a frivolous or fraudulent lawsuit can be subject to disciplinary action and is therefore discouraged from making a meritless claim.

Evaluation of the medical records involves identifying deviations from the standards of care required of the health care professional and establishing with a certain degree of probability that the deviation from the requisite standards was the proximate case of the client's injury. From the client's interview and the expert's opinion, the attorney formulates the basis of liability. At this point, the attorney is ready to draft the complaint.

Pleading

The attorney identifies all plaintiffs or parties alleging harm, and all possible defendants or alleged wrongdoers. All of the plaintiffs must bring their action in one lawsuit. A common practice is to name multiple defendants in a lawsuit. For example, a lawsuit may name the health care facility, physician, nurse, and other health care providers involved in the patient's care.

The basic purpose of pleading is to inform the court and the parties of the contentions in the lawsuit. Pleadings are used to focus and identify the issues involved in the action. The three types of pleadings are (1) the complaint, (2) the answer, and (3) the answer to a counterclaim or cross-claim.

Complaint

The complaint is a written, formal statement of the plaintiff's claim. The essential elements of the complaint are (1) the caption naming the court and the parties, (2) the elements of the cause of action, and (3) a prayer for relief, also known as the request for damages.

The complaint must allege all four elements of the negligence or malpractice claim. The allegations must state that the defendant breached a duty of care, which proximately caused the plaintiff's injury, and that the plaintiff is entitled to some relief or damages.

Duty is usually the easiest of the elements to prove. Once a nurse–patient relationship is established, a duty exists to exercise ordinary care and attention in proportion to the physical and mental condition of the patient (*Eversole v. Oklahoma Hospital Founders,* 1991). A breach of duty is established by expert testimony that the nurse deviated from the required standards of practice. The third element, causation, is the most difficult to establish. Causation refers to a causal connection between the behavior, conduct, action, or inaction of the nurse and the injury suffered by the patient. In most jurisdictions, the plaintiff does not have to plead general damages, such as pain and suffering and disability, because these are inferred as natural consequences of the tortious conduct or behavior. However, special damages such as loss of wages, loss of consortium, medical expenses, and loss of enjoyment of life must be specifically alleged in the complaint.

The lawsuit is initiated when the complaint is filed with the court. Once filed with the court, the case is assigned a case or docket number, which will be used as case identification in all future correspondence. An order is then filed with the clerk to issue a summons (Pozgar, 1993). The defendant is served with process by receiving a copy of the summons and complaint, either by certified mail or by a process server. After receiving service of process, the nurse should immediately contact the insurance carrier, hospital administrator, or nursing supervisor. Service of process allows the court to obtain jurisdiction over the person. Jurisdiction gives the court the authority to hear the case and makes the parties accountable to the court. The process server, the person serving the defendant, must give notice to the court that the defendant was properly served.

Demurrer

After service of process but before responding to the factual allegations in the complaint, the defendant can file a demurrer, or a pleading challenging the legal sufficiency of the plaintiff's claim. Although the grounds for demurrer vary according to state law, the most common grounds are the complaint is vague and ambiguous, the plaintiff lacks capacity, the facts fail to state a cause of action, another lawsuit is already pending, and there is a lack of personal or subject matter jurisdiction. If the demurrer is sustained, the court can allow the plaintiff to amend the complaint, and if the plaintiff refuses or fails to amend within a certain time, the complaint is dismissed. If the demurrer is overruled, the defendant must answer the complaint.

Answer

An answer is a written response to the allegations in the complaint. The defendant responds to each allegation with an admittance or denial and can assert affirmative defenses. The answer must be filed with the court within a certain amount of time after service of process, usually within 20 days. If the defendant fails to answer within the specified time frame the court can enter a default judgment, which is a judgment in favor of the plaintiff because the defendant failed to answer or defend the allegations. The judgment can be put aside, however, if the defendant can show adequate cause for failing to respond.

The answer serves to put at issue the factual allegations in the complaint by denying the allegations. A general denial is a statement denying the whole complaint. In many jurisdictions and especially in malpractice cases, a general denial is unacceptable because the complaint may contain some statements that are true. For example, the complaint may contain a statement that "Plaintiff was a patient in the defendant's hospital for five days from August 12–16." This particular statement in the complaint may be true, although subsequent statements alleging breach of duty may be in dispute. A general denial would have the effect of denying the true statement. To avoid this, the defendant responds to the complaints using specific denials to refute the untrue allegations and admits those that are true. If an allegation is not denied, it is deemed true or admitted.

The answer can assert defenses that can be used to negate the claim. The first type of defense, defense of law, is a legal bar against the case going forward. Examples of defenses of law include the statute of limitations and sovereign immunity doctrines. Defense of fact is asserted by stating that the care provided adhered to the requisite standards of care or that the breach of due care was not the proximate cause of the plaintiff's injury (Fiesta, 1988).

DEFENSES

Statute of Limitations

The statute of limitations refers to the time frame during which a case must be filed or the plaintiff loses the right to bring the claim. Its primary purpose is to encourage the early filing of lawsuits to enable the defendant to defend a claim while the facts and other variables can be remembered. The statute of limitation begins to run when the alleged act occurred or when the injured patient discovered or should have discovered the wrong. It may be tolled, or stopped temporarily, if the plaintiff was reasonably unaware of the existence of a wrong. For example, the statute of limitations may be tolled for the period of time a postsurgical patient was not aware that a sponge was left in his or her body.

Statutes in each state specify the time frame within which a person can file a lawsuit. The usual time period is one to three years.

The following case illustrates the intricacies of the statute of limitations doctrine. In *Perez v. Bay Area Hospital* (1992), a mother and child filed a negligence claim under the state's Tort Claim Act against the hospital, employee of Children's Service Division (CSD), and the Department of Health Resources for erroneously reporting that the child had a sexually transmitted disease. The child was taken to the hospital on January 27, 1988, and diagnosed with a vaginal infection. Two days later, a hospital employee reported to the children's service division that the 7-year-old child has tested positive for gonorrhea. The CSD employee along with a police officer went to the child's school, informed the secretary of the situation, and questioned the child. Later that day, the CSD employee informed the child's mother of the report. Upon further inquiry, the mother learned that the laboratory tests were negative for gonorrhea.

On July 13, 1989, the mother was appointed the child's guardian *ad litem* and filed a lawsuit on behalf of herself and the child. The defendants asserted the statute of limitations defense and contended that the plaintiff was barred from bringing the claim.

The court ruled in favor of the child but against the mother. The statutory period of 270 days for the child to bring the lawsuit did not run until a guardian *ad litem* was appointed. However, the statutory period of 180 days for the mother to bring the lawsuit began to run in January 1988, when she was first made aware of the erroneous report. Although she did not know the identity of the person making the false report, this does not toll the statute of limitations. She knew the person was associated with the hospital, and through discovery could have obtained the person's identity.

Sovereign Immunity

The doctrine of sovereign immunity established a legal barrier to people who sought to sue the federal or state government. It originated from the premise that the King is blameless and therefore should not bear liability. Today, the doctrine has basically been abolished by federal and state government.

Good Samaritan

Good samaritan laws refer to state laws that relieve health care professionals and laymen from liability for care rendered in emergency situations. These laws were designed to encourage health care professionals to provide assistance at accident sites without fear of reprisal. The law does not provide protection when the care rendered is grossly negligent or when the individual charges for the services rendered.

Contributory Negligence

The doctrine of contributory negligence is based on the premise that a wrongdoer cannot benefit from the wrongdoing of others. If the defendant can show a causal connection between the plaintiff's negligent conduct and the plaintiff's injury, the plaintiff may be barred from recovery of damages, even if the defendant was also negligent. In many jurisdictions, the failure of the plaintiff to exercise reasonable behavior would defeat a claim of negligence against the defendant.

Assumption of the Risk

A plaintiff assumes the risk of injury or harm inherent in a given situation when he or she knows of and understands the risks and voluntarily selects the course of behavior that can lead to harm. For example, a nurse who fails to wear a mask when caring for a patient with a known airborne communicable disease and then contracts the disease can be said to have "assumed the risks."

Counterclaim

As part of the answer, the defendant may bring any claim he or she has against the plaintiff by filing a counterclaim. In most instances the claim does not have to relate to the original claim stated in the complaint. The plaintiff is then required to file a response or answer and admit, deny, or offer defenses against the allegations in the counterclaim.

DISCOVERY

Discovery is a process used to obtain relevant information about the case prior to trial. The purposes of discovery are to (1) obtain factual information, (2) identify and gather additional evidence, (3) narrow and define the legal issues, and (4) preserve testimony for trial. To facilitate the legal process, parties must comply with discovery orders or risk court-ordered sanctions.

Privileged material, as defined by the state rules of evidence, is not discoverable. An example of privileged material is work-product doctrines that contain the attorney's thoughts, observations, legal theories, litigation strategies, and other notations made in anticipation of litigation. In many states, incident reports are not discoverable, because they are prepared in anticipation of litigation. Incident reports contain deviations from acceptable standards or "unusual occurrences" that can result in litigation. They are used to identify and correct sources of potential harm.

Methods used for discovery include (1) oral deposition, (2) written deposition, (3) interrogatories, (4) requests for admissions, (5) requests for production and inspection of documents and other items, and (6) physical and mental examinations.

Depositions

A deposition is an examination of a witness under oath with each attorney asking questions, in the presence of a court reporter who records the questions and answers. The person being deposed or questioned is called the deponent. Individuals who are likely to be deposed are those with direct knowledge of the events, such as the patient's nurse, the nursing supervisor, and the patient's physicians. The party seeking to depose a witness must give written notice to the other party identifying the date, time, and place of the deposition. A court order is usually not required, unless a party wants to depose a witness before a lawsuit is filed or immediately after service of process. These requirements protect the witness by allowing him or her time to consult an attorney. Along with the notice of deposition, the party may receive a subpoena duces tecum, which is a court order requesting that certain items be brought to the deposition. In a deposition, all parties have the right to be represented by an attorney and are subject to direct and cross-examination.

Information obtained during discovery can be introduced during the trial and can be used to impeach or discredit a witness. Therefore, the deponent must be prepared for the deposition. The nurse preparing for questioning at a deposition or trial should

1. Review the medical record before the deposition. Never attempt to answer questions from memory.
2. Answer only the question asked. The deponent should not volunteer information and should request clarification of the question when needed.
3. Remain calm. Displays of anger and hostility can make the nurse appear hostile and uncooperative.
4. Unless instructed otherwise, do not answer questions to which an attorney has raised an objection. The question may be self-incriminating, vague, irrelevant, or loaded.
5. Answer all questions honestly and truthfully. Never try to conceal or disguise information.

Written or Telephone Deposition

In a written deposition, the parties submit in writing questions that the deponent will be asked to answer, although the deponent answers the questions orally and under oath. Written depositions are used when the deponent is at a distant location, unable to travel, or the travel costs incurred are expensive (Cournoyer, 1989).

Depositions may also be taken by telephone if both parties agree. In both written and oral depositions, the deponent has the opportunity to review the deposition transcript and make corrections before signing it.

Interrogatories

Interrogatories are written questions sent from one party to another that must be answered under oath by the receiving party. Unlike written depositions, interrogatories can only be obtained from a party to the action and the answers are prepared in writing. Interrogatories must be answered within a time period established by state law. The questions are answered by the party and reviewed by the attorney before the party signs them under oath.

Requests for Production of Documents

Any party can inspect and copy materials in the possession of the other party that are not protected by the privileged rule. Requests for production of documents can be made for relevant documents, papers, photographs, records, correspondences, maps, charts, tapes, and other items from which data or information can be obtained. The party requesting the document must describe the items in sufficient detail so the other party knows which items are being requested. A court order is not required if the request for production is made of a party to the suit, but if the request involves a nonparty, a subpoena duces tecum is required.

Requests for Medical Examinations

A physical or mental examination may be ordered when the patient's condition is an issue in the lawsuit. The party requesting the examination must show *good cause*. The court has the discretion to deny an examination and will usually do so if the tests are dangerous or painful.

Requests for Admission

Requests for admission are used to eliminate issues that are not controversial. They are used to facilitate the trial process by acknowledging the truthfulness of certain facts, authenticity of documents, and applicability of legal concepts to facts. Once admitted, the matter is considered conclusive unless the court allows the party to withdraw or amend the admission.

PRETRIAL CONFERENCE

In most jurisdictions, the pretrial conference may be ordered at the discretion of the trial judge or on an attorney's request. It is used to streamline the case and to eliminate the extraneous variables before the actual trial begins. The trial judge sets a date for termination of discovery, eliminates uncontested issues, delineates the issues in dispute, and rules on pretrial procedural matters. During these conferences, the attorneys may present the judge with a list of questions to ask prospective jurors and request specific jury instructions. The goal of pretrial conference is to facilitate the trial process.

The trial judge may explore the possibility of a settlement between the parties. Although a settlement can occur any time from the beginning of a suit until a jury verdict, many cases are settled during the pretrial conference. A settlement can be reached with some or all of the defendants. If a settlement is offered, the attorney must convey the offer to the plaintiff. Once accepted, a settlement agreement is signed by the plaintiff and defendant(s). If the settlement offer is rejected, the case goes to trial.

Evidence of a settlement with some of the defendants is not admissible to establish liability of the other defendants. In *Holgar v. Irish* (1993), the personal representative of the decedent's estate brought a medical malpractice action against the surgeon, physicians, and operating room nurses for injuries incurred from surgical sponges left in the decedent's body during an operation. Prior to trial, the hospital settled with the plaintiff. Denying the plaintiff's motion to prevent the jury from hearing about the previous settlement, the court informed the jury of the plaintiff's settlement with the hospital. The jury returned a verdict for the hospital and the plaintiff appealed. The appellate court held that the trial court committed reversible error by informing the jury of the settlement. The prejudicial effects of planting in the jurors' minds that the true guilty party has already admitted liability or that the plaintiff has received compensation from other sources outweigh any beneficial effects.

MOTION FOR SUMMARY JUDGMENT

A motion is a written formal request by either party in a lawsuit asking the judge to grant the request. A motion for summary judgment requests the judge to examine the pleadings and render a judgment. Summary judgment is granted when there are no issues of facts to be tried and the rights of the parties can be determined from the affidavits and other documents submitted without the need for a formal trial. Issues of fact are decided by the jury, whereas issues of law are decided by the trial judge. Although summary judgment can avoid a long expensive trial, it is only appropriate when there are no genuine issues of fact. The court may grant full or partial summary judgment, which can result in a full final judgment or a judgment in favor of certain parties. The grant of summary judgment is appealable.

In *Hillhaven Rehabilitation & Convalescent Center v. Patterson* (1990), the center appealed the trial court's denial of summary judgment. Patterson, as executor of decedent's estate, filed a medical malpractice claim against the center alleging failure to provide reasonable care. The decedent, a resident of the home, fell out of bed, suffered a broken hip, and died from injury-related complications.

After discovery, the center filed a motion for summary judgment, and attached a supportive affidavit from its expert witness outlining adherence to the standard of care for nursing homes. In response, the plaintiff filed a physician's affidavit containing a general statement that the center had deviated from the requisite standard of care. The court ruled that the plaintiff could not prevail on an affidavit containing a general conclusionary statement from an expert. "He [the expert] must state the particulars in which the treatment was negligent, including an articulation of the minimum standard of acceptable professional conduct, and how and in what way defendant's deviated therefrom" (*Hillhaven*, 1990, p. 558). The plaintiff was allowed, however, to proceed under a general negligence theory, which does not require the opinion of an expert witness.

JURY

The United States Constitution and state constitutions preserve the person's right to trial by jury to determine issues of fact. For example, malpractice claims usually involve issues of fact and are triable to a jury.

A party can waive the right to a jury trial either directly or indirectly. The failure to make a timely request for a jury trial is an indirect waiver of this constitutional right. Once waived, the trial judge becomes the trier of both facts and law.

Although each state may devise its own system of jury selection, it cannot exclude citizens based on race or gender. Members of the jury are selected from a larger group of citizens called venire. Prospective jurors must answer questions about their biases, impartiality, and prejudices through a process known as voir dire, which means "speak the truth." Attorneys may request that a prospective juror not be allowed to serve, if the prospective juror cannot serve impartially, have an interest in the outcome, or is related to any of the parties. This process is known as a "challenge for cause." In many jurisdictions, attorneys have an unlimited number of challenges for cause. A peremptory challenge, on the other hand, allows the attorneys the right to excuse a specific number of jurors without cause. This allows attorneys to utilize their intuition of prospective jurors who "appear" wrong based on the case content or facts. The number of jurors selected for the trial depends on state law, but usually ranges from six to twelve jurors. After a full jury is empaneled or seated, the actual trial begins. The primary role of the jury is to decode the factual issues in dispute and decide which party's testimony or evidence is more credible. Therefore, both the witnesses and the attorney must make a favorable impression on the jury.

ORDER OF THE TRIAL

The plaintiff has the burden of proof with respect to the elements of negligence or malpractice. Usually the plaintiff will open the trial and present facts. The defendant then attempts to refute the evidence presented by the plaintiff.

Burden of Proof

In a civil suit, the burden of proof is the "preponderance of the evidence." Preponderance of the evidence requires the weighing of the evidence presented and ruling in favor of the party who tips the scales to his or her side. If the evidence is perfectly balanced or is tipped in favor of the defendant, the plaintiff has not sustained the burden of proof and will lose the case.

Normally the plaintiff has the burden of proving that the defendant breached the duty of care and the resultant injuries were caused by that breach. In some cases, however, the burden of proof can shift to the defendant. Where a plaintiff has presented credible, well-defined evidence to establish negligence, the burden of proof can shift to the defendant who must refute the evidence. For example, the doctrine of *res ipsa loquitur* (the thing speaks for itself) allows the plaintiff to establish a prima facie case of negligence.

Under the doctrine of *res ipsa loquitur*, the burden of proof shifts to the defendant after the plaintiff presents evidence that (1) the event is the kind that would not have occurred in the absence of negligence, (2) the agency or thing that caused the harm was in the exclusive control of the defendant, and (3) the plaintiff could not have contributed to the event.

The doctrine of *res ipsa loquitur* was applied in the case of *Dalley v. Utah Valley Regional Medical Center* (1990). After an elective cesarean section, the plaintiff had a burn on her right leg. She alleged that the burn was not present immediately before surgery. The medical records reflected that a nurse had noted the burn while transporting the plaintiff from the operating room to the postanesthesia care unit. Skin grafts were required to repair the burn. Applying the doctrine of *res ipsa loquitur*, the court noted that it is not common for a female to go into the operating room for a cesarean section and come out with a burn on a previously healthy leg without some occurrence of negligence of the operating room personnel.

Opening Statements

The opening statements set the stage for the entire trial. They are a concise, simple overview of the facts and give the jurors a perspective from which to view the case. Essential elements in opening statements are (1) a focused discussion on the evidence to be presented at trial, (2) a summary of the facts, and

(3) a listing of who will be called and the substance of the witnesses' testimony.

The defense attorney's opening statements may refute the plaintiff's story and provide the jurors with an alternative statement of the facts. The attorney denies liability, explains the facts in a manner most favorable to the defendant's case, and identifies the witnesses who will substantiate those facts.

Testimony

After the opening statements, the trial testimony begins when the first witness is called. A witness is a person who is sworn in to provide evidence about the case. There are two types of witnesses, a fact witness and an expert witness. A fact witness testifies as to what was personally observed or heard. This type of witness can only provide evidence or corroborate another's witness testimony.

Unlike a fact witness, an expert witness can render a personal opinion regarding the evidence. An expert witness is a person who has extensive knowledge and experience in a specialized area of practice. The expert reviews the medical records, transcripts of depositions, and client interviews to deduce inferences and formulate an opinion as to duty, breach of duty, causation, and in some cases damages. The primary roles of the expert are to (1) establish the standards of care, (2) assist the jurors to understand the sequence of events, and (3) interpret the technical aspects of the case. An expert must be qualified based on experience, education, and background to render a professional opinion.

Historically, physicians were used to establish whether the nurse complied with or deviated from the accepted standard of care. This scenario is changing as the legal profession continues to acknowledge that nursing is a distinct profession from the medical profession.

The witness' testimony is a form of oral evidence. The other type of evidence is called physical or demonstrative evidence. Physical evidence consists of objects or things that are allowed to be used because they help prove or disprove facts. Examples of physical evidence include pictures, objects, documents, tapes,

drawings of the human body, slides, models, textbooks, policy and procedure manuals, equipment, committee minutes, and other relevant items or objects. The admissibility of evidence, either oral or physical, is governed by the state's rules of evidence.

After the witness takes the oath, the plaintiff's attorney begins the direct examination, which consists of a series of questions designed to elicit information from the witness. As in deposition, a witness is prepared by the attorney to give trial testimony. During preparation, the attorney has informed the witness how to testify for the jury. In essence, the witness should look directly at the jurors, and speak clearly, distinctly, and with confidence. Testimony from the attorney's own witness is called direct examination. During direct examination, the attorney can not tell the story or ask questions that suggest an answer, which are called leading questions.

After the direct examination, the opposing attorney cross-examines the witness. The general purpose of cross-examination is to cast doubt on the witness' testimony, either by impeachment or attacking credibility. A witness can be impeached if statements made prior to trial, for example in the deposition, are inconsistent with the witness' trial testimony. During cross-examination, the attorney can ask leading questions. If the testimony elicited from the cross-examination is damaging, the attorney is permitted to redirect, in an attempt to alleviate or repair the damage. In some instances, the opposing attorney can re-cross-examine the witness.

A formal objection can be raised to a question asked of either party or to an answer given by a witness. If an objection is raised to a question, the witness should stop and not answer the question. If the objection is overruled, an answer is allowed and if sustained, the questions must be rephrased or eliminated. An objection to a witness' answer that is sustained will be stricken from the record and the jury instructed to disregard the answer.

After all the plaintiff's witnesses have been called to testify and have been cross-examined, the plaintiff rests his or her case. At this time, the defense will usually make a motion for directed verdict or dismissal on the premise that the plaintiff has failed to prove a cause of action and that reasonable jurors could not possibly rule in favor of the plaintiff. If the judge grants the motion, the trial ends at this point and the losing party has the right to appeal. In deciding whether to grant a motion for directed verdict, the judge considers the evidence in the "light most favorable to the nonmoving party." If denied, the defense begins to present its evidence. After the defense rests its case, either side may present a motion for a directed verdict. The court will grant the motion if no genuine issues of fact exist for the jury to decide.

The order of presentation may change for closing summation or arguments. The defense attorney proceeds first, followed by the plaintiff. Closing arguments provide the opportunity for the attorneys to summarize the points most favorable to their case. The defense counsel usually sympathizes with the plaintiff's injuries but denies any liability on the part of the defendant. The plaintiff's attorney gives the jury the last impression of the case. At this time, the attorney emphasizes the weaknesses in the defense's case, highlights the strengths in the plaintiff's case, and elaborates on what could be considered a "fair and just" damage award. Both attorneys are prohibited from introducing new evidence during closing arguments.

Jury Instructions

After closing argument, the judge instructs the jury on relevant law to be applied in the case. The instructions often include specific requests of the attorneys and applicable state law. The jury uses these instructions and the evidence presented in the case to reach a verdict. Because instructions requested by the attorneys are often favorable to their case, a judge is not obligated to word the instructions verbatim and in some instances can refuse to use the requested instructions (Cushing, 1988). Each party may object to the instructions given and the matter can be taken up on appeal.

Following instructions, the jury retires to the jury room to deliberate the guilt or innocence of the defendant(s). After a verdict is reached, the judge enters a judgment in accordance with the verdict. The verdict may take two forms: a general verdict, in which the jury decides the case for the plaintiff or defendant; or a special verdict, where the jury is requested to make special findings in regard to specific factual questions.

After the jury returns a verdict, either party can make posttrial motions. The most common motions are (1) for a judgment not withstanding the verdict, and (2) for a new trial. A judgment *non obstante veredicto* (n.o.v.) is used to overturn a jury verdict when the evidence is inconsistent with the verdict. Unlike a directed verdict, a judgment n.o.v. does not remove the decision from the jury. If the judgment n.o.v. is overturned on appeal, the jury's verdict is reinstated.

Great deference is given to a jury verdict. Courts consider the jury's verdict conclusive as to all disputed facts and conflicting testimony and therefore refrain from overturning the verdict, unless substantial evidence does not support the verdict. In *Silvis v. Hobbs* (1992), the court noted it will not "reweigh or disturb the jury's findings unless the findings are inherently impossible or improbable as not to be entitled to belief" (p. 1016).

A motion for a new trial can be made to relitigate all or some of the issues. A new trial may be granted for any misconduct, either attorney or juror, that results in bias, erroneous or prejudiced outcomes, or product consequences that erode the principles of justice. In addition, a new trial may be granted on the basis on newly discovered evidence that may alter the previous outcome. The trial judge will deny a motion for a new trial if the misconduct or error was harmless or was not significant enough to affect the outcome.

In *Bahr v. Harper-Grace Hospitals* (1993), the court remanded the case or sent it back to the trial court for a new trial based on the erroneous admission of testimony that was prejudicial. The decedent's sister was allowed to testify that a neurologist told her that the decedent should have been in an intensive care unit (ICU). Under the state's rules of evidence, the statement was considered hearsay and should be excluded, unless plaintiff's attorney established an exception to the hearsay rule, which was not done. Because one of the issues in the case was whether the decedent should have been admitted to the ICU rather than to a private room, the court ruled that the statement was prejudicial and allowing it "would be inconsistent with substantial justice" (*Bahr*, 1993, p. 529).

A jury verdict in favor of the plaintiff results in the award of monetary damages. Damages can be classified into three general categories: nominal, compensatory, and punitive. Depending on the jurisdiction, a fourth type of damages, hedonic damages, may be recognized. An award of nominal damages is a statement that a wrong has been committed but the injury or harm suffered is minimal. Compensatory damages, on the other hand, may be very significant. Included in the category of compensatory damages are pain and suffering, out of pocket expenses, loss of wages, loss of earning capacity or business profits, and medical expenses. Punitive damages are awarded to punish defendants for gross negligence or reckless disregard for the person's well-being. These types of damages are usually not covered by the defendant's insurance carrier and therefore must be paid directly by the defendant. The primary purpose of punitive damages is to deter certain types of behavior or conduct.

The case of *Manning v. Twins Falls Clinic and Hospital* (1992) illustrates conduct considered an extreme deviation from reasonable care. During a transfer to a private room, the nurse temporarily removed the supplemental oxygen of a patient with terminal COPD and refused to replace it, in spite of the family members' requests. The nurse did not attempt to obtain portable oxygen because of the short distance involved. Shortly into the move, the patient suffered extreme respiratory distress. Resuscitation efforts were discontinued after the patient was identified as a no code, and shortly thereafter, the patient died.

The plaintiffs were awarded punitive damages of $800 against the nurse and $180,000 against the hospital, although the latter was reversed on appeal. The court noted that an award of punitive damages by a jury will be sustained when "the defendant has acted in a manner that was an extreme deviation from reasonable standards of conduct, and that the act was performed by the defendant with an understanding of or disregard for its likely consequences" (*Manning*, 1992, at 1191).

Some states have placed limits on the amount of punitive damages that can be awarded. Damage awards are appealable.

Hedonic damages, recognized in certain states, provide compensation to the injured party for the loss of pleasure or enjoyment of life. Jurisdictions that allow hedonic damages value the pleasures and amenities associated with life. In *Eyoma v. Falco* (1991), the court sustained an award of hedonic damages to a patient who was comatose for over a year and thus unaware of his incapacitation. The decedent had undergone an uneventful gallbladder surgery. In the recovery room, he attempted to pull the oral airway, so the anesthesiologist removed it and instructed the recovery room nurse to monitor the patient's respirations due to the type of narcotics the patient had received during surgery. After the anesthesiologist left, the nurse asked another nurse to watch the decedent. She then left to attend another patient. Upon her return, she noted the patient's respirations were eight per minute. Shortly thereafter the anesthesiologist assessed the patient and noted that he was not breathing. Although resuscitation efforts were started immediately, the patient suffered brain damage due to oxygen deprivation.

Acknowledging the lack of consensus on whether to award hedonic damages, the court rejected the contention that loss of enjoyment of life is not compensable unless consciously experienced.

> Currently, three different views prevail among those jurisdictions that have addressed the issue of whether loss of enjoyment of life is a recognizable category of injury for which damages may be awarded. A minority of jurisdictions refuse any recovery for loss of enjoyment of life. Most of these jurisdictions, however, base their positions on decisions rendered at the turn of the century that largely have been ignored. The majority position allows consideration of loss of enjoyment of life, but only as one of the numerous factors characterizing a general damage award for pain and suffering. Finally, proponents of a third position assert that loss of enjoyment of life is a proper element of damages, separate and distinct from pain and suffering, for which compensation should be awarded (*Eyoma*, 1991, pp. 658–659).

To support the position taken, the court stated:

> We believe that the loss of pleasure and enjoyment, which as a natural and direct consequence accompanies that incapacity, is a loss that is inseparable from it and is not dependent on the ability to appreciate one's own restrictions. Thus, a plaintiff who has been comatose should, as part of disability and impairment, be compensated for the loss caused by existing in a comatose state including the resultant loss of enjoyment of normal activities (*Eyoma,* 1991, p. 662).

The defense counsel will attempt to reduce the amount of damages awarded by offering several defenses. First, the doctrine of contributory negligence, allowed in some jurisdictions, can prevent the plaintiff from recovering any amount of damages if the plaintiff in any way contributed to the injury. The defense counsel will argue that the plaintiff's conduct fell below the standards required of a reasonable prudent patient. The attorney must show that the patient was aware of and could appreciate the danger, and that there was a causal connection between the patient's behavior and the injury or harm suffered.

To counter the harsh effects of contributory negligence, many jurisdictions instituted comparative negligence. This defense lessens the plaintiff's damage award by the percentage of negligence demonstrated by the plaintiff. For example, if the damage award was $500,000 but the plaintiff was found 50% negligent, the award would be reduced by $250,000, and the defendant would only be required to pay $250,000. However, several states have modified versions of comparative negligence systems.

VERDICT FOR THE DEFENDANT

The jury usually returns a verdict for the defendant when the plaintiff has failed to prove, by the greater weight of the evidence, a breach of duty or causation or when the plaintiff assumed the risk. If the plaintiff is not successful in establishing that the nurse deviated from the standards of care and this deviation caused the injury, the verdict will be for the defense.

In rendering a verdict for the defense, the jury may have decided that the plaintiff assumed the risk associated with the situation. The assumption of the risk doctrine applies to situations in which the plaintiff failed to take reasonable precautions to prevent the harm or injury. The defense must establish that the plaintiff was aware of the dangers, understood the risks involved, and knowingly consented or engaged in the behavior that led to the injury.

APPEAL

Either party to the lawsuit can file an appeal if events during the trial may have prejudiced or biased the jury. The appeal must be based on issues of law, decided by the trial judge. Appellate courts will usually accept the jury's finding of fact and are very hesitant to overturn a jury verdict. The attorneys must identify the issues reserved for appeal and submit written briefs containing case law to support their contention of error in the trial court. The appellate court reviews the brief, asks questions of attorneys during oral argument, and renders a decision. It is not the role of the appellate court to retry the case.

CONCLUSION

Malpractice litigation from start to finish is a very lengthy and time-consuming process. The trial process is designed to ensure that the parties in a lawsuit get their day in court, and receive fair and equitable treatment.

Nevertheless, the process can be intimidating to the nurse who has never been involved in a malpractice lawsuit. Nurses should remember that the attorney is their advocate and therefore must work closely with him or her before and during the trial.

REFERENCES

Cournoyer, C. P. (1989). The nurse manager & the law. Rockville, Maryland: Aspen.

Cushing, M. (1988). Nursing jurisprudence. Norwalk, Connecticut: Appleton & Lange.

Fiesta, J. (1988). The law and liability: A guide for nurses (2nd ed.). New York: John Wiley & Sons.

Heckman, F. (1989). [Interview]. In A. Hutkin. Resolving the medical malpractice crisis:

Alternatives to litigation. <u>Journal of Law and Health,</u> <u>4</u> (1), 31.

Imershein, A., & Brents, A. (1992). The impact of large malpractice awards. <u>The Journal of Legal Medicine,</u> 13, 33–49.

Pozgar, G. (1993). <u>Legal aspects of health care administration</u> (5th ed.). Rockville, Maryland: Aspen.

CASE CITATIONS

Bahr v. Harper-Grace Hospitals, 497 N.W.2d 526 (Mich. App. 1993).

Dalley v. Utah Valley Regional Medical Center, 791 P.2d 193 (1990).

Eversole v. Oklahoma Hosp. Founders, 818 P.2d 456 (Okla. 1991).

Eyoma v. Falco, 589 A.2d 653 (N.J. 1991).

Hillhaven Rehabilitation & Convalescent Center, 392 S.E.2d 557 (Ga. App. 1990).

Holger v. Irish, 851 P.2d 1122 (Ore. 1993).

Manning v. Twin Falls Clinic & Hospital, 830 P.2d 1185 (Idaho 1992).

Perez v. Bay Area Hospital, 829 P.2d 700 (Ore. App. 1992).

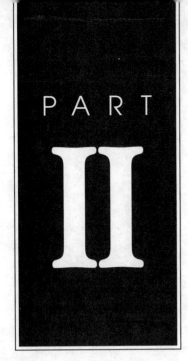

PART

II

*Specific Perinatal
Liability Issues*

CHAPTER 6

Scope of Perinatal Liability

Barbara Sinclair and Davia Solomon

Never before has it been so critical for nurses to be knowledgeable and conscientious about their responsibility in carrying out professional roles according to established standards and guidelines and to act as other reasonably prudent persons would act in the same situation. It is said that we are living in a more litigious society and perhaps that is true. However, significant changes in the health care delivery system, expansion of nurses' activities, roles, and functions within various subsystems, education of the consumer, and newer interpretations by various courts have resulted in more and more legal action being taken to correct real or perceived harm. The boundaries are somewhat blurred but the fact remains that when individual, group, or corporate conduct causes harm to another, those at fault can be held legally liable.

Liability, as broadly defined by Webster (1937), means bound or obligated by law or equity, responsible; answerable. A legal liability is one that the courts recognize and enforce when lack of responsibility causes injury and a lawsuit follows. The law is rarely static. If the results of various cases seem contradictory, it is because they come from different times and are from different courts in different states. To determine outcomes from recent situations, one must determine the applicable law at the time and place of the occurrence. Trends in the law can be discerned by examining previously decided cases of similar circumstances.

PERSONAL LIABILITY

Nurses are accountable for their actions to the same degree that any other health care professional is accountable under the rule or doctrine of personal liability. Simply put, every person is liable for his or her own tortious conduct. A tort is a civil legal wrong. Consideration must be given also to the fact that the law does not permit a wrongdoer to avoid legal liability for the wrongdoing even though someone else also may be sued for the conduct in question. However, the concept of suing multiple defendants often includes the "deep pockets" idea of including those who can afford to pay the most.

According to information from the two primary insurance carriers for nurses between 1967 and 1977, the most frequent site, by a very large margin, for alleged wrongdoing on the part of the nurse is the hospital; the areas most involved are obstetrics, patient rooms, emergency departments, and operating rooms; and the reasons for the claims are improper treatment related to birth, improper treatment, miscellaneous, and patient falls (Kelly & Joel, 1996). In 1994, current statistics from the National Practitioner Data Bank reveal that 5 nurses in 10,000 are sued in a given year with the greatest number of claims resulting from patient falls and many others from circumstances similar to those listed earlier, such as "bad baby" cases, burns, medication errors, and mistaken identity of patients (Kelly & Joel, 1996).

It is easily recognized that an individual is liable for his or her own conduct. However, under certain circumstances individuals may be responsible for others' actions. For example, a partnership can be liable for the wrongful act of one of its members or an employer may be answerable for the acts of employees.

Consider the following in terms of partnership liability. Doctors A, B, and C are partners in a medical group. Doctor A sees a prenatal patient throughout her pregnancy and anticipates no problems with the delivery. He goes on vacation, leaving Doctors B and C to handle the patient's delivery. At the time the patient entered the hospital in active labor, neither Doctor B nor C could be found. During the labor problems were encountered. Finally, Doctor B showed up and proceeded to order a cesarean section for the patient. The baby suffered severe hypoxia and it is later determined that the child has brain damage. Under the theory that the entire partnership shares in the responsibility for the care and treatment of the patient, it can be seen that the entire partnership is liable for damages rather than just Doctor B or even Doctors A and B.

To comprehend liability one must first understand the relationship among the parties involved. It is easy to understand why an individual is responsible for his or her own conduct; however, it is more difficult to understand how it is possible that an individual or group could be accountable for someone else's mistakes, or wrongful acts, yet this indeed does occur.

However, this form of liability where one person is responsible for the acts of another does not exist in the absence of identifiable relationship or circumstance that would justify such an imposition (*Rubio v. Swiridoff,* 1985). Unless such a special relationship exists, one person cannot be responsible for the conduct of another (*Robertson v. Wentz,* 1986). Thus, the *negligence* (a legal concept discussed in Chapter 4) of one person does not extend to a noninvolved person, in legal terms called a *nonparty,* except

where the interests of justice demand it. The fundamental rule is that one person, free from fault, must not be required to bear the consequences of the actions of another.

VICARIOUS LIABILITY

The exception to the above circumstance is termed vicarious liability. This is a legal concept that comes from the Latin word *vicar,* which means deputy. For example, in the Catholic faith, the Pope is considered to be the Vicar of Christ; however, having a vicar is not exclusively the prerogative of the divine. Distinct and common relationships where vicarious liability may be imposed include employer and employee, employer and independent contractor, principal and agent, parent and child, and an automobile owner who gives permission to a driver to operate his or her vehicle. In all of these relationships, the actions of the "vicar" can be attributed to the principal, even though there is no personal fault or causal relationship between the actions of the principal who is held liable and the injured. Under this concept, nurses are often held to be the agents of the hospital or physician for whom they work and, as a result, vicarious liability is imposed.

Employer–Employee

For purposes of law, an employee has been defined as anyone who is subject to the absolute control of the employer with respect to activities, labor, or work to be done as part of an assigned job. Generally speaking, a person becomes an employee when he or she is hired to perform services for wages or salary.

The legal theory upon which the courts hold employers responsible for the wrongful acts of their employees is called *respondeat superior,* literally, "let the master answer" (53 Am. Jur. 2d, Master and servant, Section 3). In each circumstance, the relationship of employer–employee must be established by the facts particular to the given case. In Ohio, the court held that a surgeon was not liable when an injury resulted to a patient because a scrub nurse had used a different machine than that which the surgeon had ordered. The court said that the nurse was an employee of the hospital, the hospital had complete control of the operating room, and the hospital could direct how any work was to be done (*Clary v. Christiansen,* 1948).

In a case in California, a hospital was held liable for the negligence of a nurse anesthetist who improperly administered an anesthetic to a child who subsequently died. Testimony at the trial revealed that the hospital provided the nurses, the anesthetist, the operating room, and "everything for the operation"; an employee of the hospital acknowledged that she was in charge of all anesthetists at the hospital, and she received no salary or payment of any kind from the surgeon or the patient (*Cavero v. Franklin General Benevolent Society,* 1950). In that case also, the hospital had to pay for the damages caused by its deputy, or vicar.

In another case involving improper administration of anesthesia, the hospital was held liable for the acts of its employee when it was determined that the nurse anesthetist was alone in the room with the patient for 10 minutes during which time she administered the anesthetic agent. Before the surgery began, she noticed a distention in the patient's abdomen and removed the anesthesia equipment. The patient suffered a great deal of pain due to the penetration of air into his stomach and intestines and sued the doctor, hospital, and nurse. The trial court ruled that the hospital was liable for the negligent acts of its employee, the nurse anesthetist (*Kemelyan v. Henderson,* 1954).

Whenever an employee is found to be not liable, the employer must also be found not liable under the doctrine of *respondeat superior.* In a case in Texas, the court found the fact that the hospital had hired foreign nurses had no bearing on the liability of the hospital in the absence of negligence or wrongful acts by the nurses (*Clark v. Harris Hospital,* 1976).

Direct Versus Vicarious Liability

An employer can also be held liable to an injured party when his or her own negligence directly contributes to the injury. The most common examples of this direct liability are found when the employer negligently hires, retains, trains, or

supervises an incompetent employee. A jury in Texas found a hospital negligent for assigning a nurse to labor and delivery on night shift:

> when it knew or should have known that the nurse was not qualified to perform the tasks required by this position and that she sometimes fell asleep at her station. They further alleged that the hospital was negligent in failing to adequately supervise the nurse. (*St. Paul Medical Center v. Cecil,* 1992)

In that case, a pregnant woman appeared at the hospital at approximately 11:00 P.M. and was placed in a labor room in a hospital gown. She advised the nurse that her water had broken. At approximately 12:10 A.M., the nurse performed a pelvic examination. At 1:30 A.M., the nurse requested a physician resident to perform a speculum examination, which revealed ruptured membranes and the presence of meconium. At 2:45 A.M., the nurse attached an external fetal monitor (EFM). At 3:20 A.M., the resident installed an internal monitor, which revealed severe fetal hypoxia and more meconium. A cesarean section was performed at 4:57 A.M. and a male infant was born with hypoxic ischemic encephalopathy. As a result, the child had severe and permanent neurological deficits, cognitive deficits, hearing loss, physical impairments, and other disabilities associated with cerebral palsy. To support the charges, the nurse's employee evaluations were introduced into evidence. About 3½ months prior to the incident, the hospital rated the nurse as an unsatisfactory employee, noting that she sometimes fell asleep while on duty, that she had trouble with electronic fetal monitoring, and that she was reluctant to seek guidance from her supervisors concerning maternal–child care and actual or potential problems in labor and delivery. This case clearly demonstrates that evaluations will be reviewed and can be used against a nurse if he or she is ever sued.

It is important to note that, as part of the doctrine of *respondeat superior,* the employer is liable for the actions of an employee when those actions are undertaken within the scope of the job (*Perez v. Van Groninger & Sons, Inc.,* 1986). In other words, the employee must be at work and carrying out duties by and for the employer in order for the employer to be liable.

In addition, liability exists for any intentional or malicious acts committed by an employee while functioning within the scope of employment. However, if personal malice is involved, the employer is not liable (*Martinez v. Hagopian,* 1986). For example, if an enemy of a nurse is admitted to the hospital and the nurse does something to harm that enemy, the hospital would not be responsible for any harm that occurred even if the patient proves that the harm was done purposely.

Captain of the Ship/ Borrowed Servant Doctrines

On occasion, doctrines that have been formulated at different times and for specific reasons may come into conflict. An example of such conflict is the doctrine of the "captain of the ship." The concept was developed on the theory that the surgeon is in complete control of all activities in the operating room, including the "borrowed servant" doctrine in which an employee of the hospital is, in essence, "loaned" to the surgeon.

The distinction between the two becomes a question of who has control over whom. In a case involving a patient burned during an operation by an x-ray device, one court said:

> It appears from our authorities that generally, when a hospital assigns its nurses to a duty for an operating surgeon in its operating room and surrenders to the surgeon the direction and control of the nurses in relation to the work to be done by them, the nurses become the servants of the operating surgeon insofar as their services relate to the work so controlled and directed by the surgeon, and the hospital is no longer liable for torts committed in such controlled and directed work. (*Synott v. Midway Hospital,* 1970)

However, in most cases, what is of critical importance is a determination of whether, at the time of the harmful act, the employee was working for the original "master" (in this case the hospital) or working for the "special master" (the surgeon). The test usually applied is whether the special master was in such control that he could at any time stop or continue the work and determine the way in which the work was to be done. In the cases involving nurses in hospitals, the question is immediately presented as to whether the hospital has surrendered the direction and control over the nurse to the surgeon so that the nurse becomes the "borrowed servant" of the hospital.

In resolving the question, some courts have been influenced by the "captain of the ship" rule that places the surgeon in complete and total control of the operating room. Other courts have taken the position that there is a difference when the acts or services performed by the nurse in assisting the surgeon are merely administrative. Still other courts have taken the premise that although the hospital may not be responsible for acts of the nurse that are "medical" in nature and involve professional skill and decision making, the hospital may be subjected to liability when the particular act of the nurse is administrative or clerical in character requiring no professional knowledge, skill, or experience.

In the following cases, general staff nurses have been held to be borrowed servants of the surgeon. In the first case, four nurses were assigned to assist a surgeon during the performance of a hysterectomy on the surgeon's private patient. During the operation, the surgeon called for hot water to irrigate the incision and one of the nurses brought water that the surgeon said was too hot. She brought more water, and even though tested by the surgeon, the patient was burned. After paying the claim, the surgeon's insurance company sued the hospital seeking recovery from them as "joint masters." The court ruled:

> [I]n the operating room the surgeon must be master and cannot tolerate any other voice in the control of his assistants; and where, as in the instant case, the evidence was clear that the surgeon had exclusive control over the acts in question, it could not be said that the hospital was a joint master or co-master. (*St. Paul-Mercury Indemnity Co. v. St. Joseph's Hospital,* 1942)

In an action against a hospital for burns suffered from hot water bottles placed at a patient's feet during labor, it was held that the nurse was a servant of the physician at the time of the injury and was not a servant of the hospital (*Jordan v. Touro Infirmary,* 1922).

A more recent situation involved a patient who was injured by an improperly applied splint to his leg following surgery on his knee. The court ruled that the surgeon was responsible and not the hospital because "it was clear from the evidence that acts of this nature performed by hospital employees were beyond their regular duties and were done with the authority and upon the instruction of the surgeon . . ." (*Shutts v. Siehl,* 1959).

Yet another situation involved the nurse who inappropriately used a solution to be injected into the patient as an anesthetic agent. The court held this to be a medical rather than an administrative act and the hospital was not held liable for the negligence of the nurse (*Steinert v. Brunswick Home, Inc.,* 1940).

In cases involving the improper counting of sponges or instruments, most courts have held that such counting is an administrative act, making the hospital liable for harmful acts by the nurses. In several instances, however, courts have ruled that sponge counting is strictly the duty of the surgeon. In the following case, the question of who the nurse worked for was left for the jury to decide. The action was for medical malpractice in which the plaintiff alleged that a sponge or "GYN tape" had been left inside her after a hysterectomy. The sponge was undiscovered for more than two years during which time serious complications arose. The sponge was removed in a second operation; however, the plaintiff required yet a third surgery to correct total bowel obstruction. The jury found that both the doctor and the hospital (as employers of the nurses) were equally responsible for plaintiff's damages. On appeal, the court found that the jury could reasonably determine that the operating room nurses were employees of the hospital at the time of their harmful act, and discussed the special employment issues presented in this case. The court noted that the "captain of the ship" doctrine upon which the trial court relied was a special application of the borrowed servant rule that is based on the theory that the

surgeon is in complete control of all activities in the operating room. In reviewing the development of this doctrine, the court noted that cases have adopted an ad hoc approach in determining whether the assistant was a temporary employee, looking to the question of actual control or direction by the surgeon over the particular function under the facts of the cases (*Truhitte v. French Hospital,* 1982).

Other cases have held that the surgeon is not liable as a special employer for harmful acts of a nurse performed while not under the surgeon's direct supervision and control, as in duties in preparing a patient for surgery (*Hallinan v. Prindle,* 1936) or postoperative care (*Sherman v. Hartman,* 1955).

During the setting up of an operating room tray, a nurse mistakenly substituted formalin for the requested solution of novocaine and the patient was severely burned at the site of the injection. The court in that case held that there was nothing in the evidence to support the plaintiff's contention that the nurse, in preparing the tray for the operation, was the servant, employee, or even the agent of the doctor. The court further held that the nurse, in performing her duties in the operating room, was acting for her employer, the hospital, and not for the operating surgeon. The court refused to hold the doctor responsible for the nurse's negligent acts because the nurse's acts were not performed under conditions where, in the exercise of ordinary care, the doctor could have or should have been able to prevent their injurious effects and did not (*Hallinan v. Prindle,* 1936, pp. 661–662).

Therefore, in cases involving the question of whether the physician or hospital is responsible for the nurse's acts, the jury will hear all the facts as to what the nurses were doing and decide as a jury who he or she was working for in order to find the superior who would be responsible for any acts causing injury.

Independent Contractors

An employer may be liable for the actions of employees, but that is not the case with an employer and an independent contractor. Independent contractors are individuals with special skills who are hired for specific tasks or specific periods of time. The distinction in this instance has to do with the amount of control imposed by the employer. Independent contractors complete their activities according to their own discretion. The employer has no right of control over the means by which results are obtained. However, they do establish the expected results or outcomes. An employer may have some liability for the acts of an independent contractor if there should have been prior knowledge of incompetence and as a result the employer was negligent in its duty of selection.

There are situations in which a nurse would be considered an independent contractor. For example, private duty nurses are professionals acting in an independent capacity and contracted by the patient or family. As such, any negligence attributed to them while at a hospital will generally not subject a hospital to liability. However, if a private duty nurse works for a registry, the registry may be held liable.

An example of a case involving an independent contractor was an action resulting from burns occurring after an operation. It was shown that electric pads placed upon the patient were placed by a special duty nurse, not a regularly employed nurse, and as a result the hospital was found not at fault. When the nurse is held to be an independent contractor, hired to and legally responsible for fulfilling job duties, the hospital is not liable even when it pays the nurse and collects the money from the patient (*Kamps v. Crown Heights Hospital, Inc.,* 1937).

Contemporary situations where nurses might be held to be independent contractors are especially significant. Advanced practice nurses with their own practices are at potential risk for lawsuits and should carry their own liability insurance to protect themselves. Even though nurse practitioners and certified nurse midwives in most states must operate within guidelines set by a physician or provide services in consultation with a physician, it is usual that the physician will be held liable only when he or she knew or should have known of potential inadequacies with a particular nurse practitioner or certified nurse midwife. Advanced practice nurses today are treated as business owners who are essentially liable for their own actions.

Agents

An agent may be an employee or an independent contractor depending on the type of relationship entered into with the principal (principal here means the main person or organization to whom the public would look for responsibility, for example, the hospital or physician). If no control was exercised by the principal over the way in which the details were carried out, the agent would be an independent contractor. However, at any given time, one cannot be both an agent and an independent contractor (Creighton, 1986).

According to the Civil Code in most states, an agency relationship can either be *actual,* as previously discussed, or *ostensible.* An ostensible agency occurs when the principal intentionally, or by lack of ordinary care, causes people to believe that an individual is an agent or employee when there is no employment relationship (California Civil Code, Sections 2298, 2300). This theory of liability is most common when a hospital is held liable for the negligent acts of an independent contractor physician.

> A patient today frequently enters the hospital seeking a wide range of hospital services rather than personal treatment by a particular physician. It would be absurd to require such a patient to be familiar with the law of *respondeat superior* and so to inquire as to each person who treated him whether he is an employee of the hospital or an independent contractor. (*Capan v. Divine Providence Hospital,* 1980)

A Michigan court stated that a hospital generally is not liable for the negligence of a physician who is an independent contractor and merely uses the hospital's facilities to provide treatment to private patients. However, if the patient looked to the hospital to provide services and there was a representation by the hospital that medical treatment would be provided by physicians working there, an agency could be found. The court also stated that factors to be considered in determining whether an agency exists include whether or not the plaintiff had an independent relationship with the physician prior to entering the hospital and whether the hospital was really the site for treatment by the plaintiff's own physician (*Brackens v. Detroit Osteopathic Hospital,* 1989).

It is conceivable that advance practice nurses could face this dilemma if they utilize health care agencies as a locale to provide services to patients. The issue may become more obvious as more certified nurse midwives and nurse practitioners obtain hospital privileges.

Students

Liability for students who utilize health care facilities as settings for clinical learning activities is virtually the same as for registered nurses. Students must be responsible for their own actions (Feutz-Harter, 1991). They are expected to comply with the same standards of care as registered nurses who perform the same clinical activities. Obviously, they need appropriate supervision and should not be assigned to activities beyond their abilities.

If the clinical instructor is making student assignments and providing supervision, it is the responsibility of the instructor to assess the students' capabilities and provide direction, assistance, and evaluation as needed. If a nurse from the institution is making assignments and/or providing supervision, the instructor is responsible for providing the nurse with information about the students' capabilities and the nurse should then assess these capabilities (Feutz-Harter, 1991).

The interaction between instructor and unit nurse is often blurred regarding student experiences. As a result, there may be a question as to who is actually liable should a legal situation arise. It may be that the nurse (and the health care institution employer) and the instructor (and educational institution employer) are all named in an action. Frequently, contractual agreements between the health care agency and educational institution will explicate the responsibilities of each.

In all events, patients should be apprised that the care giver is a student nurse from a given school and is not in the employment of the health care institution.

CORPORATE LIABILITY

Generally, when one addresses corporate responsibility, it is in terms of the liability of officers and directors of that corporation to the shareholders of the corporate stock. However, in speaking specifically of corporate responsibility in hospitals, the law recognizes that the hospital is no longer merely the building that houses the physician's equipment and medical supplies but is the entity providing health care to many communities. Therefore, when a person is injured in a hospital and can prove that a policy of the hospital corporate board was at fault, the corporation itself can be held liable for sustained injuries.

Types of Hospitals

In a discussion on hospital liability, it is worth mentioning that there are different types of institutions, each with its own particular set of responsibilities. To be examined here are hospitals categorized by ownership: government or public hospitals, charitable nonprofit hospitals, and for-profit proprietary hospitals.

Government or Public Hospitals

In the past, government or public hospitals had immunity from lawsuits because one could not sue governments (sovereign immunity). In recent years this freedom from liability gradually is being reversed. In the case of federal government employees, the Federal Tort Claims Act confers a general waiver of immunity from suits for wrongs arising from the negligence of federal government employees (60 Stat. 812; 28 U. S. C.). In the case of state or local governments, some require that employees answer their own charge of negligence against them.

Charitable Nonprofit Hospitals

Until fairly recently, nonprofit hospitals enjoyed immunity from lawsuits based upon the rationalization that (1) the hospitals were not health care providers but merely buildings housing equipment for physicians; (2) public policy supported the immunity; (3) the assets of the hospital could be used only for charitable purposes; and (4) patients who entered these hospitals did so at their own risk and with a waiver of claims for injuries (*Cook v. John N. Norton Memorial Infirmary,* 1918).

When courts abandoned the concept of charitable immunity they did so because it was deemed inequitable to allow certain institutions to escape liability merely because of their designation as nonprofit entities. The change did not occur based on the recognition that the hospital's role as a health care provider was changing (*Flagiello v. Pennsylvania Hospital*, 1965).

This opened an interesting prospect for the future. As immunities weakened, courts were quick to enter and apply the doctrine of ostensible agency (discussed earlier) to hospitals, thereby permitting recovery against a hospital for the negligent acts of its independent contractor physicians. Soon, thereafter, the doctrine of *corporate negligence* was formulated, which declared that a hospital may be held directly liable to patients for breaches of certain duties separate from those by its nonemployee physicians.

Corporate Negligence

In discussing corporate negligence, one must be aware first that the intent of most courts in formulating this doctrine was to hold the hospital liable as an administrator of hospital services. Only as the administrator of such services could a hospital be held directly liable for patient injuries occurring within its walls. The corporate negligence doctrine was first adopted by the Illinois Supreme Court, which concluded that the concept that hospitals do nothing more than furnish facilities and hire physicians was no longer valid. The court found that present-day hospitals hire large staffs of physicians who collaboratively provide treatment and charge patients for the care received and, as a result, are holding themselves out as health care providers. The court then looked at the hospital's regulations, standards, and bylaws to determine whether it failed in its self-appointed role as health care administrator (*Darling v. Charleston Community Hospital*, 1965).

Even though the court in that Illinois case did not explicitly say what it was that the hospital did wrong, it was the first case to hold that a hospital has an independent duty to supervise the physicians who practice within its walls. The next case fastened a duty upon the hospital to review the qualifications of their physicians in order to ensure that only qualified physicians practice there. In that case, a patient was subjected to improper colon surgery, following which he pro-

duced evidence that this particular doctor had performed similarly improper procedures on two other patients (*Purcell v. Zimbleman*, 1972).

In a later case, the Pennsylvania Supreme Court identified the duties owed by the hospital to its patients (*Thompson v. Nason Hospital*, 1991):

1. A duty to use reasonable care in the maintenance of safe and adequate facilities and equipment. This was essentially a restatement of the law of premises liability, which states that owners of property are responsible for events that occur on their property and for which hospitals were always liable.

2. A duty to select and retain only competent physicians. A hospital has an independent duty to take reasonable steps to ensure that its medical staff is qualified. This would include peer review committees and JCAHO (Joint Commission on the Accreditation of Health Organizations) review for licensure. In addition to physicians, advanced practice nurses who apply for hospital privileges would be considered under this duty. The concept has created some problems for hospitals and for plaintiffs alike. Whereas the hospital must accept and implement the results reached by the peer review committees, the hospital itself cannot do anything other than check an applicant's resume for accuracy, check references, and act as an administrator. The hospital would not be liable under a theory of corporate negligence if an unqualified physician is practicing because the administrative staff (usually not physicians) are not competent to judge the propriety of medical procedures.

3. A duty to oversee all medical care in the facility. This duty entails investigating potential staff members, including physicians, nurses, and assistive personnel. In a Texas case, a valid claim was asserted against the hospital alleging that it was liable in recklessly hiring an orderly. This orderly injured a patient when attempting to remove a catheter without first deflating the balloon (*Wilson N. Jones Memorial Hospital v. Davis*, 1977). In another case

in California (*Elam v. College Park Hospital,* 1982), the court found that the hospital was liable under a theory of corporate negligence by inappropriately screening the competency of its medical staff to ensure the adequacy of medical care for patients at its facility. In that case, a podiatrist admitted a patient to the hospital with the concurrence of a medical doctor and the plaintiff was injured as a result of surgery to correct bilateral bunions and bilateral hammer toes. The plaintiff alleged that the hospital knew of three other cases involving the same podiatrist and yet took no action to investigate, recommend revocation of surgical privileges, or suspend the privileges.

4. A duty to formulate, adopt, and enforce adequate rules and policies to ensure quality care for the patients. This duty to oversee involves taking "reasonable steps to implement general guidelines and directives designed to coordinate the many arms of the hospital" (*Rohe v. Shivde,* 1990). The distinction between reviewing medical decisions and implementing guidelines was demonstrated when a hospital was found to be negligent for violation of a hospital bylaw. A physician refused to provide a consultation to another physician. The hospital's bylaws imposed a duty upon the hospital to use "reasonable efforts to assist physicians in obtaining consultations from other staff physicians." The court stated:"

[T]his duty does not amount to unlawful practice of medicine because it requires not medical expertise but administrative expertise to enforce rules and regulations which were adopted by the hospital to insure a smoothly run hospital routine and adequate patient care and under which the physicians have agreed to operate. (*Johnson v. St. Bernard Hospital,* 1979)

For-Profit Proprietary Hospitals

For-profit hospitals have all of the previously listed doctrines applied equally and probably with greater effectiveness in some jurisdictions.

In these institutions, there are no governmental or charitable immunities to prevent a plaintiff from suing for corporate negligence.

CONCLUSION

All of the these theories of liability have been used successfully against doctors, hospitals, and nurses. What the perinatal nurse needs to know and understand regarding these theories is how certain actions can lead to liability and what can be done to prevent it. Using common sense, one's educational expertise, and good judgment; maintaining currency; and following approved standards and guidelines will probably suffice in most instances in allowing a nurse to practice a lifetime of delivering good care to patients without the threat of a lawsuit.

REFERENCES

53 Am. Jur. 2d, Master and servant, Section 3.
California Civil Code, §§ 2298, 2300.
California Corporations Code, §§ 15013, 15014.
Creighton, H. (1986). Law every nurse should know (5th ed.). Philadelphia: W. B. Saunders.
Feutz-Harter, S. (1991). Nursing and the law (5th ed., p. 19–20). Eau Claire, WI: Professional Education Systems.
Kelly, L., & Joel, L. (1996). The nursing experience (p. 484). New York: McGraw-Hill.
Restatement, Agency. 1933 § 2(3); see also §§ 220, 250, 251.
60 Stat. 812; 28 U. S. C. §§ 1291, 1346, 1402, 1504, 2110, 2401, 2402, 2411, 2412, 2671, 2680.
Webster's new international dictionary of the English language (2nd ed.) (1937). Cleveland: William Collins.

CASE CITATIONS

Brackens v. Detroit Osteopathic Hospital, 174 Mich. App. 290, 435 S.W.2d 472 app. den. 433 Mich. 857 (1989).
Capan v. Divine Providence Hospital, 430 A. 2d 647, 649 (Pa. Sup. 1980).
Cavero v. Franklin General Benevolent Society, 36 Cal. 2d 301, 223 P.2d 471 (1950).
Clark v. Harris Hospital, Tex. Civ. App. 2 Dist., 543 S.W.2d 543 (1976).

Clary v. Christiansen, 83 N.E. 2d 644 (Ohio Ct. App., 1948).

Cook v. John N. Norton Memorial Infirmary, 180 Ky. 331, 202 S.W. 874 (1918).

Darling v. Charleston Community Hospital, 211 N.E.2d 253 (Ill. 1965).

Elam v. College Park Hospital, 132 Cal. App. 3d 332, 183 Cal. Rptr. 156 (1982).

Flagiello v. Pennsylvania Hospital 208 A.2d 193 (Pa. 1965).

Hallinan v. Prindle, 17 Cal. App. 2d 656, 62 P. 2d 1075 (1936).

Johnson v. St. Bernard Hospital, 399 N.E.2d 198 (Ill. App. 1979).

Jordan v. Touro Infirmary, 123 So. 726 (L.A. App. 1922).

Kamps v. Crown Heights Hospital, Inc., 251 App. Div. 849, 296 N.Y.S 776, aff'd 277 N.Y. 86 (1937).

Kemalyan v. Henderson, 45 Wash. 2d 693, 277 P.2d 372 (1954).

Martinez v. Hagopian, 182 Cal. App. 3d 1223, 227 Cal. Rptr. 763 (5th Dist. 1986).

Perez v. Van Groninger & Sons, Inc., 41 Cal. 3d 1223, 227 Cal. Rptr. 106, 719 P.2d 676 (1986).

Purcell v. Zimbleman, 500 P.2d 335 (Ariz. App. 1972).

Robertson v. Wentz, 187 Cal. App. 3d 1281, 232 Cal. Rptr. 634 (1st Dist. 1986).

Rohe v. Shivde, 560 N.E.2d 1113 (Ill. App. 1 Dist. 1990).

Rubio v. Swiridoff, 165 Cal. App. 3d 400, 211 Cal. Rptr. 338. (5th Dist. 1985).

St. Paul Medical Center v. Cecil, 842 S.W.2 808 (Tex. App. Dallas 1992).

St. Paul-Mercury Indemnity Co. v. St. Joseph's Hospital, 212 Minn. 558, 4 N.W.2d 637 (1942).

Sherman v. Hartman, 137 Cal. App. 2d 589, 290 P.2d 894 (1955).

Shutts v. Siebl 109 Ohio App. 145, 10 Ohio Ops. 2d 363, 164 N.E.2d 443 (1959).

Steinert v. Brunswick Home, Inc., 259 App. Div. 1018, 20 N.Y.S.2d 459, app. den. 260 App. Div. 810, 22 N.Y.S.2d 822 (1940).

Synott v. Midway Hospital, 287 Minn. 270, 178 N.W.2d 211 (1970).

Thompson v. Nason Hospital, 591 A.2d 703 (Pa. 1991).

Truhitte v. French Hospital, 128 Cal. App. 3d 332, 180 Cal. Rptr. 152 (1982).

Ware v. Culp, 24 Cal. App. 2d 22, 74 P.2d 283 (1938).

Wilson N. Jones Memorial Hospital v. Davis, 553 S.W.2d 180 (Tex. Civ. App. Waco 1977), writ. ref. nre. (Oct. 26, 1977) and rehg. of write of error overr. (Nov. 30, 1977).

CHAPTER

7

Critical Care Obstetrics

Suzanne McMurtry Baird

Over the last decade, critical care obstetric nursing has emerged as a subspecialty of perinatal nursing. Perinatal services throughout the country are currently developing programs to meet the needs of pregnant patients requiring critical care. This broadened scope of practice has developed in response to changes in the obstetric patient population that increase the likelihood for complications. Perinatal nurses are well acquainted with these changes, which are often cited in the literature (Zuspan & Sachs, 1988).

Due to advancements in health care and technology, women with preexisting conditions, such as congenital heart defects and cystic fibrosis, now survive childhood and become pregnant. Additionally, certain chronic conditions are no longer considered contraindications to pregnancy. Women with diabetes, hypertension, and renal disease now have the opportunity to conceive, continue the pregnancy, and achieve optimal outcomes. Finally, the complex nature of our society has increased the likelihood that pregnant patients will be involved in substance abuse and trauma, both of which can result in serious consequences for mother and fetus.

The change in the scope of nursing practice was preceded by the identification of maternal/fetal medicine as a subspecialty by the American College of Obstetrics and Gynecology (ACOG) in 1972. This, along with the evolution of neonatal intensive care units, facilitated the creation of ter-

tiary care centers equipped to care for pregnant patients with complex needs. Many areas of the country established referral systems, which resulted in clustering of pregnant women with complications in these high-risk centers, facilitating the research that led to the creation of the first critical care obstetric unit in 1986 (Mabie & Sibai, 1990). Since this time, the obstetric community has recognized the need for availability of an enhanced level of care, and critical care obstetrics (CCOB) is a service in a growing number of hospitals.

In the past, and as is often still the case, these patients were managed in traditional intensive care units (ICU) by intensivists. In the ICU the patients received the benefit of technology in the form of hemodynamic monitoring and ventilatory support but lost the family-centered approach common to most perinatal units. In addition, the admission of pregnant patients to the ICU often caused anxiety for the staff, who were unfamiliar with the unique physiologic changes associated with pregnancy, pregnancy-related disease processes, and the special needs of the fetus. The development of obstetric critical care services bridged the gap between traditional intensive care and obstetrical management. Regardless of whether the nursing care is delivered in a dedicated obstetrical intensive care unit or in a surgical or medical intensive care unit, staff must possess the knowledge base and have the experience necessary to care for these complex patients. The standards for patient care follow the patient regardless of where the care is delivered. Critical care and perinatal nurses will be held to the same standard of care for maternal and fetal assessment, intervention, and evaluation. It is essential that all nurses involved in the care of critically ill pregnant patients take steps, personally and professionally, to acquire and maintain the skills necessary to meet this level of care. In the majority of hospitals, there is no dedicated obstetric critical care unit and these patients are managed from a medical perspective, through collaboration between the obstetricians and critical care specialists. In this situation, perinatal and ICU nurse specialists must collaborate to meet the needs of both the mother and her fetus.

SOURCES OF LIABILITY

The expanded scope of nursing practice present in the delivery of critical care is associated with a greater degree of liability for professional malpractice and negligence (Salatka, 1992). Perinatal nurses have historically experienced increased liability exposure as well. The combination of these two areas of specialty practice adds a new dimension to risk management efforts of nurses and health care organizations.

Because the specialty of obstetric critical care nursing is new, there is little in the nursing literature reflecting pertinent legal principles. In addition, due to the lengthy process involved in liability litigation, case law precedents have not been established. Consequently, we must turn to information concerning traditional critical care nursing and perinatal nursing in an attempt to identify sources of liability. Potential and actual sources of liability include failure to assess, failure to intervene, failure to document, failure to validate informed consent, failure to appropriately use technology and equipment, improper use of restraints, failure to adhere to advanced directives, and improper administration of medication.

Failure to Assess

A major area of liability for nurses is the failure to assess and monitor patient status. Patients are hospitalized so that they may be monitored either continuously or intermittently. In most settings, this responsibility belongs to the nurse. Perinatal nurses have struggled with this source of liability for years. In *Dobrzenieck v. University Hospital of Cleveland* (1984), a labor and delivery nurse was found liable for damages arising from her failure to adequately monitor a high-risk patient. The nurse failed to properly assess the fetus of a preeclamptic patient and to interpret signs of fetal compromise. As a result, the fetus was delivered by cesarean section in an asphyxiated state and was born with total blindness and mental retardation. A settlement of $2.2 million was reached for the plaintiff. In *Alvis v. Henderson Obstetrics* (1992), nurses were found liable for their failure to determine the breech presentation of an infant that was delivered vaginally at 34½ weeks and suffered severe kidney damage due to prolonged hypoxia. The plaintiff was awarded $2 million in a shared verdict against the hospital and the attending physician.

In *Wheeler v. Yettie Kersting Memorial Hospital* (1993), the patient was taken to a small, community hospital in Texas for evaluation prior to transfer to a facility in Galveston. Nursing assessment at the small hospital revealed that the patient was 4 cm dilated, 70% effaced, and had bulging membranes. There was no mention in the medical record of the presenting part. Fetal monitoring and labor assessment were not performed. The nurses obtained permission from the physician on call at their hospital and the physician in Galveston to transport Ms. Wheeler. En route, Ms. Wheeler's membranes ruptured and she proceeded to deliver the lower extremities and body of a breech infant. Head entrapment occurred and the fetus subsequently expired prior to complete delivery. The Texas Court of Appeals found the nurses responsible, in part, for their failure to completely assess the patient's condition and fetal presentation.

The process of assessing a critically ill pregnant patient requires an understanding of the complex relationship between maternal and fetal physiology. This is best accomplished by staff who possess knowledge of the high-risk pregnant patient and who have acquired specific critical care skills such as invasive hemodynamic monitoring, respiratory support, advanced resuscitation, and drug therapy. This comprehensive knowledge base provides the foundation for both initial and ongoing assessment. In settings where nurses do not possess both perinatal and critical care skills, ongoing collaboration between nurses from both areas is essential in order to adequately assess and intervene on behalf of the mother and fetus.

Due to the nature of obstetric care and the potential for rapid change in patient status, it is often the perinatal nurse who identifies patients in need of critical care services. Display 7-1 lists the indications for invasive hemodynamic monitoring in the pregnant patient as outlined by ACOG (1988). Although it is the decision of the physician whether or not to utilize available technology, nurses must provide a comprehensive, noninvasive assessment to assist in management decisions. Assessment of the critically ill pregnant patient should include particular attention to cardiovascular and respiratory status, neurologic and renal function, as well as indications of fetal well-being.

Frequency and scope of assessment depend on maternal and fetal conditions, and are suggested by current recommendations from the American Association for Critical Care Nurses (AACN, 1989) and the Association of Women's Health, Obstetric, and Neonatal Nurses (AWHONN, 1991). Failure to follow established assessment parameters places the patient at risk and increases the nurse's liability. Currently, AWHONN recommends that the nurse responsible for the care of high-risk patients assess the maternal and fetal status every 15 minutes during the first stage of labor and every 5 minutes during the second stage. The most appropriate method of surveillance remains in question. In 1986, the Nurses' Association of the American College of Obstetrics and Gynecology (NAACOG), now known as AWHONN, and the American College of Obstetrics and Gynecology (ACOG) issued a joint statement concerning electronic fetal monitoring (EFM), which recommended the use of continuous EFM for high-risk patients (ACOG/NAACOG, 1986). However, in 1990, NAACOG published practice guidelines that allow the nurse to choose between auscultation and EFM (NAACOG, 1990). If auscultation is

DISPLAY 7-1

Indications for Invasive Hemodynamic Monitoring During Pregnancy

- Shock of unknown etiology
- Adult respiratory distress syndrome
- Massive blood loss or fluid replacement
- Conditions refractory to treatment or of unknown etiology:
  - Sepsis
  - Pulmonary edema
  - Oliguria
  - Heart failure
- Preexisting chronic conditions, such as New York Heart Association class III or IV cardiac disease
- Pregnancy-induced hypertension complicated by pulmonary edema or oliguria

Source: American College of Obstetricians and Gynecologists (1988). Invasive hemodynamic monitoring in obstetrics and gynecology. ACOG Technical Bulletin (p. 121)

selected as the method for fetal surveillance the nurse must realize that changes in maternal hemodynamic status and oxygen transport will influence oxygen delivery to the fetus, which may result in subtle changes in fetal status that could go unrecognized by auscultation. In the case of a critically ill pregnant woman, the prudent approach seems to favor continuous EFM as the mode of fetal assessment.

Failure to Intervene

Nurses also experience increased liability exposure for failure to appropriately intervene on behalf of their patients. Interventions consist not only of appropriate actions based on assessment data, such as maximizing oxygen delivery to the fetus through the administration of oxygen and maternal position changes, but also include timely communication with the physician regarding patient status. In the case of *Fairfax Hospital System, Inc. v. McCarty* (1992) the nurse was found liable for her failure to intervene in the case of nonreassuring fetal status as well as for her failure to communicate the extreme nature of the situation to the attending physician. The court held that her actions proximately caused the neurologic injuries suffered by the infant. The jury awarded the plaintiff $3.5 million, which was later reduced by the court as required by statutory law.

Failure to communicate was also a central feature in *Baptist Medical Center v. Wilson* (1993). In this case, the nurses neglected to notify the obstetrician of patient complaints indicative of uterine rupture, resulting in intrauterine fetal death. The jury found for the plaintiff and awarded $600,000.00. In the case of *Henry v. Felici* (1988), a 3-year-old female suffered an accidental blow to the head that resulted in severe injury. The admitting hospital was unable to provide a CT scan to evaluate the extent of the child's injury. The neurologist secured permission from a neurosurgeon at another facility to transfer the child immediately for evaluation. The transfer order was given at 2:00 P.M. Due to a series of circumstances, the transfer was not accomplished until 4:00 P.M. At this point in time, damage to the child's brain was so severe that surgery was unsuccessful

and she died. Her parents brought suit against all of the care providers involved. The ICU nurse at the original hospital was found liable for the delayed transport and the hospital settled with the plaintiffs.

Performance of critical care interventions for pregnant women requires that the attending nurse possess a thorough knowledge base of the disease process and pharmacotherapeutics, advanced clinical skills involving the use of complicated equipment and devices, and the ability to interpret patient data including laboratory test results and physical examination findings. Common diagnoses that are associated with the need for critical care services for the obstetric patient are listed in Display 7-2.

Technology, equipment, and procedures tend to be the focus of concern for perinatal nurses expanding their scope of practice into critical care. Although the mastery of these skills is very important, it is the interpretation of the information obtained that has the greatest impact on the plan of care. Conversely, critical care nurses caring for pregnant women must possess the same skills in fetal assessment and have the same understanding of the unique relationship between the mother and the fetus that the perinatal nurse has. If these requirements are not available in a single nurse, then collaboration between nurse specialists is essential.

According to professional standards set forth by AACN, critical care nurses have the responsibility to diagnose and treat actual or potential life-threatening illness (Sanford & Disch, 1989). The critical care nurse interprets patient data, identifies actual or potential problems, plans needed interventions, and, finally, responds with appropriate treatment. Depending upon patient status and physician availability, the critical care nurse may be required to diagnose and perform necessary treatment while avoiding the practice of medicine. An example in clinical practice involves the nurse who implements Advanced Cardiac Life Support (ACLS) protocols following the identification of a pulseless dysrhythmia. Hospital and unit practice guidelines help facilitate independent nursing interventions and decision making while decreasing liability.

Failure to Document Accurately and Appropriately

"If it wasn't documented, it wasn't done." Documentation errors and omissions continue to be a significant source of liability for nurses. In *Ketchum v. Overlake Hospital Center* (1991), the Appellate Court of Washington noted that the lack of documentation by an ICU nurse revealed that critical assessment data indicating a deterioration in the patient's neurological status was overlooked. The patient suffered severe neurological impairment and the medical records did not reflect the nurse's assessment or interventions.

The lack of documentation is not the only source of liability with which nurses must contend. In the case of *Broodover v. Mary Hitchcock Memorial Hospital* (1990), a jury verdict against the hospital resulted, in part, from inappropriate documentation by the nurse that contained speculation as to the cause and admission of responsibility for the fall of a postoperative patient that resulted in a fractured hip. In her documentation, the nurse speculated that the fall resulted from an attempt by the patient to reach the bathroom when his calls for assistance went unanswered.

One purpose for the nursing documentation is to demonstrate the application of the nursing process in a way that will provide a retrospective reflection of the care of the patient. Whether the documentation tool represents an integration of perinatal and ICU content or whether collaborative nursing documentation is maintained using separate perinatal and ICU tools, all pertinent information must be present in the patient record. The use of flowsheets and innovative documentation systems such as documentation by exception are appropriate in caring for critically ill pregnant women. It is essential, however, that the record demonstrate the entire continuum of nursing care and provide explicit information regarding salient events. This includes not only assessment data and interventions but also the interpretation of data and the plan of care for the patient as well as an evaluation of the patient's response to interventions and the ability and success of the patient in achieving specific outcomes.

Failure to Validate Informed Consent

The responsibility of obtaining informed consent for medical procedures rests with the physician. However, nurses are not immune from legal action in cases where patients contend that they lacked specific information regarding a treatment or procedure. In Pennsylvania (*Foflygen v. Zemel*, 1992), a hospital nurse was implicated in a suit in which a patient, who underwent gastric stapling, suffered major postoperative complications. The patient's legal counsel alleged that because the nurse obtained the patient's signature on the actual consent, the nurse, as well as the physician, committed battery. The court disagreed and dismissed the charges against the nurse.

Physicians and hospitals have the legal duty to the patient of obtaining informed patient consent. The dialogue surrounding the informed consent process must include information concerning the nature of the procedure, the risks associated with the treatment or procedure (both inherent and potential), alternative treatments, and the potential sequelae if the patient

DISPLAY 7-2

Frequent Diagnoses Leading to Admission to the Critical Care Obstetrics Unit

Hypertension
- Chronic
- Severe preeclampsia
- HELLP syndrome

Eclampsia

Cardiac disease

Diabetic ketoacidosis

Renal disease

Liver disease

Asthma

Lupus

Hemorrhage

elects not to proceed with the treatment. Treatments performed without the patient's informed consent, absent a few exceptions, constitute battery and theoretically may subject the care providers to criminal charges as well as civil action.

The role of the nurse in the informed consent process consists of validating that informed consent was provided by the physician and obtaining the patient's voluntary signature on a consent form. The nurse must not encourage the patient to sign the informed consent document unless the nurse is absolutely satisfied that the patient has a clear understanding of the information presented by the physician. In an advocacy capacity, the nurse has an ethical duty to the patient to facilitate complete understanding of pertinent information but must not assume responsibility for providing specific content.

Care of critically ill pregnant women is a relatively unusual occurrence and often takes patients and their families by surprise. In this environment where urgent care may be necessary, the informed consent process may be rushed and incomplete. Ideally, nurses attending the patient, either in the labor and delivery area or in ICU, should be present when the physician explains the procedure to the patient and family. It is appropriate for the nurse to validate the patient's understanding of the information. The nurse's signature as a witness on a consent form simply verifies that the patient's signature is not forged.

An emergency exception to the requirement for obtaining informed consent has been traditionally acknowledged. This permits the medical staff to provide emergent care for patients who are unable to consent, when family members are not available or if significant harm will occur if treatment is not initiated. Health care providers are permitted to assume that patients would all consent to treatment if they could. In some cases due to the clinical condition or specific treatment modalities, the patient will be unable to engage in informed consent and participate in management decisions. The best case scenario is that she has advanced directive documents that present her wishes prior to incapacitation. These situations often necessitate direct involvement of the next of kin in making critical decisions involving the mother and the fetus. The dialogue that occurs should involve the next of kin in a supportive environment to allow family members to adequately explore care options.

Failure to Appropriately Use Technology and Equipment

Advancements in technology and equipment also increase the liability of nurses caring for critically ill pregnant women and often result in large awards. Potential sources of liability include failure to utilize equipment according to the manufacturer's recommendations and hospital policy, the use of defective equipment, and the inappropriate use of equipment. In the case of *Mather v. Griffin Hospital* (1988), the labor and delivery nurses failed to provide appropriate intubation equipment for support of a newborn experiencing respiratory distress. The jury believed the infant suffered asphyxia during the prolonged time that it took to secure an adequate airway and awarded the plaintiff $9 million. The judgment was upheld on appeal.

In *Davenport v. Ephraim McDowell Memorial Hospital* (1988), a postoperative patient suffered cardiac and respiratory arrest that went unnoticed by staff members because the cardiac monitor alarms were turned off or the volume was adjusted so low that the warning was not audible. A jury originally ruled in favor of the defendants, but on appeal, the court allowed testimony that indicated the hospital changed its alarm policy following this incident. Testimony for the plaintiff alleged that failure to use existing alarms constituted a deviation from the accepted standard of care.

Caring for critically ill pregnant women often necessitates the use of sophisticated monitoring techniques and equipment with which the perinatal nurse may be unfamiliar. If the patient is cared for in the ICU, critical care staff may be unfamiliar with the use of the fetal monitor. The ideal situation would allow an OBICU nurse trained in the use of various technology and equipment to provide total care for the patient. However, in the majority of settings this is not possible, and perinatal and ICU nurses must collaborate in the use of equipment to prevent injury.

Improper Use of Restraints

Another source of liability for nurses involves the use of restraints. Use of physical and chemical patient restraints may be necessary in certain critical care clinical situations to limit patient movement and prevent patient injury. Research conducted by the Health Care Financing Administration (HCFA) reports that 42% of extended-care patients are restrained and that restraints are used in 13% of all acute-care admissions (Health Care Financing Administration, 1992). The use of restraints to prevent injury may actually create risk for the patient by contributing to the development of confusion, agitation, decubitus ulcers, contractures, and other problems associated with immobility (Stolley et al., 1993).

Concerns about the use of restraints were originally addressed in the Nursing Home Reform Act, which was part of the legislative package known as the Omnibus Budget Reconciliation Act (OBRA) enacted in 1987. OBRA restricts the use of restraints in long-term care facilities and requires that all alternative measures to modify a patient's behavior be used by the care providers before restraints are placed. OBRA also mandates that physical restraint devices may only be applied with a physician's written order specifying why the restraint was used and the length of time that the physician anticipates that this intervention will be necessary (Omnibus Budget Reconciliation Act of 1990). The Food and Drug Administration (FDA, 1991) has made similar recommendations.

In 1992, the Joint Commission of Accreditation of Healthcare Organizations (JCAHO) issued specific criteria for the use of restraints in the acute care setting (JCAHO, 1992). The commission defined restraints as "a physical or mechanical device to involuntarily restrain the movement of the whole or a portion of a patient's body as a means of controlling his/her physical activities in order to protect him/her or others from injury." JCAHO regulations only include guidelines for physical restraints. Intubated patients and those undergoing invasive hemodynamic monitoring are often mechanically restrained. Continuous intravenous sedation may also be used to control behavior; however, there is little in the legal literature addressing the use of chemical or pharmacologic restraining. Despite the development of these guidelines by official regulating agencies, restraining devices are often misapplied and mismanaged. Nurses utilizing restraining devices must be aware of the regulations regarding their use and take care to appropriately document adherence to existing hospital policy.

Failure to Follow Advance Directives

An additional area of nurse liability involves failure to follow advance directives. In *Anderson v. St. Francis-St. George Hospital* (1992), the Ohio Court of Appeals held that, in the presence of an advance directive, resuscitative efforts constitute battery. In this case the patient suffered ventricular fibrillation and was defibrillated by the nurse despite the presence of a "Do Not Resuscitate" order on the chart. The patient survived the episode but subsequently died. The original contention of the administrator of the patient's estate was that the actions of the nurse resulted in "wrongful life" for the decedent; however, the court found that no legal cause of action exists for wrongful life. The court, although unwilling to recognize this cause of action, acknowledged that the interventions of the nurse caused pain and suffering, emotional distress, disability, and medical expenses and that these injuries were consistent with the act of battery.

The Patient Self-Determination Act (PSDA), federal legislation enacted in December 1991, requires institutions to ask patients if they have previously prepared an advance directive and to notify patients about the process for initiating advance directives (Omnibus Budget Reconciliation Act of 1990). The purpose of the PSDA is to promote the opportunity for patients to discuss treatment options and plans with their health care providers, leading to the promotion and consummation of advance directives prior to illness. Most states have enacted legislation that promotes living wills and/or a durable power of attorney. Living wills express the patient's wishes for the initiation of life-saving interventions in the event of imminent death or permanent vegetative state. A durable power of attorney allows for designation of a particular individual to make decisions on behalf of the patient if the patient is unable to express his or her wishes (Teno et al., 1994).

Acquiring an advance directive from a critically ill pregnant patient during hospitalization is a controversial issue for several reasons. Enhancement of patient anxiety and mistrust may occur if discussions occur during the hospital admission process. Additionally, the admission process is often chaotic, thereby preventing patients from grasping information needed to make a comprehensive decision on advance directives. Finally, patients may be unable to engage in a thoughtful decision-making process due to illness. If these events occur, the purpose of the PSDA is not fulfilled.

Currently 47 states have passed legislation allowing advance directives (see Display 7-3). A person executing a formal advance directive must be 18 years of age or older. The directive must be written, signed, and witnessed. Because many statutes forbid the patient's health care providers from witnessing a document for their patient, the critical care nurse should not act as a witness. Generally, a living will is not required when a patient is competent and can communicate a refusal of treatments. In states that do not possess current statutes for living wills, if the patient has a witnessed document with clear and convincing language expressing his or her wishes, the patient still has the constitutional right to be free from medical intervention.

The decision to forego resuscitative measures is ideally made jointly among the patient, family,

Display 7-3

Jurisdictions That Have Living Will Statutes*

Alabama	Hawaii	Missouri	South Carolina
Alaska	Idaho	Montana	South Dakota
Arizona	Illinois	Nebraska	Tennessee
Arkansas	Indiana	Nevada	Texas
California	Iowa	New Mexico	Utah
Colorado	Kansas	North Carolina	Vermont
Connecticut	Louisiana	North Dakota	Virginia
Delaware	Maine	Oklahoma	Washington
District of Columbia	Maryland	Ohio	West Virginia
Florida	Minnesota	Oregon	Wisconsin
Georgia	Mississippi	Rhode Island	Wyoming

*Information as of November 1998. To update this information, or to receive end-of-life decision-making publications or state-specific information, please contact the Society for the Right to Die at (212) 366-5540.

and medical staff. If the patient is incompetent the decision may be made between the family and the physician. Failure to document and adhere to advance directives places the nurse in a precarious position if the patient's wishes are not respected.

If life support measures have been initiated, when can they be terminated? This has been an issue in many court cases and opinions vary from state to state. The Harvard criteria, established in 1968, defined a reliable benchmark for determining brain death as noted in Display 7-4 (Harvard Medical School, 1968). There have been no case reports of patients regaining brain function once they have met these criteria. The President's Commission for the Study of Ethical Problems in Medicine, Biomedical and Behavioral Research issued a report entitled *Defining Death* in 1981. The recommendation from the commission was that the legal and medical communities should attempt to establish a uniform statute that defines death by physiologic measures rather than by rapidly changing medical criteria and tests. The death of a critically ill pregnant woman is a difficult situation with which to deal. In most cases, a maternal death is the last event that anyone anticipates. Although there are women who enter into pregnancy with preexisting conditions, such as cardiac disease, that greatly increase the risk of morbidity, this is not the case for the vast majority of women. There have been numerous case reports of the indefinite extension of life for a pregnant woman who legally meets the criteria of death, usually to extend the gestational period and facilitate fetal lung maturity so that the baby can live.

Improper Administration of Medication

Medication errors continue to create a source of liability for nurses. In the case of *Dessauer v. Memorial General Hospital* (1981), an OB nurse was transferred to the emergency room where she inadvertently administered 850 mg of lidocaine instead of the prescribed 50 mg dose to a patient experiencing chest pain. The patient suffered

DISPLAY 7-4

The Harvard Criteria for Determining Brain Death

1. Complete unresponsiveness: total unawareness of external stimuli (that is, irreversible coma)

2. No spontaneous muscular movements, including respiration. If the patient has been on a mechanical ventilator, one can turn it off for 3 minutes to observe whether the patient breathes spontaneously. For this criteria to be valid, the patient must have a normal carbon dioxide tension and must breathe room air for at least 10 minutes before the test.

3. Absent reflexes, spontaneous or elicited, except those that are spinal cord reflexes (for example, knee jerk).

4. A flat EEG for at least 10 and preferably 20 minutes is a confirmatory rather than essential criterion.
   a. There are further procedural criteria for the way the test should be done.
   b. EEG data are not valid when there is hypothermia or CNS depression from medications.

Source: Harvard Medical School. (1968). Ad hoc committee of the Harvard Medical School to examine the definition of brain death: A definition of irreversible coma. Journal of the American Medical Association, 205, 337.

severe complications and required life support. Eventually the patient was removed from life support at the request of his wife. The court found the nurse and the hospital liable for Mr. Dessauer's injury and awarded the plaintiff $225,000.00. In the critical care of pregnant women, nurses must always remember that many medications directly effect uterine blood flow, cross the placenta, and may cause hemodynamic changes in the fetus as well as the mother. Multiple infusions of a variety of drugs increase the likelihood of drug incompatibilities and adverse outcomes. Nurses caring for patients in this situation must be knowledgeable concerning all facets of pharmacological therapeutics including medication names, adverse reactions, appropriate dosage, expected therapeutic response, techniques for administration, and duration of treatment.

STRATEGIES TO LIMIT LIABILITY

Untoward events may occur in the course of caring for critically ill pregnant women and their fetuses. Increasingly, the medical and nursing communities are held accountable, not only by the courts, but by the payers as well, for patient outcomes. Although it is impossible to eliminate all sources of liability exposure, there are specific strategies that organizations can use to limit risk. These include the development of standards of care, collaboration among providers to establish standing orders, measures to ensure the availability of adequate and appropriately educated staff, and consultation among providers.

Standards of Care

The Joint Commission for the Accreditation of Healthcare Organizations (JCAHO) mandates that critical care units must meet specific program requirements that outline the delivery of quality care (JCAHO, 1992). Standards for nursing practice were first developed by the American Nurses Association (ANA) in order to establish a minimum level of care that each patient should receive (ANA, 1975). Specialty areas of nursing, such as those represented by AACN and NAACOG, followed the lead of ANA with the development of practice standards outlining the

important aspects of care for the major patient populations within each specialty (Alspach, Bell, Canobbio, et al., 1986; AWHONN, 1993).

AACN established standards of nursing practice for the care of critically ill patients in 1989 (Sanford & Disch, 1989) and identified three specific types of standards. The first type, structure standards, provides information regarding the environment in which care is delivered and the educational requirements of care providers. The second type, process standards, addresses the recommended interventions performed in the delivery of patient care. The nursing process provides the foundation for these standards and includes patient assessment, the development of a plan of care, implementation of the plan, and evaluation of the patient's response to interventions with appropriate revisions to the plan of care. The third type of standard, outcome standards, represents the anticipated result of care delivery.

Multidisciplinary collaboration is essential for the successful treatment of seriously ill pregnant women and ideally should be reflected in practice guidelines that address both medical and nursing management. If this level of cooperation is not available in your facility, specific nursing standards or guidelines need to address all facets of the nursing process including assessment, intervention (independent, interdependent, and dependent), and documentation. Standards of care must reflect current literature, allowing the nurse to use research-based practice. Because critical care obstetric nursing is a new subspecialty, specific nursing research dealing with this population is limited. Practice standards outlined by AWHONN and AACN apply to critically ill pregnant and postpartum patients. Liability surrounding failure to assess, intervene, and document may be limited by utilization of comprehensive, research-based practice guidelines. Nurses caring for these patients must be cognizant of applicable critical care and perinatal standards. If this level of practice is not available within a single provider, collaboration between specialty nurses is essential.

Standing Orders

Standing orders operationalize practice guidelines. It is expected that critical care nurses will collect data and make diagnoses. It may also be necessary that they use independent judgment and treat life-threatening situations even in the absence of a physician. The identification of appropriate standing orders ideally reflects collaboration between physicians and nurses, taking into consideration the organization's practice environment, the expertise of the nursing staff, and availability and proximity of physicians and anesthesia personnel.

Organizational Support for Staffing and Staff Development

Caring for critically ill pregnant women requires the availability of skilled nurses 24 hours a day, 7 days a week. According to the AACN standards, members of the professional nursing staff must have a current license to practice, demonstrate competency in essential skills, have a patient-centered philosophy, and possess the ability to problem solve as well as the ability to practice within established guidelines (Sanford & Disch, 1989). Organizational support must be expressed through the adherence to acceptable staffing ratios. Care providers often express fear of liability resulting from inadequate numbers of staff.

In the case of *Leavitt v. St. Tammany Parrish Hospital* (1981) the hospital was found negligent for failing to provide adequate staffing to meet a patient's needs. In this case, the plaintiff, a 57-year-old woman suffering from congestive heart failure and diabetes, notified the nurses station by using her call light that she needed assistance to ambulate to the bathroom. Because the patient was experiencing weakness and impaired thought processes from her medication, the nursing staff had previously instructed the patient to request assistance prior to getting out of bed. After making her request, Ms. Leavitt waited for 15 minutes and when she received no response walked to the bathroom unassisted and fell. The court found in favor of the plaintiff, stating that the hospital breached its duty to the patient by inadequate staffing. Staffing ratios need to reflect patient acuity and staff competency. A critically ill pregnant woman may need the skills of several nurses during the acute phase of her treatment. If, in the judgment of the nurse, safe staffing ratios are not being maintained, that nurse is responsible for notifying supervisors of the situation. Staffing problems should never be recorded in the medical record, but are more appropriately dealt with via the use of incident reports.

Organizational support is also important in terms of staff development and continuing education. When creating a dedicated critical care obstetric (CCOB) program, careful attention should be paid to the identification of competencies necessary to create a safe practice environment. The theoretical basis for this enhanced level of practice should be presented in a consistent and organized fashion and should be accompanied by the opportunity for clinical practice in a supervised setting. Preceptor arrangements work well in accomplishing this goal.

Consultation

If a dedicated CCOB program is not available in your hospital or organization, consultation among nurses and other providers caring for the patient is essential. The philosophy of critical care obstetrics maintains that there is a baseline level of care to which critically ill pregnant women are entitled. In most hospitals this level of practice will be met collaboratively between a perinatal nurse and a critical care nurse. This collaboration needs to be evident in the plan of care and should represent the best practice of these specialists. It may also be necessary to consult with additional nurses, such as psychiatric or dialysis specialists, if particular problems arise.

Maternal Stabilization and Transport

Caring for critically ill obstetric patients often requires maternal transport to either an intensive care environment or a tertiary care facility in order to provide comprehensive maternal or neonatal care. Transporting critically ill pregnant patients should be a thoughtful, proactive system to prevent patient injury. Prior to transport, maneuvers to stabilize the mother and fetus should be accomplished.

Maternal transport to perinatal centers began in the 1970s. The two types of transport systems described in the literature are one-way and two-way. One-way transport requires staff from the referring hospital to escort the patient during transport to the perinatal center. The transporting nurse and physician assume responsibility for the mother and fetus until arrival at the perinatal center. Two-way transport requires the perinatal center staff to travel to the referring hospital, assuming responsibility for the patient and providing care during transport.

CONCLUSION

As critical care obstetric nursing continues to develop as a specialty, nurses practicing in this area must implement standards of practice integrating both critical care and obstetric skills. Critical care obstetric nurses face numerous areas of potential liability, but can take steps to decrease their risk. The most important risk management strategies are education and collaboration, which prepare the nurse to deal with the complex needs of the critically ill obstetric patient.

REFERENCES

Alspach, J. F., Bell, J., Canobbio, M., et al. (1986). AACN education standards for critical care nursing. St. Louis, MO: C.V. Mosby.

American College of Obstetrics and Gynecology/Nurses' Association of the American College of Obstetrics and Gynecology. (1986, March). Joint statement on fetal monitoring. ACOG Newsletter.

American College of Obstetrics and Gynecology. (1988). Hemodynamic monitoring in obstetrics and gynecology. ACOG Technical Bulletin, No. 121.

American Nurses Association. (1975). A plan for implementing of the standards of nursing practice (pp. 11–17). Kansas City, MO: ANA.

Association of Women's Health, Obstetric, and Neonatal Nurses. (1991). NAACOG: Standards for obstetric, gynecology, and neonatal nursing (4th ed.). Washington, DC: AWHONN.

Association of Women's Health, Obstetric, and Neonatal Nurses. (1993). Didactic content and clinical skills verification for professional nurse providers of basic, high–risk and critical care intrapartum nursing. Washington, DC: AWHONN.

Food and Drug Administration. (1991). Potential hazards with protective restraint devices. FDA Medical Alert (pp. 91–93). Rockville, MD: FDA.

Harvard Medical School. (1968). Ad hoc committee of the Harvard Medical School to examine the definition of brain death: A definition of irreversible coma. Journal of the American Medical Association, 205, 337.

Health Care Financing Administration. (1992). State operations manual. Baltimore, MD: United States Department of Health and Human Services.

Joint Commission on Accreditation of Healthcare Organizations. (1992). Accreditation manual for hospitals. Oakbrook Terrace, IL: JCAHO.

Mabie, W. C., & Sibai, B. M. (1990). Treatment in an obstetric intensive care unit. American Journal of Obstetrics and Gynecology, 162(1).

Nurses' Association of the American College of Obstetrics and Gynecology. (1990, March). Fetal heart rate auscultation. OGN Nursing Practice Resource.

Omnibus Budget Reconciliation Act of 1990, P.L. 101-508, Sec. 4206, 4751.

President's Commission for the Study of Ethical Problems in Medicine and Biomedical and Behavioral Research. (1981, July). Defining death (p. 25).

Salatka, M. A. (1992). Professional liability in critical care nursing. Ohio Northern University Law Review, 19, 85–98.

Sanford, S., & Disch, J. (Eds.) (1989). AACN standards for nursing care of the critically ill (2nd ed.). Reston, VA: Reston Publishers.

Stolley, J. M., et al. (1993). Developing a restraint use policy for acute care. Journal of Clinical Ethics, 23 (12), 49–54.

Teno, J. M., et al. (1994). Do formal advance directives affect resuscitation decisions and the use of resources for seriously ill patients? The Journal of Clinical Ethics, 5(1), 23–29.

Zuspan, F. P., & Sachs, L. (1988). The impact of subspecialties on obstetrics and gynecology. American Journal of Obstetrics and Gynecology, 158, 747–753.

CASE CITATIONS

Alvis v. Henderson Obstetrics, 592 N.E.2d 678 (S.C. 1992).

Anderson v. St. Francis-St. George Hospital, 614 N.E.2d 841 (Oh. 1992).

Baptist Medical Center v. Wilson, 618 S.2d 1335 (Ala. 1993).

Brookover v. Mary Hitchcock Memorial Hospital, 893 F.2d 411 (N.H. 1990).

Davenport v. Ephraim McDowell Memorial Hospital, 769 S.W.2d (Ky. 1988).

Dessauer v. Memorial General Hospital, 628 P.2d 337, N.M. Ct. App. (1981).

Dobrzenieck v. University Hospital of Cleveland, No. 17, 843 Cyahoga City. Court of Common Pleas (May 1984).

Fairfax Hospital System, Inc. v. McCarty, 419 S.E.2d 621 (Va. 1992).

Foflygen v. R. Zemel, M.D., 615 A.2d 1345 (Pa. 1992).

Henry v. Felici, 758 S.W.2d 836 (Tex. 1988).

Ketchum v. Overlake Hospital Medical Center, 804 P.2d 1283 (Wash. 1991).

Leavitt v. St. Tammany Parish Hospital, 396 S.2d 406 (La. 1981).

Mather v. Griffin Hospital, 540 A.2d 666 (Conn. 1988).

Wheeler v. Yettie Kersting Memorial Hospital, 866 S.W.2d 32 (Tex. 1993).

CHAPTER 8

Assessment of the Patient in Labor

Susan Drummond

The intrapartum period begins with the onset of labor, is characterized by uterine contractions and progressive cervical dilation, and ends with the delivery of the placenta and membranes (Nurses' Association of the American College of Obstetricians and Gynecologists, 1991). This time may be marked with a variety of occurrences resulting in increased risk status for mother and/or fetus. The nurse traditionally monitors the two patients on a minute-by-minute basis throughout the intrapartum period. It is important for the nurse to understand this encompassing role and how to protect oneself from legal action. This chapter discusses the roles and responsibilities of the intrapartum nurse, addresses areas of potential legal liability, and discusses strategies to decrease liability.

ROLE OF THE INTRAPARTUM NURSE

The American Nurses Association (ANA) has defined the practice of nursing as the "diagnosis and treatment of human responses to actual or potential health problems" (American Nurses Association, 1980). The Nurses' Organization for Obstetric, Gynecologic and Neonatal Nurses (NAACOG) further describes intrapartum nursing as directed toward providing quality nursing care through the use of the nursing process;

facilitating an emotionally and socially satisfying experience for the patient and family; promoting a physically safe birth experience for the mother, fetus, and family; and collaborating with health care team members in the delivery of quality patient care (NAACOG, 1988a).

Providing quality care within a holistic framework is the very foundation of nursing. In the 1990s the challenge is to provide the highest quality care within a budget-constrained setting. Nurses need a strong educational base to provide theoretical knowledge and clinical expertise and develop interpersonal and communication skills (Wiltse, 1992). They must be able to adapt to rapidly changing environments and stressors to maintain quality and may be faced with accepting a variety of responsibilities in the intrapartum setting.

Triage Responsibilities

A role emerging across the nation is that of the triage nurse in an obstetric setting. Patients presenting to a labor and delivery unit may first be assessed by a triage nurse. Nursing triage skills are needed in the labor and delivery unit to obtain an accurate history, decrease patient waiting time, prioritize patient needs, and assign risk status (Angelini, Zannieri, Silva, Fein, & Wand, 1990). One study demonstrated that triage nurses had a positive impact on clinical services by minimizing congestion in waiting areas, avoiding duplication of services, and decreasing patient waiting time (Zwicke, Bobzien, & Wagner, 1982).

The role of triage nurse has been utilized in Emergency Departments for some time, but is still a relatively new concept for many labor and delivery units. However, as numbers of nursing staff decrease in some units due to budget constraints and as patient acuity levels increase, the need exists for nursing triage skills. The nursing functions could include evaluating patient acuity, prioritizing the order in which patients are seen, evaluating patients for labor, placing them in labor rooms, assigning a primary nurse, and initiating electronic fetal heart rate monitoring. This concept also could include an expanded role for an advanced practice nurse. The advanced practice nurse could perform sterile speculum exams to rule out rupture of membranes and perform nonstress tests and contraction stress tests in addition to the previously mentioned functions.

Admission Assessment

Once admitted, the patient should be assessed by a qualified professional nurse (Nurses' Association of the American College of Obstetricians and Gynecologists, 1991). The prenatal record, if available, should be carefully reviewed. Display 8-1 lists information that should be obtained either from the prenatal record or through patient interview.

The nurse may perform a physical examination. Appropriate areas of assessment are listed in Display 8-2. The nurse should also assess the patient's labor progress through cervical exam and status of the amniotic membranes. This may be accomplished by sterile speculum exam, utilizing the nitrazine, fern, and pool assessment criteria. Careful interview history may provide the necessary information regarding membrane status.

Obstetrics has the unique distinction and responsibility of providing care to two patients in one (Nurses' Association of the American College of Obstetricians and Gynecologists, 1991). The admitting nurse must also assess fetal status. For the intrapartum patient, this assessment may include fundal height assessment;

abdominal palpation for position, presentation, and fetal size; and fetal heart rate assessment by fetoscope, Doppler, or electronic fetal monitor (Nurses' Association of the American College of Obstetricians and Gynecologists, 1991).

Other responsibilities during initial assessment include risk identification; assessing the patient's support system, sociocultural, and economic needs; and documentation and communication of findings. The nurse then uses the assessment data to develop a plan of care and initiates the plan in accordance with written hospital policies and protocols.

In *Dent v. Perkins* (1993), a nurse failed to adequately assess the patient's condition and appropriately notify the physician. The patient's physician had just gone off-call and failed to inform the obstetric nursing staff that another physician was covering. The patient arrived at the hospital in labor and was examined by an obstetrical nurse. The patient was admitted to a nonobstetrical unit as no rooms were available in the labor and delivery area. The patient ultimately delivered approximately 4 1/2 hours later in that room, assisted only by an obstetrical nurse. The birth was complicated by a fetal face presentation. Further, the nurse's notes indicated that the child was trapped in the birth canal for 15 minutes. The record also stated that no physician was called until after the child was born. The child expired two days later.

A physician expert testified that if the patient was admitted to the labor and delivery unit where a physician was present, the infant would have survived. A nursing expert testified that the nurse did not assess the patient's condition adequately or notify the physician appropriately. The court found that combined physician and nursing negligence caused the infant's demise.

As the health care environment changes, so must staffing patterns. Economic constraints have caused many units to employ nonlicensed personnel to work with licensed nurses in providing care. Certainly specific functions exist that nonlicensed personnel can perform adequately. These may include vital sign assessment, initiating electronic fetal monitoring, meeting comfort and hygiene needs of the

DISPLAY 8-1

Admission Assessment: Information to Be Obtained by Nurse

Reason for admission as stated by patient and events leading up to hospitalization

Date of last normal menstrual period, frequency of periods, and results of early pelvic examination findings (to estimate the date of delivery)

Obstetric history, starting with the first pregnancy and including all pregnancies up to the current pregnancy

Past medical illnesses and/or surgeries

Family history, including
- Genetic and congenital abnormalities
- Mental retardation
- Metabolic problems
- Multiple births

Menstrual and sexual concerns related to conception

A systems review

Past or present systemic and genital infections, including sexually transmitted diseases

Exposure to viruses

Bleeding problems

Persistent nausea and vomiting

Allergies or drug sensitivities

Gynecologic anomalies, including
- Uterine anomalies
- Fibroids
- Exposure to diethylstilbestrol

Exposure to hazardous agents

Substance abuse history, including past or present use of
- Alcohol
- Caffeine
- Tobacco
- Drugs, including prescription, over-the-counter, and illicit drugs

Dietary habits before and during pregnancy

Significant weight changes

Prepregnancy weight

Exercise pattern

Elimination patterns

Sleep patterns

Any significant stress

Relationships with significant others, including the potential for abusive relationships

Socioeconomic, cultural, and environmental factors

Source: NAACOG. (1991). *Standards for obstetric, gynecologic and neonatal nursing* (4th ed.). Washington, DC: NAACOG.

DISPLAY 8-2

Admission Assessment: Physical Examination

Review of prenatal history

Review of diagnostic testing, blood work, procedures, and biophysical monitoring

Evaluation of the condition for which the patient is hospitalized

Measurements of height and weight

Vital signs

Abdominal palpation for estimated fetal size, position and presentation, and determination of fundal height

Pelvic exam, as indicated

Comprehensive physical assessment of body systems

Source: NAACOG. (1991). <u>Standards for obstetric, gynecologic and neonatal nursing</u> (4th ed.). Washington, DC: NAACOG.

patient, and other functions. It is important that staff in these two roles work as a team, as it is the ultimate responsibility of the professional nurse to assimilate the information, develop the plan of care, and respond to any changes in maternal or fetal status.

STAGES OF LABOR

Labor is divided into four stages, (1) cervical dilation, effacement, and downward movement of the fetus; (2) birth; (3) expulsion of the placenta; and (4) the immediate postpartum time.

First Stage of Labor

The first stage of labor begins with the onset of regular contractions and ends with complete cervical dilation (10 cm). This stage is comprised of two phases: the latent phase and the active phase. The latent phase begins with regular uterine contractions and ends when the cervix is dilated 3–4 cm. Typically this is the longer phase of the two. The contractions during this phase are milder, and the woman may prefer ambulating throughout or even remaining at home. The length of the latent phase varies greatly among women; however, a prolonged latent phase is defined as one exceeding 20 hours in the nullipara and 14 hours in the multipara (Friedman, 1978).

The active phase of the first stage of labor begins at approximately 4-cm dilation and ends when the cervix is completely dilated. This phase is characterized by stronger, more frequent contractions and more rapid cervical change. An "adequate labor" describes a wide range of uterine activities; the amplitude of each contraction varies from 25 to 75 mm Hg, and contractions occur over a total of 2–4.5 minutes in every 10-minute window, achieving from 95 to 395 Montevideo units. The time between 8 and 10 cm is also called the transition phase. The patient typically experiences increased pain and the urge to bear down during contractions. Dependent upon the size and type of institution in which one works, the nurse may be asked to perform many interventions independent of the physician or nurse-midwife. Standards upon which the nurse may base care during the first stage of labor have been developed and are listed in Display 8-3.

Fetal monitoring and uterine activity assessment should be performed throughout the active phase of labor. Timing of assessment is

DISPLAY 8-3

Accepted Standards of Nursing Care During First Stage of Labor

Assess maternal physical and psychological responses and plan nursing care from data obtained

Explain nursing interventions and their rationale to the patient and her support persons

Monitor fetal heart rate and its characteristics at specified intervals by the selected methods and document findings using appropriate terminology

Perform vaginal examinations to evaluate effacement and dilation of the cervix, station of the presenting part, and fetal presentation and position

Assess and record status and progress of labor

Monitor uterine activity patterns using palpation and/or the electronic fetal monitor

Assess and record color, amount, and odor of amniotic fluid at spontaneous rupture of membranes

Confirm rupture of membranes with nitrazine or fern test

Assist with artificial rupture of membranes and record the color, amount, and odor of amniotic fluid

Perform and document maternal surveillance per hospital protocol, including measures of

    Blood pressure

    Temperature

    Pulse

    Respirations

Obtain cultures, if indicated

Assess for signs of infection and dehydration

Initiate fluid replacement therapy, including blood and blood products

Differentiate between normal and abnormal rate of cervical effacement and dilation, and descent of the presenting part

Apply direct fetal electrode and/or intrauterine pressure catheter in accordance with nurse practice acts, institutional policy, and medical orders

Recognize normal and abnormal fetal heart rates or nonreassuring characteristics and promptly initiate appropriate nursing interventions

Recognize normal and abnormal uterine activity and intervene accordingly

Perform ultrasound examinations in accordance with institutional policy, competency validation, and nurse practice acts

Monitor mother and fetus for desired and deleterious effects of administered medications

Promote family involvement in the birth process to the extent desired by the patient and within the guidelines of the health care facility

Provide care and comfort measures for the laboring patient

Position the mother to promote uteroplacental perfusion

Assist with anesthesia procedures and monitor mother and fetus for the desired and undesired response to obstetric analgesia and anesthesia during labor

Prepare patient for general anesthesia (if indicated)

Communicate information to the primary health care provider as indicated

Document all care according to hospital guidelines

Source: NAACOG. (1991). <u>Standards for obstetric, gynecologic and neonatal nursing</u> (4th ed.). Washington, DC.

based on assignment of risk status. Table 8-1 illustrates the frequency of fetal monitoring and uterine assessment that meets the minimal standards of care.

Second Stage of Labor

The second stage of labor begins with complete cervical dilation and ends with the birth of the infant. This stage is usually brief, normally averaging only 20 minutes for parous women and 50 minutes for nulliparous women. A prolonged second stage is defined as one that exceeds 2 hours. However, adequate pushing is usually demonstrated by descent and expulsion of the fetus, rather than the actual time involved. Uterine contractions combined with intra-abdominal pressure from the patient's bearing down effort result in descent of the presenting part of the infant. Effective bearing-down efforts will result in steady descent of the fetal head, and then distention and bulging of the perineum. With each contraction a larger portion of the presenting part is visualized at the introitus. This is referred to as crowning. The nurse should observe the head advancing with bearing-down efforts. Although the head retreats slightly between contractions, it should make steady noticeable progress toward the perineum. The nurse should help the patient into a comfortable position, usually semi-sitting with legs flexed or a squatting or kneeling position. Following the birth of the head is a sudden sense of relief, and generally the shoulders and the rest of the body are delivered quite rapidly.

The intrapartum nurse provides one-to-one care for the labor patient at this time, and has much responsibility for managing the patient's pushing efforts, assessing maternal and fetal physiologic well-being, and providing emotional support for the patient and family. The nurse should be in constant attendance at this time. Appropriate nursing care during the second stage of labor is described in Display 8-4.

Third Stage of Labor

The third stage of labor begins with birth of the infant and ends with delivery of the placenta. Following delivery of the infant, the walls of the uterus contract, which decreases uterine size, resulting in a decreased area for placental attachment. The placenta is forced to accommodate to the decreased surface area by separating from the uterine wall. Following separation, expulsion is generally accomplished by gravity and maternal pushing efforts.

Nursing responsibilities in the third stage of labor include ongoing assessment of maternal and neonatal status, implementation of nursing interventions, completion of delivery records, and encouraging early parent–infant contact. Maternal physiologic status during this stage is determined primarily through monitoring vital signs, the process of placental separation and delivery, and blood loss. If uterine bleeding is excessive, an elevated pulse rate may be the first sign, followed by hypotension.

The nurse is generally responsible for the initial assessment of the normal newborn, which begins with the Apgar score. Apgar scores are officially assigned at 1 and 5 minutes after birth and reflect the newborn's adaptation to extrauterine life. The scoring system assesses heart rate, respiratory effort, muscle tone, reflex irritability, and color. Each category is assigned a value from

TABLE 8-1. Frequency of Monitoring Necessary to Meet Minimal Standards of Care		
	Low-Risk	High-Risk
First stage labor-active phase	q 30 min	q 15 min
Second stage labor	q 15 min	q 5 min

Source: NAACOG. (1991). *Standards for obstetric, gynecologic and neonatal nursing* (4th ed.). Washington, DC: NAACOG.

0 to 2, with 10 being the highest total score. If the infant remains with the parents for a period of time after birth, the nurse will observe frequently for abnormal skin color or respiratory difficulty and will promote thermoregulation.

The nurse also observes the parents' first response to their new infant. If the infant is immediately placed on the mother's abdomen after delivery, the nurse can encourage the parents in their early contact with the newborn and observe their reactions. This is usually a time of excitement, wonderment, and pleasure, but occasionally the nurse may observe ambivalent or negative feelings. Although this stage is quite short, the nurse can verbalize any concerns regarding parental–infant bonding to caregivers in the nursery or postpartum unit.

Fourth Stage of Labor

The fourth stage of labor encompasses the first 4 hours postpartum. During this stage the uterus should be firm and the fundus should be palpable at or below the umbilicus. The first hour especially is a time when the patient is at increased risk for bleeding complications (Wheeler, 1991). Immediate postpartum hemorrhage is the result of uterine atony in most instances. Factors that increase risk for uterine

atony in the immediate postpartum period include a precipitous labor, uterine overdistension, prolonged labor, grand multiparity, oxytocin induction or augmentation, and large-for-gestational-age infants (Creasy & Resnick, 1984).

Fundal massage is used to avoid excessive blood loss and is often initiated by the nurse. Massage stimulates the myometrium to contract and promotes hemostasis. The nurse places one hand facing the patient's head with the thumb resting on one side of the uterus and the fingers along the opposite side; the other hand massages the uterus (Zwicke, Bobzien, & Wagner, 1982). Only the amount of force needed to stimulate uterine contractions is used. Excessive aggressive massage may result in uterine prolapse. In less emergent cases, the patient can be instructed to participate in fundal massage.

When uterine atony does not respond to fundal massage, other interventions are indicated. Intravenous fluids should be started or continued to prevent hypotension. Medications used to combat uterine atony include synthetic oxytocin, ergonovine maleate, and prostaglandins (Zwicke, Bobzien, & Wagner, 1982). All result in rhythmic uterine contractions.

The nurse must also monitor the patient's bladder during this time. A full bladder prevents

DISPLAY 8-4

Nursing Responsibilities During Second Stage of Labor

Assess and record the fetal heart rate and its characteristics per hospital protocol

Assess and record maternal vital signs as appropriate

Assist with positioning to optimize uteroplacental blood flow, promote comfort, and promote fetal descent

Assist with pushing efforts

Mobilize resources for neonatal resuscitation and stabilization

Prepare the equipment and the environment for the delivery

Provide support and encouragement

Source: American Nurses Association. (1980). <u>Nursing: A social policy statement.</u> Kansas City, MO: American Nurses Association.

the uterus from contracting effectively, which may contribute to increased blood loss. If the patient does not have sensation to notice a full bladder, the nurse can empty the bladder with a catheter.

Occasionally, bleeding continues despite all efforts at control and may become life-threatening. The patient may then require surgical intervention such as dilation and curettage (D & C) or possibly hysterectomy.

Nursing assessment includes vital signs, palpation of the uterine fundus, and observation of bleeding. Typically this assessment is done every 15 minutes during the first hour following delivery.

ONGOING ASSESSMENT

The nurse is responsible for ongoing assessment of the mother and fetus throughout the stages of labor. Maternal physiologic status, labor progress, and fetal well-being should be continuously monitored. Also, maternal comfort level and any educational needs of the patient or family should be assessed. The patient who is admitted in labor and classified as "low-risk" may not maintain that status throughout the labor and delivery process. The nurse must assess regularly according to established standards and change the plan of care in order to meet the needs of the patient.

Fetal monitoring may be accomplished by auscultation with a Doppler or by continuous electronic fetal monitoring in accordance with hospital policy and regardless of risk status. It has been demonstrated that with a 1:1 nurse/patient ratio, intermittent auscultation at intervals of 15 minutes during the active phase of the first stage of labor and 5 minutes during the second stage is equivalent to continuous electronic fetal heart rate monitoring (American Association of Pediatricians & American College of Obstetricians and Gynecologists, 1992). More specific information regarding fetal heart rate monitoring is included in Chapter 9.

Uterine assessment should include frequency, duration, and quality of contractions and uterine resting tone. The assessment may be accomplished simply by palpation. The tocody-

namometer on the electronic fetal monitor or an intrauterine pressure catheter may also be utilized. Uterine assessment is performed and documented at the same intervals as the fetal heart rate.

Uterine contractions that result in "adequate labor" have been described. The intrapartum nurse should be alert to abnormal patterns. Contractions that are constant (with intervals of less than 30 seconds between contractions) or prolonged (lasting more than 90 seconds) require further evaluation. Strong constant uterine contractions may result in uterine rupture. Vasoconstriction occurs during the contractions due to the pressure of the surrounding tissue resulting in a decreased oxygen exchange with the fetus. The interval between contractions allows the flow of oxygenated blood to the fetus to resume. If the intervals between contractions are short, the fetus is at risk for anoxia. Thus regular assessment of uterine resting tone is very important.

Regularly used standards manuals for OBGYN services do not identify specific intervals for vital signs assessment for the laboring patient; they only state that they should be done "regularly . . . and according to hospital policy" (Friedman, 1978; Nurses' Association of the American College of Obstetricians and Gynecologists, 1991). Hospitals should develop protocols that adequately assess the status of their patient population and are reasonable for the nursing staff to perform.

One example protocol states that the nurse should (1) assess pulse, respirations, and blood pressure every 30–60 minutes depending on phase and stage of labor and possible presence of risk factors; and (2) assess temperature every 4 hours if membranes are intact, or every 2 hours if membranes are ruptured. For the patient with significant risk factors or one who is unstable, vital sign assessment may be as frequent as every 5 minutes.

Although a comprehensive list of all conditions that would elevate a patient to a "high-risk" status does not exist, a variety of conditions are found in published texts that label a pregnancy as "high-risk." These include but are not limited to preterm labor, preterm rupture of membranes, pregnancy-induced hypertension, insulin-dependent diabetes, other preexisting medical conditions, placenta previa, substance abuse, and psychosocial problems. It is important to remember that assignment of risk status is an ongoing dynamic process. The patient who is admitted in labor at 40 weeks gestation without identifiable risk factors from the prenatal record might still develop complications. For example, she may have a precipitous delivery and a postpartum hemorrhage requiring fluid and blood products resuscitation. At this point the patient's risk status would be elevated, requiring a change in the nursing plan of care. Her condition might warrant an increase in the nurse/patient ratio, requiring an alteration in the staffing pattern. The frequency of vital sign assessment would increase, and the use of other monitoring equipment, such as a pulse oximeter, may be indicated.

It is important for the nurse at the bedside to be alert to changes in risk status and use nursing judgment to determine whether increased assessment and intervention are necessary, as these actions may not be specifically set forth in a hospital protocol.

Nursing units should develop protocols that encompass current standards in accordance with general hospital policy and particular nurse practice acts that vary among the states. Nurses who perform functions that are outside or in addition to the general guidelines of national standards, hospital policy, and state nurse practice acts should realize that they increase their liability risk. A nurse who accepts responsibility for additional practice needs clearly written policies and procedures to govern that practice (Nurses Association of the American College of Obstetricians and Gynecologists, 1988b).

SITUATIONS OF RISK

Uterine Rupture

Although rare, uterine rupture is associated with high rates of maternal and fetal morbidity and mortality. Women at risk for uterine rupture include those with a previous uterine incision, high parity, uterine hyperstimulation, uterine overdistention, and pathologic retraction bands.

Women with an obvious uterine rupture describe severe abdominal pain, possibly with a sensation of tearing, followed by a cessation of uterine contractions. Vaginal bleeding is also noted. The fetal heart rate pattern frequently demonstrates a pattern consistent with acute distress. On vaginal examination, the fetus is ballotable, and the fetus may be palpable outside the uterus. The treatment is immediate cesarean delivery and possible transfusion of several units of packed red blood cells.

Nursing management includes a thorough history of the patient's description of abdominal pain, uterine contraction activity, amount of vaginal bleeding, and presence or absence of fetal movement. Immediate assessment includes vital signs, current amount and type of vaginal bleeding, and fetal monitoring. Intravenous access should be obtained.

The nurse is also responsible for accurate ongoing assessment, including monitoring the mother and fetus for any change in condition and implementing an appropriate plan of care.

Failure of a nurse to properly assess and intervene in the presence of uterine rupture is illustrated in the case of *Baptist Medical Center Montclair v. Wilson* (1993). The patient, a VBAC candidate, was admitted to the labor and delivery unit in early labor. Hours later, the patient experienced a sharp pain in her abdomen. Within moments, the patient and her husband noticed vaginal bleeding. The patient told the nurse that she felt as though her stomach had ripped open and the baby had moved up toward the ceiling. Approximately 20 minutes later, the nurse performed a cervical exam and determined that the patient's cervix was completely dilated. The fetal heart rate had dropped to 60 beats per minute. The nurse then notified the physician of her assessment, but did not report that the patient had experienced the sharp abdominal pain, "as though her stomach had ripped open." Fifteen minutes later, the physician examined the patient, and found that she was not dilated. An emergency cesarean delivery followed. The delivery occurred almost one hour following the patient's first reports of sharp abdominal pain. The patient had suffered a uterine rupture. Fetal distress resulted as the baby was pushed into the abdominal cavity causing placental abruption. The infant died at 5 months of age, as a result of brain damage sustained at birth.

Several deviations from the standard of care were noted. The standard of care required the nurse to notify a physician of anything that deviated from the regular course of labor such as the complaint of sharp abdominal pain and a sensation of abdominal tearing. The standard of care also required a proper, accurate nursing assessment. The nurse assessed the patient as being completely dilated when the cervix was not dilated at all. This improper assessment caused the physician to manage the patient differently. Finally, the standard of care required the nurse to start oxygen as soon as the fetal heart rate dropped. However, oxygen was not started until about 15 minutes following the drop in fetal heart rate.

Fundal Versus Suprapubic Pressure

A nurse may be called upon to provide fundal or suprapubic pressure during the second stage of labor. Obstetricians and nurses frequently do not agree on the need or technique used when the request for fundal pressure is made. The situation may be urgent; therefore, nurses need to be clearly aware of their role and the potential liability they incur.

Fundal pressure is the application of gentle steady pressure on the fundus of the uterus. Suprapubic pressure is steady pressure on the suprapubic area of the body to direct the anterior shoulder of the infant posteriorly behind the pubic bone and under the symphysis (Kline-Kaye & Miller-Slade, 1990; Penney & Perlis, 1992).

One of the most common indications for the use of some type of extrauterine pressure is shoulder dystocia. This condition is diagnosed when, after delivery of the fetal head, further progress toward delivery of the infant is prevented by impaction of the fetal shoulders within the maternal pelvis, requiring specific efforts to relieve the obstruction and allow delivery (Seeds, 1989). Shoulder dystocia is associated with several clinical conditions: multiparity, macrosomia (infant larger than 4,000 grams), prolonged second stage, and previous delivery of a fetus larger than 4,000 grams (Bowes, 1994).

Many uncertainties exist regarding the use of fundal pressure. Most obstetric nurses do not receive clinical instruction in this area of practice. The amount of force to apply is not clearly described. Some have expressed the effort required as "firm but not too forceful" or "moderate pressure" (Resnick, 1980). These terms are too vague to provide clinically useful information leaving the one applying the pressure to gauge the appropriate amount of force. When a clear distinction between suprapubic pressure and fundal pressure is made, the literature generally favors the use of suprapubic pressure to disimpact the anterior shoulder (Nurses' Association of the American College of Obstetricians and Gynecologists, 1988b).

Using fundal pressure may only impact the anterior shoulder against the symphysis pubis. Other undesirable or adverse fetal and maternal consequences may also result from the use of fundal pressure. One study of 24 cases of shoulder dystocia showed that fundal pressure in the absence of other maneuvers resulted in a 77% complication rate, particularly neonatal orthopedic and neurologic damage (Gross, Shime, & Farine, 1987). These findings are a logical result of fundal pressure, which increases the risk of injury to the brachial plexus (Seeds, 1986). However, the actual contribution of fundal pressure to fetal injury is unclear.

Reports of uterine rupture have been proposed in relation to severe fundal pressure. However, using isolated reports to attribute uterine rupture to only one factor may be inappropriate, as a combination of factors (such as parity, fetal size, and previous uterine surgery) could all contribute to uterine rupture (Nurses' Association of the American College of Obstetricians and Gynecologists, 1988b).

The intrapartum nurse is responsible for providing quality care that is in accordance with standards of practice. National standards giving specific guidelines for nursing practice regarding fundal pressure during the second stage of labor do not exist. A nurse with limited clinical experience may be asked to act in an urgent situation and may feel unprepared. Some obstetric units may choose to develop a protocol to provide the nurse with guidelines regarding application of fundal pressure. However, because much confusion still exists with the issue of application of fundal pressure, many hospitals have no written protocol or guideline for nursing practice in this area.

Umbilical Cord Prolapse

Umbilical cord prolapse (UCP) is an obstetric emergency and is defined as the protrusion of the umbilical cord alongside (occult) or ahead of the presenting part of the fetus (Buckley, 1990). UCP may be diagnosed when the cord can be visualized externally or palpated in the vagina or alongside the presenting part by the intrapartum nurse, nurse-midwife or physician (Griese & Pickett, 1993). The appearance of severe variable decelerations or bradycardia in the fetal heart rate tracing that do not respond to maternal position change, oxygen therapy, or intravenous hydration should alert the nurse to the possibility of cord prolapse (Levy, Meier, & Makowski, 1984).

UCP is more likely to occur in situations where the fetal presenting part does not fully descend into or occupy the pelvis. Traditionally included in this risk category are fetal malpresentation, cephalopelvic disproportion, multiple gestation, grand multiparity, abnormal placentation, hydramnios, and prematurity. One study (Critchlow, Leet, Benedetti, & Daling, 1994) identified prematurity, breech presentation, and being a second-born twin as risk factors for cord prolapse. Another study found that obstetric interventions such as amniotomy, cervical ripening labor induction and amnioinfusion did not increase the risk for UCP (Roberts, W. E., Martin, R. N., Roach, H. H., Perry, K. G. Jr., Martin, J. N. Jr., Morrison, J. C., 1997).

On admission, nurses should identify patients at risk for developing cord prolapse. Through careful assessment, health care providers may be able to predict those at high risk for UCP and possibly avoid it. Although not all cases are predictable, the nurse can recognize interventions that place the patient at unnecessary risk for UCP (Gross, Shime, & Farine, 1987).

In *Province v. Center for Women's Health and Family Birth* (1993), a nurse was found negligent for failing to properly assess and intervene in a birth involving umbilical cord prolapse. The patient notified the nurse that she felt something "like a heartbeat in my vagina," and that it was "pulsating." The patient also asked the nurse to call her doctor, but the nurse did not because she felt the complaint was insignificant.

The patient was later permitted to ambulate to the restroom where she noticed the umbilical cord protruding. An emergency cesarean delivery was performed, but the infant suffered severe brain damage.

Nursing management of UCP traditionally included placing the patient in Trendelenburg or knee–chest position, manually elevating the fetal presenting part to relieve compression on the cord, administering oxygen, notifying the physician, and preparing the patient and family for probable cesarean section delivery.

An alternative management plan when delivery is not imminent involves bladder filling. Katz, Lancet, Blichstein, Mogilner, and Zalel (1988) describe one such plan, which included rapidly infusing 500–700 ml of sterile 0.9% saline into the bladder via Foley catheter and concomitant intravenous infusion of ritodrine hydrochloride. If the cord protruded from the vagina, it was gently returned, and a warm wet gauze tampon was inserted. Fetal heart rate monitoring was continued while preparations were made for a prompt cesarean section delivery.

Although both methods result in cesarean section delivery, the bladder filling method might be especially useful for nurses in rural or outpatient settings who anticipate greater length of time until delivery or potential transport of a patient to another location.

In accordance with state nurse practice acts and hospital policies, nurses can be credentialed to perform a variety of obstetric assessments. For example, nurses could be certified to perform limited ultrasound assessments (AWHONN, 1993). Ultrasound performed by a qualified nurse could ascertain the presence or absence of fetal heart motion in a patient presenting with the absence of cord pulsation or inaudible fetal heart tones (Gross, Shime, & Farine, 1987). Having this information immediately available would aid the health care team in determining the most effective management plan for the mother and infant.

Abruptio Placentae

Abruptio placentae is a premature separation of the normally implanted placenta prior to the delivery of the fetus. The incidence is approximately 1 in 90 pregnancies (Iyasu, Saftlas, Rowley, Koonin, Lawson, & Atrash, 1993) with associated perinatal mortality ranging between 20 and 40% (Karegard & Gennser; 1986; Krohn, Voigt, McKnight, Daling, Starzyk, & Benedetti, 1987; Hurd, Miodovnik, Hertzburg, & Lavin, 1983). For those infants who survive, an increased occurrence of neurologic impairment exists.

The etiology of abruptio placentae is uncertain, but many maternal risk factors are well documented in the literature, including maternal age, cigarette smoking, cocaine use, overdistension of the uterus, abdominal trauma, and hypertension. One study found that teenagers and women 35 years old and older were more likely to develop abruptio placentae than other age groups (AWHONN, 1993). Another found significantly increased risk for placental abruption and fetal distress among third trimester cocaine users (Cohen, Green, & Crumbleholme, 1991). Maternal hypertension seems to be the most consistently identified factor predisposing to placental abruption. It has been demonstrated that 50% of patients with a fetal demise caused by an abruption have hypertension as well (Abdellah, Sibai, Hayes, & Anderson, 1984).

Abruptio placentae is initiated by retroplacental hemorrhage, which occurs in the decidua basalis and originates from degenerative changes in the small arteries of the placenta. This bleeding leads to clot formation, which results in progressive separation of the placenta from the uterus. Decreased placental surface area causes diminished oxygen availability to the fetus.

Placental abruption can be broadly classified into three grades that correlate with clinical and laboratory findings (Benedetti, 1991). Grade 1 is associated with slight vaginal bleeding and some uterine irritability. Maternal physiologic status is stable and the fetal heart rate pattern is normal. In Grade 2 abruption vaginal bleeding is mild to moderate. The uterus is irritable, and tetanic contractions may be present. Maternal pulse rate may be elevated and fibrinogen level generally is below normal. The fetal heart rate pattern typically shows signs of distress. Grade 3 abruption is associated with moderate to severe bleeding, which may be concealed. The uterus is tetanic, rigid, and painful. Maternal hypotension happens frequently, and fetal death may occur. Fibrinogen levels are often reduced to less than 150 mg percent, possibly with other coagulation abnormalities present.

Clinical presentation varies widely and is related to the severity of the abruption. The classic symptoms are abdominal pain, a firm tender uterus, and dark vaginal bleeding. The patient may report sharp, severe pain that persists or becomes dull and achy. However, any or all of these symptoms may be absent. Many cases of abruptio placentae are diagnosed upon examination of the placenta after delivery.

Careful continuous assessment by the intrapartum nurse may help identify a placental abruption. The contraction pattern characteristic of an abruption demonstrates frequent, low-amplitude contractions with elevation of resting tone (Dorman, 1989). In severe cases the uterus may become rigid and be very painful to palpation. Signs of fetal stress or distress are generally evident in the fetal heart rate pattern.

Management is dependent on the degree of abruption, gestational age, and fetal status. Inpatient management with frequent fetal heart rate monitoring, possible tocolysis, and timely use of cesarean delivery are advocated to prolong pregnancy in cases of extreme prematurity, without a resulting increase in perinatal mortality rates (Sholl, 1987). Vaginal delivery is possible in cases where maternal and fetal physiologic states are stable. However, cesarean delivery is indicated in cases of severe bleeding that might place the mother or fetus in jeopardy, fetal distress, or failure to progress rapidly in labor.

Nursing management includes frequent assessment of vital signs, amount of vaginal bleeding, uterine contractions and resting tone, and fetal heart rate monitoring. The patient should be maintained in a lateral position to optimize uteroplacental perfusion and oxygen delivery to the fetus.

Placental abruption is one of the most common causes of disseminated intravascular coagulation

(DIC) due to increased release of thromboplastin into the maternal circulation and a resulting consumption of clotting factors. Intravenous access should be maintained at all times. The patient should be typed and cross-matched for several units of packed red blood cells in the event that bleeding complications occur.

Lambert v. Sisters of Mercy Health Corporation (1985) illustrates the role of the intrapartum nurse in assessing for uterine rupture. The patient's history indicated that her doctor planned a repeat cesarean delivery. The patient had a sudden onset of sharp pain that continued but became milder and dull. She reported the symptoms to her physician, but was told not to worry and to stay home. After several hours of continued pain, the patient went to the hospital. At this time, the fetal heart rate tracing showed no signs of distress. The patient told her nurse that the pain she was experiencing was now moderate and constant. The nurse suspected that the patient might be in labor and notified the physician. The pain continued to increase in intensity and the physician recommended by phone that the patient be given Valium. Some time later the physician arrived, examined the patient, and ordered a cesarean section. The infant suffered severe brain damage and subsequent demise from oxygen deprivation caused by abruptio placentae. The nurse, hospital, and physician were found liable for the injury that occurred.

STRATEGIES TO DECREASE LIABILITY

The role of the intrapartum nurse is very involved, and places the nurse at risk for legal liability in many areas. The health care consumer today demands high quality care. Obstetrics has traditionally been a highly emotionally charged area of practice. Parents expect to take home a perfect baby. When intrapartum events result in a less than optimal outcome, families frequently pursue legal action. The nurse should be armed with all possible defenses to avoid a malpractice suit.

Standards of Care

Familiarity with the standards of care is essential. Standards reflect current knowledge in the field and are always changing as knowledge changes. These standards, which govern practice, protect both the patient and the nurse. They prevent the nurse from providing care that is more appropriately provided by another member of the health care team. Thus, the patient's welfare is safeguarded.

Ignorance of a standard is not a valid defense. Nurses who are new to obstetric nursing are held to the same standard of practice as those with years of clinical experience. Therefore, all intrapartum nurses should know the current standards and apply them to their clinical practice through use of hospital protocols.

Documentation

Documentation of care can decrease liability risk. One of the most important responsibilities of a nurse is providing an accurate account of all events related to the care of the patient (Blackwell, 1993). With decreased nursing staff and resultant increased tasks involved in patient care, documentation may unfortunately become less of a priority than it should be.

The intrapartum nurse must document according to standards of care and must follow the nursing process. Initial history and physical exam of the patient in labor as well as documentation of fetal status should be included in the nurse's notes. Documentation through the stages of labor includes maternal and fetal physiologic status, labor progression, risk status, and the meeting of educational needs. Many institutions prefer using a flow-sheet format to decrease the amount of time spent in long, handwritten notes.

A nurse may not be asked to testify in a malpractice case until several years after the event occurred. If the nurse has documented all aspects of care, carefully recalling the events will be much easier. Documentation is of vital importance in defending oneself against a malpractice claim. This concept will be discussed in greater detail in Chapter 18.

Communication

Communication of information is vital in the health care field. The intrapartum nurse must effectively communicate with the patient and other members of the health care team. The initial nurse–patient interview is a necessary step in establishing open communication. The patient must feel that her words are understood and that her concerns are being heard and dealt with in a timely and sensitive manner (Farrell, 1993).

The nurse must also communicate with other members of the health care team, especially the birth attendant. Communication should be frequent and include information regarding labor progress, maternal and fetal physiologic status, conditions placing the patient at risk, and any emergent situations.

The health care team should work together in reassessing the patient and updating the plan of care. A healthy working relationship between providers generates enthusiasm and intellectual interchange of ideas, thus enhancing the quality of care given. Legal risk is therefore decreased.

SUMMARY

The responsibilities and duties of the nurse working with intrapartum patients are numerous. The nurse is responsible for meeting physiological, emotional, and educational needs as well as being a patient advocate. Nurses come to the obstetric arena from a variety of educational backgrounds; yet they provide the same type of care to similar patients. Professional organizations have provided standards to govern care; however, different institutions apply these standards in different ways when designing protocols. Some hospitals allow more independent nursing practice than others. To decrease the risk of malpractice, the nurse must be careful to accurately assess the patient, follow a developed plan of care, and be alert for sudden changes in maternal or fetal status.

REFERENCES

Abdellah, T. N., Sibai, B. M., Hayes, J. M., Jr., & Anderson, G. D. (1984). Relationship of hypertensive disease to abruptio placentae. Obstetrics and Gynecology 63(3), 365–370.

American Association of Pediatricians and American College of Obstetricians and Gynecologists. (1980). Guidelines for Perinatal Care (3rd ed.). Washington, DC: American Association of Pediatricians and American College of Obstetricians and Gynecologists.

American Nurses Association. (1980). Nursing: A social policy statement. Kansas City, MO: American Nurses Association.

Angelini, D. J., Zannieri, C. L., Silva, V. B., Fein, E., & Wand, P. J. (1990). Toward a concept of triage for labor and delivery: Staff perceptions and role utilization. Journal of Perinatal and Neonatal Nursing, 4, 1.

AWHONN. (1993). Nursing practice competencies and educational guidelines for limited ultrasound examinations in obstetric and gynecologic infertility settings. Washington, DC: AWHONN.

Benedetti, T. J. (1991). Obstetric hemorrhage. In S. G., Gabbe, J. R. Niebyl, & J. L. Simpson, (Eds.), Obstetrics: Normal and problem pregnancies. New York: Churchill Livingstone.

Blackwell, M. K. (1993). Documentation serves as invaluable defense tool. American Nurse, 25(7), 40–41.

Bowes, W. A. (1994). Clinical aspects of normal and abnormal labor. In R. K. Creasy & R. Resnick (Eds.), Maternal-fetal medicine: Principles and practice (rev. ed.). Philadelphia: W. B. Saunders.

Buckley, K. (1990). Recognition of fetal distress. In K. Buckley & N. W. Kulb (Eds.), High risk maternity nursing manual. Baltimore: Williams & Wilkins.

Creasy, R., & Resnick, R. (1984). Maternal-fetal medicine: Principles and practice. Philadelphia: W. B. Saunders.

Critchlow, C. W., Leet, T. L., Benedetti, T. J., & Daling, J. R. (1994). Risk factors and infant outcomes associated with umbilical cord prolapse: A population-based case-control study among births in Washington state. American Journal of Obstetrics and Gynecology, 170(2), 613–619.

Dorman, K. F. (1989). Hemorrhagic emergencies in obstetrics. Journal of Perinatal and Neonatal Nursing, 3(2), 23–32.

Farrell, E. (1993). Communication: A critical part of nursing. American Nurse, 25(7), 40–42.

Friedman, E. A. (1978). Labor: Clinical evaluation and management (2nd ed.). New York: Appleton-Century-Crofts.

Griese, M. E., & Prickett, S. A. (1993). Nursing management of umbilical cord prolapse. Journal of Obstetrical, Gynecological, and Neonatal Nursing, 311.

Gross, S. J., Shime, J., & Farine, D. (1987). Shoulder dystocia: Predictors and outcome. A five year review. American Journal of Obstetrics and Gynecology, 156(2), 334–336.

Hurd, W. W., Miodovnik, M., Hertzberg, V., & Lavin, J. P. (1983). Selective management of abruptio placentae: A prospective study. Obstetrics and Gynecology, 61(4), 467–473.

Iyasu, S., Saftlas, A. K., Rowley, D. L., Koonin, L. M., Lawson, H. W., & Atrash, H. K. (1993). National trends in the incidence of abruptio placentae, 1979 through 1987. Obstetrics and Gynecology, 168(5), 1424–1429.

Karegard, M., & Gennser, G. (1986). Incidence and recurrence rate of abruptio placentae in Sweden. Obstetrics and Gynecology, 67(4), 523–528.

Katz, Z., Lancet, M., Blickstein, I., Mogilner, B. M., & Zalel, Y. (1988). Management of labor with umbilical cord prolapse: A 5-year study. Obstetrics and Gynecology, 72(2), 278–281.

Kline-Kaye, V., & Miller-Slade, D. (1990). The use of fundal pressure during the second stage of labor. Journal of Obstetrical, Gynecological, and Neonatal Nursing, 4, 511.

Krohn, M., Voigt, L., McKnight, V., Daling, J. R., Starzyk, P., & Benedetti, T. J. (1987). British Journal of Obstetrics and Gynaecology, 94(4), 333–340.

Levy, H., Meier, R., & Makowski, E. L. (1984). Umbilical cord prolapse. Obstetrics and Gynecology, 64(4), 499–502.

NAACOG. (1991). Standards for obstetric, gynecologic and neonatal nursing (4th ed.). Washington, DC: NACOG.

Nurses' Assocation of the American College of Obstetricisn and Gynecologists (1988a). The nurse's role in induction/augmentation of labor. Washington, DC: Nurses' Organization for Obstetric, Gynecologic and Neonatal Nurses.

Nurses' Association of the American College of Obstetricians and Gynecologists (1988b). Practice competencies and educational guidelines for nurse providers of intrapartum care. Washington, DC: NAACOG.

Penney, D. S., & Perlis, D. W. (1992). Shoulder dystocia: When to use suprapubic or fundal pressure. MCN: American Journal of Maternal Child Nursing, 17(5), 276–277.

Resnick, R. (1980). Management of shoulder girdle dystocia. Clinical Obstetrics and Gynecology, 23(2), 559-564.

Roberts, W. E., Martin, R. W., Roach, H. H., Perry, K. G. Jr., Martin, J. N. Jr., & Morrison, J. C. (1997, June). Are obstetric interventions such as cervical ripening, induction of labor, amnioinfusion, or amniotomy associated with umbilical cord prolapse? American Journal of Obstetrics and Gynecology, 176(6), 1181–1185.

Seeds, J. (1986). Malpresentations. In S. G. Gabbe, J. R. Niebyl, & J. L. Simpson (Eds.), Obstetrics: Normal and problem pregnancies. New York: Churchill Livingstone.

Sholl, J. S. (1987). Abruptio placentae: Clinical management in nonacute cases. American Journal of Obstetrics and Gynecology, 156(1), 40–51.

Wiltse, B. (1992). Promoting quality nursing care. In L. K. Mandeville, & N. H. Troiano (Eds.), High-risk intrapartum nursing (pp. 7–29). Philadelphia: Lippincott.

Wheeler, D. (1991). Intrapartum bleeding. NAACOG's Clinical issues 2. Washington, DC: NAACOG.

Zwicke, D. L., Bobzien, W. F., & Wagner, E. H. (1982). Triage nurse decisions: A prospective study. Journal of Emergency Nursing, 8(3), 132–138.

CASE CITATIONS

Baptist Medical Center v. Wilson, 618 So.2nd 1335 (Ala. 1993).

Dent v. Perkins, 629 So.2nd 1354 (La. App. 1993).

Lambert v. Sisters of Mercy Health Corp., 369 N.W.2d 417 (1985).

Province v. Center for Women's Health & Family Birth, 20 Cal. App. 4th 1673 (Cal. 1993).

CHAPTER 9

Fetal Heart Rate Monitoring and Interpretation

Donna Miller Rostant and Michelle L. Murray

For the perinatal nurse, there is no greater challenge than determining the appropriateness of fetal heart rate monitoring and accurately interpreting fetal heart rate patterns. Fetal monitoring is useful for many purposes including the establishment of fetal well-being, identifying the fetus at risk for asphyxia and other difficulties before and during labor, and providing an evaluation of the response of the uterus and fetus to the forces of labor. Allegations of inappropriate fetal heart rate monitoring or misinterpretation of the fetal heart rate data lie at the core of many obstetrical lawsuits. Unrecognized continued fetal asphyxia is devastating to the fetus, mother, and health care provider.

Beckman (1996) examined malpractice claims with allegations of nursing negligence filed from 1988 through 1993. Of 747 cases alleging nursing negligence, 17.14% (128 of 747) experienced an adverse outcome (including maternal injury, fetal injury, and maternal and fetal death) in the labor and delivery area. While the primary cause of fetal/newborn injury was inadequate communication of nursing assessment data to the physician, failure to detect fetal distress in a timely manner because of infrequent assessment of fetal monitor tracings was the cause of over half of the injuries in cases alleging nursing negligence. Failure to inform the physician promptly of fetal distress caused serious injury to 35 newborns and

resulted in the death of 16 others. Other causes of injury included failure to timely implement the chain of command when the physician did not respond appropriately to fetal distress, inadequate fetal nursing assessment, and medication errors.

The perinatal nurse is expected to perform in a prudent, reasonable manner. Labor, delivery, and labor triage nurses are usually the first to assess a pregnant patient and often have a tremendous impact in the subsequent intrapartal course. In most cases, an abbreviated prenatal history is at the hospital when the pregnant patient first presents to the labor and delivery suite. In addition to thoroughly and accurately assessing the pregnant woman upon her presentation to the hospital, the reasonable, prudent labor and delivery nurse should be able to accurately and adequately interpret fetal heart rate patterns. To do so, the nurse must have a thorough understanding of the physiology involved in the labor and delivery process as well as a practical understanding of fetal monitoring equipment and its functions.

The perinatal nurse should also possess appropriate communication skills. Communication skills are necessary to convey the patient status and solicit appropriate assistance from other members of the health care team. Inappropriate or inadequate communication between health care providers is a common finding in malpractice lawsuits.

This chapter provides an overview of the nurse's role in monitoring the fetus and interpreting fetal heart rate patterns and a synopsis of essential oral and written communication skills. Various legal cases are presented to illustrate the danger of inadequately trained and poorly educated perinatal nurses who become unwilling defendants in a nursing negligence action.

FETAL HEART RATE MONITORING

Methods to monitor the fetus were in place long before the development of electronic fetal heart rate monitoring. Prior to the advent of electronic fetal monitoring, auscultation of the fetus was used to identify fetal well-being.

In the early 1970s, machines became available to monitor the fetal heart rate. In order to use the devices, nurses and physicians had to obtain advanced knowledge of the monitors as well as a thorough understanding of the underlying physiology of the fetus and mother. One without the other was meaningless.

As the use of fetal monitoring became widespread, it soon became apparent that standards of practice for both physicians and nurses were needed to identify responsibilities involved in the process of fetal monitoring. Throughout the years, fetal heart rate monitoring standards have been developed and refined. Currently, there are many standards or guidelines for fetal heart rate monitoring. Some standards are local; some are national. Standards enable the perinatal nurse to understand the expectations involved while performing fetal monitoring. Appropriate standards also provide a benchmark upon which to evaluate clinical practice and quality of patient care. Finally, standards provide predictability to plan appropriate interventions when a particular fetal heart rate pattern is seen. The most accepted standards for fetal heart rate monitoring are those set forth by the American College of Obstetricians and Gynecologists and those by the Association of Women's Health, Obstetric and Neonatal Nursing (formerly NAACOG). Both of these voluntary organizations represent the collective opinions of experts in the field of obstetrics, gynecology, and women's health and have earned widespread respect in the medical and legal community. The standards are published and readily available to obstetrical personnel.

THE STANDARD OF CARE FOR FETAL HEART RATE MONITORING— AWHONN

AWHONN is a voluntary nursing association that sets forth appropriate recommendations, guidelines and standards for obstetrical, neonatal, and gynecological nurses. Although they are not legal mandates, AWHONN standards possess great weight when presented as evidence of the appropriate standard of care for nurses in those areas of practice.

AWHONN identifies educational preparation and clinical skills necessary for fetal heart rate monitoring in the antepartum and peripartum periods (AWHONN, 1998). Although AWHONN asserts that the nurse performing fetal heart rate monitoring should complete a minimum, eight hours of didactic instruction in the core competencies, acquisition of knowledge and clinical skills will vary from nurse to nurse. Thus the nurse's ultimate ability to interpret fetal heart rate monitoring should be the focus rather than the number of hours he or she spent in fetal heart rate monitoring classes.

The perinatal nurse should make every effort to periodically update his or her knowledge of fetal heart rate monitoring. AWHONN suggests a number of methods for continuing education in fetal health surveillance including formal classroom educational programs, computer software packages, videotape series, teaching rounds, and self-study packages, although there is little scientific evidence to evaluate the effectiveness of knowledge acquisition or retention (AWHONN, 1998). No matter which method of continuing education is selected, all nurses involved in fetal monitoring and surveillance should remain current with changes in technology.

Antepartal Period

Although the labor and delivery setting is usually the most active in terms of fetal heart rate monitoring, AWHONN suggests that nurses be competent in the use of fetal monitoring equipment and interpretation of data in the antepartal setting as well.

> One of the responsibilities of nurses who perform antepartum fetal surveillance should be demonstrated competency in the application and use of external electronic and auscultatory fetal monitoring equipment and interpretation of data. (AWHONN, 1998)

Before assuming responsibility for antepartal surveillance, the nurse should be able to demonstrate the skills set forth in Display 9-1. Although AWHONN does not mandate a set time period to accomplish the skills in Display 9-1, supervised clinical experience combined with simultaneous instruction should be the primary source of education. The time period needed to train a nurse to function independently is variable and will depend to a large degree on the setting within which the nurse will practice and the skills needed to develop. The clinical learning experience should be developed to meet the needs of the individual learner. Practice sessions should include a policy, procedures, and protocol manual review. Other helpful learning experiences may include electronic fetal monitoring tracing review sessions, small group discussions or case study presentations, clinical conferences, computer simulation, or programmed self-study. The nurse should be evaluated to validate the ability to function independently and accomplish the skills necessary for fetal surveillance (AWHONN, 1998).

Intrapartum Fetal Monitoring

AWHONN makes it abundantly clear that nurses should acquire necessary educational preparation and skills before implementing fetal heart rate monitoring, although a thorough knowledge base does not always guarantee the ability to use that knowledge as a skilled practitioner (Simpson, 1994).

AWHONN identified standards for intrapartum fetal heart rate monitoring and states that to be skilled in intrapartum fetal health surveillance, the nurse should be able to accomplish those goals set forth in Display 9-2. In

DISPLAY 9-1

Antepartal Surveillance Skills

A. Describe antepartum testing criteria and indications for testing, for example, high-risk pregnancy, and indicate which tests to use

B. Provide patient education regarding the procedure and its purpose.

C. Prepare the patient (perform complete assessment including Leopold's maneuvers, palpation of the fundus) and correctly apply the external electronic fetal monitor

D. Recognize indications and contraindications with each test, including the use of oxytocin and nipple stimulation

E. Recognize reassuring and nonreassuring patients according to gestational age

F. Conduct the prescribed antepartum test

G. Implement interventions per protocol for nonreassuring findings

H. Communicate the content of electronic fetal monitoring data for final interpretation in accordance with institutional policy

I. Discontinue electronic fetal monitoring according to institutional policy, procedure, and protocol

J. Communicate appropriate follow-up information to the patient

DISPLAY 9-2

Intrapartum Fetal Health Surveillance Skills

A. Implement the appropriate fetal heart rate monitoring method based on patient status, hospital policy, and current standards of practice recommended by professional organizations

B. Explain the principles of the chosen method of fetal heart monitoring to the patient and her support person(s)

C. Identify the limitation of information produced by each method of monitoring

D. Demonstrate skill in fetal heart surveillance by auscultation

    1. Perform a complete assessment including Leopold's maneuvers to determine fetal position and determine the appropriate site for auscultation

    2. Apply a fetoscope or Doppler device to the appropriate site

    3. Palpate uterine contractions for frequency, duration, and intensity; confirm resting tone between contractions; determine if abnormal findings are present

    4. Identify the presence of the baseline fetal heart rate and rhythm

    5. Identify the presence of fetal heart rate changes with or between uterine contractions

    6. Classify the findings and implement appropriate nursing interventions, including additional fetal surveillance methods as indicated

    7. Identify the clinical situations, based on fetal surveillance findings, in which immediate notification of the primary health care provider is appropriate

    8. Communicate the findings to the patient and support person

    9. Communicate the findings and resulting nursing interventions in written and verbal form in an appropriate and timely manner

    10. Document appropriate entries on the written or computerized patient record

    11. Demonstrate appropriate maintenance of auscultation equipment

E. Demonstrate skill in electronic fetal monitoring

---

addition to AWHONN, the American College of Obstetricians and Gynecologists (ACOG) also publishes various opinions, standards, and guidelines related to electronic fetal monitoring.

Intermittent auscultation of the fetal heart rate with a 1:1 nurse–patient ratio at 15-minute intervals during the active phase of the first stage of labor and at 5-minute intervals during the second stage has been shown to be equivalent to electronic fetal monitoring (American Academy of Pediatrics and the American College of Obstetricians and Gynecologists, 1992). Currently, the AWHONN and

ACOG standard for the low-risk patient is to evaluate and record the fetal heart rate following a contraction at least every 30 minutes in the active phase of the first stage of labor and at least every 15 minutes in the second stage of labor (NAACOG, 1990/AWHONN, 1993). For the patient with risk factors, the heart rate should be auscultated every 15 minutes during the active phase of the first stage of labor and every 5 minutes during the second stage of labor (NAACOG, 1990/AWHONN, 1993). Electronic fetal heart rate monitoring is not required for all patients, and in fact the uncompli-

DISPLAY 9-3

Documentation in Labor and Delivery

Observations and events that precipitated interventions

Actions taken

Maternal and fetal responses to actions taken

Maternal and fetal response to epidural anesthesia

Results of vaginal examination, pushing

Loss of variability with pushing

cated labor and delivery patient is generally monitored by intermittent auscultation. However, the perinatal nurse must be aware of factors that warrant continuous electronic fetal monitoring. When such monitoring is used, appropriate personnel are required to accurately interpret and identify fetal heart rate monitors. The assessment and documentation guidelines to use when risk factors are present during labor or when intensified monitoring is chosen are set forth in Display 9-3.

Selection of the appropriate method for fetal heart rate monitoring is important. Although the standard for low-risk patients permits auscultation, the nurse should recognize factors that warrant electronic fetal heart rate monitoring. Care should be taken to abide by institutional policy. For example, if the hospital policy mandates electronic fetal heart rate monitoring for all patients, the nurse would be unreasonable to ignore it. The more appropriate approach is to revise the institutional policy to comport with current standards.

The nurse should be able to explain the principles of the method of fetal monitoring chosen for the patient. Most women are familiar with electronic fetal heart rate monitoring and may believe it to be more accurate and reassuring than auscultation. Careful explanation will help allay the patient's concerns, should auscultation be chosen as the method to monitor the fetal heart rate. The nurse should also describe the

rationale for fetal heart rate monitoring in language easily understood by the patient.

The nurse should recognize the limitations of each method of fetal monitoring. Electronic monitoring impedes unrestricted movement and ambulation whereas auscultation provides only a snapshot of the events occurring during labor. Other factors impinging on the accuracy of electronic fetal heart monitoring may include maternal weight, fetal position, multiple births, and the degree to which the woman in labor moves about in bed.

The nurse should be able to demonstrate proficiency in auscultation by being able to perform Leopold's maneuver to locate the most appropriate site to monitor the fetal heart and to apply the auscultatory device correctly using gel or other conduction aids as appropriate. The nurse should be familiar with assessment and interpretation of contractions by palpitation. The nurse should be able to auscultate the fetal heart rate with and after a contraction to determine the effects of the contraction on the fetus and intervene appropriately after classifying the findings. The nurse should be familiar with situations that require prompt notification of the primary health care provider. Communication should be clear, concise and ongoing between the nurse, the patient, and her significant others. Documentation is essential and should be done in a timely fashion with appropriate nursing interventions and the patient's response noted (AWHONN's 1998).

Standards for fetal monitoring and documentation can also be found in the *Guidelines for Perinatal Care* (AAP/ACOG, 1992). According to the Guidelines for Perinatal Care:

> When electronic fetal heart monitoring is selected as the mode of fetal assessment, the physician and obstetric personnel attending the patient should be qualified to identify and interpret abnormalities. It is appropriate for physicians and nurses to use the descriptive terms that have been given to fetal monitoring patterns (e.g., accelerations and early, late, or variable decelerations) in chart documentation and verbal communications.

Finally, each institution must also have policies and procedures for electronic fetal monitoring (Joint Commission of the Accreditation of

Healthcare Organizations). To ensure protection from liability, institutional policies and procedures must be in accordance with national standards of care.

In addition to accurately interpreting and identifying fetal heart rate patterns, the perinatal nurse must communicate information regarding the fetal status or EFM tracings, either antepartal or intrapartum, to the physician or midwife in a timely manner in accordance with national standards and institutional policy. The physician or midwife who is responsible for the patient's care should be kept informed of her progress and notified immediately of any abnormality. He or she should be readily available when the patient is in the active phase of labor (AAP/ACOG, 1992).

COMMUNICATION

Specific nurse–physician problems of communication are addressed in Chapter 20. Regarding electronic fetal heart monitoring, communication is essential to the safe provision of perinatal nursing care. Problems specific to communication incident to fetal heart rate monitoring include the urgency with which the nurse may convey patient information, the use of terminology, and patient communication. Because of the intensity and the urgency of the situation, the nurse may communicate information about the fetal heart rate pattern in what appears to be a "panicky" tone. There may be difficulty in finding correct terminology to describe the pattern in detail. Fear of "bothering the physician" or appearing incompetent may hinder a nurse's efforts to seek medical assistance for the patient. Unfortunately, many lawsuits arise out of the failure to adequately communicate pertinent patient information (Beckman, 1996).

Effective Communication

Perinatal nurses should feel safe in communicating with physicians and other members of the health care team. They should be encouraged to solicit second opinions for questionable fetal heart rate patterns. Support by hospital administrators and physicians is important to encourage nurses to promptly notify physicians or midwives when abnormal patterns, abnormal findings, or meconium are noted, even during the night or early morning.

After calling a physician or midwife with the potential problem, the perinatal nurse should identify how long it will take before one or the other sees the patient. If the midwife or physician refuses to come to the hospital after the nurse's request, the nurse should discuss the reasons for the refusal and document them in the patient's medical record.

After the initial request, if the nurse still feels that the patient's physician or midwife should be present on the unit, and the patient's physician or midwife again refuses, it is the nurse's duty to make sure that a physician or midwife sees the patient. The physician or midwife should be cognizant of the nurse's plight and request a patient status report including interventions that have been implemented. The nurse should, at a minimum, communicate the information set forth in Display 9-3 to a physician, midwife, or other nurse. The nurse should follow the institution's chain of command policy to ensure that a physician or midwife sees the patient as soon as possible (Murray, 1996).

Terminology

Appropriate communication is needed to convey accurate information regarding the fetal status. Various problems arise when health care providers try to communicate verbally. Communication of the fetal heart rate pattern is hindered when different terminology by different health care providers is used to describe the same image. For example, type 1 and type 2 decelerations are now called early and late decelerations. Variable decelerations have been described by some as having a "late component," and baselines have been described as "wandering." Although verbal communication describing a fetal heart rate pattern is the usual mode of transferring information between health care providers who are not at the bedside, the advent of modern technology has enhanced the ability to effectively transfer the actual labor pattern. Facsimile machines and modems can immediately transmit the tracing in question to almost any location. The nurse can then review the fetal monitor strip with the physician or midwife who is not at the patient's bedside (Murray, 1996).

Nurse–Patient Communication

In addition to effective communication between health care providers, the nurse should be able to effectively communicate with the patient. In order to allay patient anxiety, the nurse should educate the patient about the fetal monitor. A clear and concise explanation of the monitor, its use, and its functions helps to decrease the patient's anxiety. Patients and families tend to focus on the fetal heart rate monitor. Nurses should be careful to explain that the fetal heart rate often accelerates and decelerates without any serious consequence. Audible alarms should also be explained so the patient does not panic should the alerts be triggered.

COMMON PROBLEMS WITH FETAL HEART RATE INTERPRETATION

Fetal heart rate interpretation, although based on sound, scientific principles, is nonetheless an art with a subjective component. Although there is usually consensus regarding the more common fetal heart rate patterns, it is not unusual for interpreters to disagree. Different educational backgrounds, experiences, and clinical skills can result in wide variations in interpretation between experienced nurses and physicians. The problem of inconsistent interpretation rests, in part, on the varying educational programs teaching fetal heart rate monitoring skills and principles. Some educational programs are provided by well-known experts with noted expertise and solid clinical skills. Other programs are taught by less credible instructors. In an attempt to minimize the variation in educational preparation, AWHONN identified "Clinical Competencies and Educational Guidelines," which identify specific areas of competency of each nurse whose practice includes the use of fetal surveillance techniques. Computer programs have also been developed to standardize the educational content.

Various studies have confirmed a lack of consistency in interpretation of fetal heart rate patterns by physicians. For example, a study by Borgatta (Borgatta, Shrout, & Divon, 1988) revealed that when five perinatologists reviewed 50 monitor strips from NSTs and then re-reviewed the same monitor strips, only 11 of the tracings were classified as the same at both readings by the same perinatologist.

Nurses have some of the same difficulty with interpretation in the antepartum period. Although the NST is the most widely used screening test for fetal well-being, Chez found that 16% of nurses interpreted a NST tracing as reactive when it was not (Chez, B. F., Skurnick, J. H., Chez, R. A., et al., 1990). Murray discovered that physicians do not necessarily have greater accuracy in interpreting fetal monitor strips than do nurses. Both nurses and physicians have been known to have difficulty in agreeing on interpretation when reviewing the same fetal monitor tracing (Murray, 1996).

As a practical matter, in a lawsuit experts often disagree on the interpretation of a particular fetal heart rate pattern and will so testify to a jury. The plaintiff's expert will testify that the defendant did not correctly interpret the fetal heart rate pattern or respond appropriately. The defendant's expert will testify that the defendant acted appropriately. The jury is then faced with the task of determining which expert is correct. Clinical expertise and educational preparation play an important role in determining an expert's credibility in this area.

INDIVIDUAL AND INSTITUTIONAL RESPONSIBILITY

In 1986, NAACOG (now known as AWHONN) recommended that "competency in electronic fetal monitoring should be documented in writing before the nurse functions independently on the intrapartum unit." NAACOG also mandated that "maintaining the quality of individual practice . . . remains inherent in the responsibilities of the professional nurse" (NAACOG, 1986). Thus although the nurse is responsible for obtaining the educational and skill preparation, the institution is responsible for ensuring that the nurse has the minimum level of competency necessary for safe, appropriate patient care. Failure to do so places the institution at risk for breaching the duty to provide skilled caregivers to its patients, leading to a possible corporate negligence action.

In 1993, McRae stated that "the lack of attention paid to proficiency in EFM is alarming" (McRae, 1993). Undoubtedly, in inexperienced or uneducated hands EFM becomes a liability. McRae suggested that hospitals ensure competency of the nurses performing fetal heart rate monitoring by including documentation of orientation programs for newly hired staff; documentation of competencies and how these are taught, measured, and maintained; developing and implementing policies regarding the nurse's role in intrapartum care; and identifying criteria for documentation in the medical record and on the EFM tracing. Fetal monitoring courses should be provided to all nurses who will be responsible for implementing fetal heart rate monitoring.

In a lawsuit, the expertise of the defendant nurse will undoubtedly be at issue. The plaintiff's attorney will attempt to prove to the jury that the nurse was unskilled or ill prepared to perform electronic fetal heart rate monitoring. Educational preparation, skills, and experience of the nurse will be closely scrutinized. The plaintiff may ask questions of the defendant nurse such as the following:

1. What is your educational background?
2. What programs have you attended having anything to do with electronic fetal monitoring?
3. Do you keep a record of the educational programs you have attended?
4. Does your institution maintain a list of programs you have attended?
5. What training have you had for the reading of monitor strips?
6. What, if anything, did your unit orientation provide for electronic fetal heart rate monitoring education?
7. How did your head nurse/supervisor assess your readiness to implement fetal heart rate monitoring?
8. Have you taken any additional training regarding electronic fetal heart rate monitoring?

Through these directed questions, the plaintiff gains an understanding about the nurse's knowledge and expertise in antepartal and intrapartal fetal heart rate monitoring (Murray, 1996).

Many plaintiff's attorneys recognize that national professional associations have identified standards of practice. Unfortunately, these same attorneys are often more familiar with the existing standards than is the practicing nurse. The attorneys will question the nurse regarding his or her membership in these organizations and the nurse's knowledge of the existence of such standards. Such questions may include the following:

1. Are you a member of AWHONN?
2. What standards, if any, are you familiar with regarding fetal heart rate monitoring?
3. What books do you consider authoritative on the subject of fetal monitoring?

The purpose of these questions is to understand the nurse's knowledge regarding the existence of standards and to identify whether he or she practices in accordance with such standards. Perinatal nurses should never underestimate a skilled plaintiff's attorney. The attorney will develop a sound knowledge base regarding the applicable standards in use and will carefully scrutinize the nurse's knowledge thereof.

Standardized Educational Programs

To minimize variation in interpretation and confusion, fetal heart rate monitoring classes should be standardized. Murray and Catanzarite developed a computer-assisted instructional program, known as Fetal Monitor Interpretation Version 2.0, to achieve this goal. Likewise, AWHONN identified core competencies and educational guidelines to identify minimal educational requirements needed for the nurse performing fetal monitoring.

In addition to physiology, basic fetal monitoring courses should include the rules of recognition for the concepts of baseline, accelerations, and decelerations. To recognize the baseline, one must be taught the concepts of range, stability, and variability (short-term and long-term). Murray believes that to recognize accelerations and decelerations, the learner should be taught the shape or configuration of the two types of accelerations (spontaneous and uniform), and shape or configuration and timing in relation to contractions of the four basic types of decelerations (early, late, variable, and prolonged) (Murray). The features of these decelerations, however, must be evaluated within the appropriate physiological context (Murray, 1996).

Murray suggests that controversial areas of fetal heart rate monitoring should also be addressed in fetal heart rate monitoring classes. Such controversies include assessment of short-term variability with an external monitor; the definitions of accelerations and reactivity; typical versus atypical variable decelerations; periodic versus nonperiodic as adjectives that describe patterns of accelerations and decelerations; and the use of the terms mild, moderate, and severe variable decelerations (Murray, 1996).

Other controversies include using the labels variable deceleration with a "late component" and "late/variable" decelerations. There are many misconceptions about late decelerations. Many nurses believe that late decelerations cannot occur if accelerations also appear on the tracing. Others believe that late decelerations do not fall below 100 bpm. Both are untrue. Late decelerations can and often do appear in the presence of accelerations and can also be very deep, even falling below 70 bpm. An instructor should understand fetal physiology and be able to correctly teach the critical characteristics of accelerations and decelerations as well as emphasize signs of fetal well-being and compromise. All of these issues should be discussed in a fetal monitoring course (Murray, 1996).

DOCUMENTATION

The FHR tracing is of utmost importance and often is the single most important documentary evidence in a medical malpractice case. Concerns of documenting the same information twice on a background of serious time constraints cause perinatal nurses to debate whether to document patient information in the medical record, on the fetal monitor strip, or both. Some nurses debate whether to document on the fetal monitor strip at all. Others believe

that only critical events should be noted on the strip. Some advocate initialing the strip at regular time intervals, usually every 15 to 30 minutes, indicating the nurse has been in the room and reviewed the strip. However, initials on a strip do not mean it has been accurately interpreted. If a nurse initials the tracing, there should also be evidence in the notes that the tracing was interpreted and that appropriate actions were taken in response to the FHR pattern and/or uterine activity pattern.

Because fetal strips may be lost, the perinatal nurse should interpret the fetal heart rate strip on a regular basis and document the findings in another part of the patient's medical record such as the flowsheet. Interventions should also be documented as well as the patient's response thereto.

Documenting crucial information in the nurses' notes is more important than documenting on the fetal heart monitor strip as the strips are more likely to be lost than the hospital record. If the nurse does not document in the record and the FHR strip is lost or misplaced, there is little chance the nurse will be able to accurately recall the events occurring during the labor. Documentation should include, at a minimum, the information set forth in Display 9-3 (Murray, 1996).

When continuous electronic fetal monitoring is used, the following should be documented:

1. Baseline—range, stability, variability (long- and short-term)
2. Acceleration types, including amplitude and duration of the largest acceleration
3. Deceleration types, including depth, duration, time to recovery, completeness of recovery (for example, resumption of previously normal rate and variability)
4. Contractions—frequency, duration, intensity peak pressure, tone (resting pressure between contractions)
5. Actions taken
6. Maternal and fetal response to actions
7. Communications

Signs of fetal well-being should be assessed and documented if they are present, for example, accelerations, short-term variability, fetal movements, and the presence of clear, non-foul-smelling amniotic fluid. The FHR should also be evaluated immediately after spontaneous or artificial rupture of membranes and the response documented. In addition, the amount, color, and odor of the amniotic fluid should be recorded.

The nurse should document baseline changes and other occurrences on the strip using the proper terminology. For example, decelerations should be based on specific criteria for onset, offset, and nadir (lowest point) of the deceleration in relation to the peak of the contraction. Late decelerations always begin after the contraction begins, their nadir is past the peak of the contraction, and they recover after the contraction ends (Murray, 1996).

ILLUSTRATIVE CASES INVOLVING FETAL MONITORING AND STRATEGIES TO MINIMIZE LIABILITY

Failure to Respond Appropriately

Nurses must accurately interpret abnormal fetal heart rate patterns and respond appropriately. In *John Doe v. ABC Hospital,* (1994), a $2.05 million settlement was reached between the hospital and an injured newborn where it was alleged that the nurses failed to respond to an abnormally low fetal heart rate. The newborn's mother went into labor on December 31, 1992. For over an hour, the fetal heart rate monitor showed an abnormally low fetal heart rate. The nurses took no action and did not notify the physician. Later, the fetal heart rate demonstrated tachycardia and late decelerations. Still no action was taken although the obstetrician saw the mother during the period the fetus was in distress. The infant was born not breathing. There was not a pediatrician available. A respiratory therapist was called to intubate the baby but was unsuccessful. The infant suffered severe deficits in mental and motor function.

In *Maxwell Davis v. Carolyn Garcia and St. Joseph Medical Center* (1995), allegations of failure to adequately monitor the fetus during labor resulted in an $8.5 million settlement. In that case, the plaintiff mother claimed that the nursing staff failed to adequately monitor the fetus during labor, failed to keep proper notes, and

failed to timely notify a physician. The child was born with cerebral palsy. In *Wareing v. U.S.A.* (1996), the plaintiff, an 11-year-old boy born at the United States Naval Hospital in Guam, claimed that the physicians and nurses mismanaged his mother's labor and delivery. The woman was 3-weeks postterm when an ultrasound revealed minimal amniotic fluid. The woman was sent home. That night the woman went into labor but waited until the contractions became regular the next morning before going to the hospital. Although the medical staff was aware of the postterm status and decreased amniotic fluid, no heightened assessment was performed. By the next morning, signs of fetal distress included poor beat-to-beat variability and the presence of profound late decelerations were noted. Once ordered, a cesarean delivery was delayed for over an hour and a half. The child was born with severe neurological deficits. The defendants did not dispute the fact that the cesarean section was untimely, but instead argued that the neurological injury suffered by the boy was as a result of intrauterine trauma occurring at or around the thirty-eighth week of pregnancy. A judge found for the plaintiff and awarded $3.6 million, which included $2.1 million in economic damages and $1.5 million in pain and suffering.

Nurses should be aware of factors that require heightened assessment and monitoring. In the case of *Wareing,* clearly the postterm status of the patient placed her at high risk for fetal or maternal complications. Nurses must be vigilant to adequately monitor the mother and fetus and intervene in a timely, appropriate fashion. Failure to do so may be devastating to the patient and newborn.

Chain of Command

Once abnormal FHR patterns have been identified, nurses are expected to timely implement appropriate nursing interventions. If the physician has been called and refused to come in, the nurse should expect to explain why he or she did not repeat the request for the physician to come to the hospital or why he or she did not implement the chain of command. Documentation of the events contemporaneously with their occurrence will solidify the nurse's credibility should a malpractice case arise many years later.

Nurses may be asked questions in deposition to determine how well they understood or utilized their chain of command. Questions may focus on the chain of command and the nurse's knowledge of the appropriate source for assistance. The attorney will question the nurse about whom he or she would turn to according to institutional policy and then ask whether the nurse contacted the appropriate person.

Nurses hesitate to document a physician's lack of response in the medical record. They are usually told by risk management personnel not to "advertise" potential conflicts in the medical records and thus some nurses may be unwilling to memorialize an unsuccessful interaction with a physician. Nurses may also believe the interaction was of little significance, preferring to forget about it rather than document the exchange. Finally, nurses may choose to affirmatively protect the doctor by not documenting an inappropriate or untimely response in the patient's chart. Some nurses may keep their own personal notes regarding a potentially adverse interaction to refer to should the need arise. Such notes are often subject to discovery rules and can be devastating evidence in subsequent litigation.

In a medical malpractice lawsuit, the nursing care will also be carefully scrutinized. Because it is maintained contemporaneously, the medical record is often the most reliable piece of documentary evidence in a medical malpractice action. If there is no documentation regarding the conversation that transpired between the nurse and physician, the nurse will be called upon to explain why she did notify the physician. The old adage, "if you didn't document it, you didn't do it" is very influential to a lay jury. Even though most nurses know that key events are often omitted from the medical record, an opposing attorney will try to convince a jury that the nurse did not record the telephone conversation because it did not take place. The physician may forget that the nurse ever called.

To illustrate this point, suppose that a nurse notified a physician at home of her concern about late decelerations on the fetal monitor. The nurse requested that the physician come to the hospital to assess the patient and fetus. The physician dismissed the nurse's concerns and told the nurse to "call if the pattern gets worse." The nurse did not document the substance of the conversation or even that the call took place.

If there is a lawsuit, the nurse is in a "no-win" situation. The nurse will be questioned as to whether she interpreted the fetal heart rate strip as abnormal. If the nurse did interpret the strip as abnormal, then clearly she deviated from the applicable standard of care by failing to communicate the information to the physician. If the nurse did communicate the information to the physician and the physician refused to attend to the patient, the nurse would be negligent for failing to implement the chain of command. If the nurse did not interpret the strip as abnormal, then she is negligent in her interpretation of the strip. The nurse should never attempt to protect the physician or midwife who is unresponsive to patient needs. Furthermore, the nurse must implement the chain of command to protect the safety of the patient and to avoid liability for his or her own failure to act (Murray, 1996).

Failure to Interpret Fetal Distress

In *Fairfax Hosp. System, Inc. v. McCarty* (1992), a nurse was sued by the parents of Luke McCarty, who was born with permanent neurological and developmental impairments. Luke's mother, Janet McCarty, was 31 years old when she was admitted to Fairfax Hospital to deliver her first child. Ms. McCarty was placed on an electronic fetal heart rate monitor at about 7:30 A.M., after spontaneous rupture of her membranes. A nurse began attending to Ms. McCarty at about 6:10 P.M. that evening and was to be with her until 9:00 P.M. The evidence presented to the court established that the fetal heart rate monitor demonstrated a broad-based deceleration at approximately 8:27 P.M. The mother began demonstrating an abnormal labor pattern and the fetal heart rate monitor demonstrated that the fetus was experiencing more and more difficulty. In spite of the fetal distress apparent on the monitor strip as early as 8:27 P.M., the nurse did not seek to notify the physician until 8:50 P.M. The obstetrician, testifying for the plaintiffs, indicated that the nurse did not tell him an emergency situation was present. He testified that a cesarean delivery could have been accomplished within 12 minutes and that had he seen the fetal monitor, he would have moved to deliver the infant shortly before 8:40 P.M. The obstetrician further testified that the nurse's failure to take action or notify him delayed the delivery and contributed in a causative manner to the eventual outcome of the infant.

Expert witness testimony established that the neurological injury was inevitable after 8:53 P.M. The jury returned a verdict in excess of $3.5 million, which was subsequently reduced to the statutory cap of $1 million.

Nurses should promptly notify physicians of nonreassuring signs in labor. The nurse is often hesitant to notify a physician or midwife for fear of "bothering" them. As seen in *Fairfax Hosp. System, Inc.,* minutes are crucial when faced with potential neurological injury. Additionally, nurses should remember that some physicians, when named as defendants, would testify to nursing negligence, especially if it tends to exculpate them.

CONCLUSION

The perinatal nurse works in a dynamic, energetic environment with constant new stimulation. In an instant, an uncomplicated labor can become complicated. The nurse must be ever vigilant for potentially adverse outcomes. Fetal monitoring is the communication link between the fetus and the external environment. The nurse performing and interpreting fetal monitoring must possess the requisite skills and educational preparation to do so. Clinical skills should be updated consistently. The nurse should also possess communication skills including the ability to convey information in a clear, precise, and comprehensive manner. Policies, procedures, and guidelines for fetal heart rate monitoring should be explicit and available to all personnel in the labor and delivery unit. National standards of care should be followed. The perinatal nurse has the duty and the responsibility to deliver appropriate nursing care. Anything less is unacceptable and potentially injurious to the mother and fetus.

REFERENCES

American Academy of Pediatrics and American College of Obstetricians and Gynecologists. (1992). Guidelines for Perinatal Care (3rd ed.). Elk Grove Village, IL: American Academy of Pediatrics and American College of Obstetricians and Gynecologists.

AWHONN. (1993a). Didactic content and clinical skills verification for professional nurse providers of basic, high-risk, and critical-care intrapartal nursing. Washington, DC: Association of Women's Health, Obstetric and Neonatal Nurses.

AWHONN. (1993b). Fetal heart monitoring principles and practices. Washington, DC: Association of Women's Health, Obstetric and Neonatal Nurses.

AWHONN. (1998). Nursing practice competencies and education guidelines antepartum fetal surveillance and intrapartum fetal heart monitoring. (2nd ed.). Washington, DC.

Beckman, J. P. (1996). Nursing negligence. Thousand Oaks: Sage Publishing.

Borgatta, L., Shrout, P. E., & Divon, M. Y. (1988). Reliability and reproducibility of nonstress test readings. American Journal of Obstetrics and Gynecology, 159, 554.

Chez, B. F., Skurnick, J. H., Chez, R. A., & Verklan, M. T., et al. (1990). Interpretations of nonstress tests by obstetric nurses. Obstetric and Gynecological Nursing, 19, 227.

General Accounting Office (GAO). (1987). Medical malpractice characteristics of claims closed in 1984. GAO/HRD-87-55. Washington, DC: U.S. Government Printing Office.

McRae, M. J. (1993). Litigation, electronic fetal monitoring, and the obstetric nurse. Journal of Obstetrical, Gynecological and Neonatal Nursing, 22, 410.

Medical malpractice verdicts, settlements and experts. 1994; 10:

Murray, M. L. (1996). Electronic fetal monitoring: Role of the nurse. In Donn & Fischer (Eds.). Risk management techniques in perinatal and neonatal practice (pp. 213–239). Armonk, NY: Futura Publishing Co.

Murray & Catanzarite. (1996). Fetal Monitor Interpretation Version 2.0. Baltimore, MD: Williams & Wilkins.

NAACOG. (1986). <u>Electronic fetal monitoring nursing practice competencies and educational guidelines.</u> Washington, DC: Nurses Association of the American College of Obstetricians and Gynecologists.

NAACOG. (1991a). <u>NAACOG standards for the nursing care of women and newborns</u> (4th ed.). Washington, DC: NAACOG.

NAACOG. (1991b). <u>Nursing practice competencies and education guidelines antepartum fetal surveillance and intrapartum fetal heart monitoring.</u> Washington, DC: Nurses Association of the American College of Obstetricians and Gynecologists.

Risk Management Foundation. (1986). Fetal monitoring problems during labor associated with most serious OB claims. <u>Forum 1986, 7,</u> 19.

Simpson, K. R. (1994). Electronic fetal monitoring competency—To validate or not to validate: The opinions of the experts. <u>The Journal of Perinatal and Neonatal Nursing, 8</u>(3), 1–16.

Trepanier, M. J., Niday, B., Davies, B., Sprague, A., Nimrod, C., Dulberg, C., & Watters, N. (1996). Evaluation of a fetal heart rate monitoring education program. <u>Journal of Obstetrical, Gynecological and Neonatal Nursing, 25</u>(2), 137–144.

CASE CITATIONS

John Doe v. ABC Hospital, Ashtabula County (Oh.), Court of Common Pleas, Case No. 93CV00357.

Fairfax Hosp. System, Inc. v. McCarty, 419 S.E.2d 621 (1992).

Maxwell Davis v. Carolyn Garcia and St. Joseph Medical Center, Medical Malpractice Verdicts, Settlements & Experts (May 1995).

Miles v. Box Butte County, 489 N.W.2d 829 (1992).

Wareing v. U.S.A., U.S. District Court, Southern District of Florida, Ft. Lauderdale Division, Case No. 93-6306-CIV-MARCUS Medical Malpractice Verdicts, Settlements & Experts (October 1996).

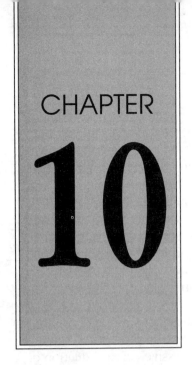

CHAPTER 10

The Use of Pitocin in Labor

Debi Law

The onset of labor is thought to be initiated by the interaction of several hormones (Bobak, 1993). Historically, one of the first hormones to be identified was oxytocin, a pituitary hormone that had an effect on the contractility of the uterus. It was first synthesized in 1953 by du Vigneaud as a means to effect uterine activity, which would produce cervical change along with fetal descent (Petrie & Williams, 1993). Prior to the synthetic availability of this hormone, induction of labor was limited to amniotomy and stripping of the membranes.

REVIEW OF LABOR

Labor is divided into two stages. The first stage of labor is regarded as the time from onset of regular contractions to full dilatation of the cervix. The second stage of labor is from the time of full dilatation of the cervix to the delivery of the fetus.

The first stage of labor is further broken down into three phases: latent, active, and transition. The latent phase of labor is referred to as the preparatory phase. It is the time the cervix effaces, or thins, from its starting point to the point of being 90–100% effaced and dilates to 4 cm. Contractions in this phase are usually regular and range between 5 to 12 minutes apart.

These contractions are often not painful to the patient but can lead to exhaustion before the active phase of labor, especially if the woman is losing sleep (Keller-Bronte, 1986). Nulliparous labor in the latent phase usually lasts 8–10 hours, 4–6 hours in the multiparous labor (Vogler, 1993). However, this phase is said to be prolonged if it lasts greater than 20 hours in nulliparas and greater than 14 hours in multiparas (Gilbert & Harmon, 1993).

The active phase of labor occurs when the cervix is between 4 and 7 centimeters dilated. Contractions are more regular, usually every 3–5 minutes, and last approximately 30–45 seconds. Active labor usually lasts 3 hours for nulliparas and 1–2 hours for multiparas (Vogler, 1993).

The transition phase lasts about 1–2 hours. It is the time when the cervix goes from 7 cm to complete dilation.

The Friedman curve is the clinical tool most often used to plot the progress of labor. To make a labor graph you need square-ruled graph paper. The left ordinates represent cervical dilatation and are numbered from 0 cm at the bottom to 10 cm at the top. The right ordinates represent the station of the presenting part and are numbered from –5 at the top to +5 at the bottom. The bottom of the graph is used to note the time of onset of contractions or the start of oxytocin induction. The patient is usually examined every 2 hours while in the latent phase of labor and every hour during the active phase. The time of the exam is noted on the bottom of the graph and cervical dilatation is represented by the letter "X". The maternal station of the presenting part is represented by the letter "O". It is important to remember two questions when interpreting the graph:

A. In what phase of labor is the patient?

B. Is labor progressing normally for that phase (Sokol, 1987)?

DYSTOCIA

Dystocia is defined as a long, difficult, or abnormal labor. Proper management requires assessment of the 5 P's: *powers* (uterine contractility and expulsive effort), *passage* (the pelvis), *passenger* (the fetus), maternal *position* during labor and birth, and the *psychologic* responses such as culture, preparation, or past experience (Lowdermilk, 1997).

Currently, dystocia is a leading indicator for cesarean delivery. Proper identification of abnormal labor and correction of abnormal contraction patterns, fetal malpresentation, and inadequate expulsive efforts may reduce unnecessary cesarean deliveries without compromising mother or fetus (ACOG, 1995).

INDUCTION AND AUGMENTATION

Induction of labor is defined as the stimulation of uterine contractions prior to the onset of spontaneous labor resulting in delivery of the fetus (ACOG, 1995). Chemical and mechanical methods used to induce labor include administration of intravenous oxytocin, artificial rupture of membranes, nipple stimulation, and soap suds enema. Oxytocin is a hormone excreted from the posterior pituitary gland. It acts in the myometrium to produce smooth muscle contractions of the uterus. Oxytocin is given in its synthetic form as Pitocin or Syntocinon for labor induction or augmentation.

The uterus responds to oxytocin in three phases. The first phase is known as the incremental phase and is the time period where the uterine activity steadily increases as the oxytocin dose is increased. The second, or stable phase, is reached when the uterine activity remains constant in spite of the increasing oxytocin dosage. It is important to remember that in this phase the contraction frequency will increase but the intensity of the contractions will decrease; therefore, quality is better than quantity (Marshall, 1985). Increases in the uterine baseline tone, hyperstimulation, and tetanic contractions are possible in the third phase when oxytocin dosages continue to increase. Identifying the uterine phase is essential for appropriate titration of oxytocin.

Augmentation implies that spontaneous labor has occurred but there are inadequate contractions to produce progressive cervical dilation or descent of the fetal presenting part. Therefore, contractions must be stimulated by performing an amniotomy, initiating oxytocin therapy, or a combination of both (ACOG, 1995).

Maternal and Fetal Indications for Oxytocin Administration

The maternal indications for oxytocin administration include, but are not limited to, pregnancy-induced hypertension, diabetes mellitus, renal disease, chronic obstructive pulmonary disease, premature rupture of membranes, postterm gestation, and chorioamnionitis.

The fetal indications for oxytocin administration are, among others, fetal demise, intrauterine growth retardation, isoimmunization, postterm gestation, and major congenital anomalies. With the exception of the demised fetus, each of these has an unusual sensitivity to stress, hypoxia, and trauma (Petrie & Williams, 1993).

Generally speaking, any contraindication for a vaginal delivery is a contraindication for induction or augmentation of labor. These include placenta previa, vasa previa, previous classical uterine incision, active genital herpes infection, invasive cervical carcinoma, abnormal fetal lie, cord presentation, pelvic structural deformities, hypertonic uterine activity, and fetal distress.

Pharmacokinetics of Pitocin

Oxytocin is a hormone excreted by the posterior pituitary (Gilbert & Harmon, 1993). Oxytocin increases the intracellular concentrations of calcium in the myometrial tissue, thereby promoting uterine contractions. The uterus responds with increasing excitability, which has been described as triphasic in nature. The incremental phase allows the uterine response to evenly increase as the dosage of oxytocin is increased. During the stable phase, uterine response remains unchanged despite the continuing increase of oxytocin. Ineffective contraction patterns can occur during the third phase because the intensity of the contractions decrease despite their increase in frequency (Gilbert & Harmon, 1993). Due to its effect on uterine activity and without other available therapeutic agents, oxytocin rapidly became the therapy of choice for induction of labor.

Risks of Oxytocin Infusion

One of the many risks of using oxytocin is decreased uteroplacental perfusion. A healthy fetus has adequate oxygen reserves to endure the impeded uterine blood flow that occurs with normal labor contractions. However, increasing the frequency, strength, and duration of contractions with the use of oxytocin can further impede the uterine blood flow, resulting in a compromised fetus. This is evidenced by a nonreassuring fetal heart rate pattern. Some of the fetal heart rate changes seen in nonreassuring patterns include tachycardia, bradycardia, and decelerations.

Uterine hyperstimulation may result from increased sensitivity to oxytocin or from a dosage that is too high. Strong tetanic contractions that occur less than 2 minutes apart or have a duration of greater than 90 seconds are considered to be a pattern of hyperstimulation. An increased resting tone above 20 mm Hg may also be considered hyperstimulation.

Tetanic contractions create excessive and extreme tension of the uterus, resulting in an increased risk for amniotic fluid embolus, cervical lacerations, uterine rupture, and decreased uteroplacental perfusion.

The second most frequent cause of uterine rupture is overstimulation of the uterus with oxytocin. The major cause is previous cesarean section (Hayshi & Castillo, 1993). Maternal tachycardia is the most common physical sign in diagnosing uterine rupture. This sign is often overlooked when terbutaline has been used in response to hyperstimulation. Other signs are fetal bradycardia, vaginal bleeding, and abdominal pain (Sweeten, Graves, & Athanassiou, 1995).

Because oxytocin has a weak antidiuretic effect, water intoxication can result if the patient is given a large volume of fluid during oxytocin administration. The antidiuretic effect is increased when large amounts of electrolyte-free dextrose solution are used to administer the oxytocin (Gilbert & Harmon, 1993). In the event of water intoxication, patients may become hyponatremic and develop signs of circulatory overload resulting in convulsions, coma, and even death.

Intravenous bolus injections of oxytocin relax the smooth muscle vasculature, resulting in severe maternal hypotension and tachycardia. Bolus injections may also result in an increase in cardiac output and/or venous return, and produce electrocardiogram changes associated with cardiac ischemia. These cardiac effects are especially dangerous in women with valvular heart disease and in those who are hemorrhaging. For these reasons, oxytocin is diluted before administration, especially after the delivery of the placenta.

A risk to the fetus that can occur from the use of oxytocin is hyperbilirubinemia. Hyperbilirubinemia occurs in the neonate from the frequently overworked hepatic system responding to the breakdown of increased red blood cells. There are a variety of factors that contribute to the etiology of hyperbilirubinemia, including Rh or ABO incompatibilities, maternal infections, fetal hypothermia, perinatal asphyxia, and prolonged administration of oxytocin during labor. Neonates who are exposed to oxytocin during labor are 1.6 times more likely to develop hyperbilirubinemia than those neonates who are not exposed to oxytocin (American Society of Hospital Pharmacists, 1990). This occurs because of the fetal hypoxia from excessive uterine contractions often seen with labors induced with oxytocin (Gilbert & Harmon, 1993). Hyperbilirubinemia is the rapid destruction of fetal erythrocytes caused from osmotic swelling. This side effect is more pronounced when the patient receives an increased amount of oxytocin, such as happens in prolonged inductions.

ASSESSMENT

Fetal maturity should be assessed prior to the induction of labor unless the benefits of induction outweigh the risks of prematurity. Methods used to determine fetal maturity include assessment of the amniotic fluid for L/S ratio and analysis of phosphatidylglycerol (PG). The L/S ratio is the most valuable test for the assessment of fetal lung maturity (Gabbe, 1987). Values of 2.0 or greater indicate pulmonary maturity.

Prior to the beginning of induction, a vaginal exam to determine cervical status is performed by a qualified registered nurse, certified nurse midwife, or physician. The Bishop score can be used to evaluate the cervical preparedness for induction by evaluating the cervical dilation, effacement, consistency, position, and station of the fetal presenting part. A Bishop score of 5 or greater represents a cervix that is favorable to induction (Display 10-1).

It is important to know the fetal presentation or the part of the fetus that will be delivered first. This can be determined by vaginal exam, Leopold's maneuvers, or ultrasound.

Fetal status is determined by evaluating a number of factors including the presence of variability, whether the fetal heart rate pattern is reassuring or nonreassuring, and the presence or absence of decelerations. Variability is assessed in two forms: long-term (LTV) and short-term (STV). LTV is described as absent, minimal, moderate, or marked. STV is described as being absent or present. Fetal heart rate patterns are considered reassuring when accelerations are present in response to contractions or fetal movement. Nonreassuring fetal heart rate patterns include variable decelerations that fall below 90 beats per minute (bpm), and have a loss of variability between contractions, the presence of late decelerations, or prolonged decelerations that fall below 90 bpm for 2–10 minutes. At least 20 minutes of tracing via electronic fetal monitoring should be obtained and evaluated prior to induction (Gilbert & Harmon, 1993).

It is important to assess the baseline fetal heart rate. Although the normal fetal heart rate is 120–160 beats per minute, each fetus must be assessed individually. A preterm fetus may have a baseline fetal heart rate in the high normal range due to the immaturity of the parasympathetic nervous system. This immaturity also accounts for the decreased variability seen in the preterm fetus. The postterm fetus may have a decreased baseline fetal heart rate such as 110–120 beats per minute, which reflects maturity of the parasympathetic nervous system. As long as nonreassuring patterns are absent and the rate remains stable, this lower baseline may be normal for this fetus.

DISPLAY 10-1

Bishop Score				
Factor	Score 0	Score 1	Score 2	Score 3
Cervical dilation (cm)	Closed	1–2	3–4	5+
Cervical effacement (%)	0–30	40–50	60–70	80+
Fetal station	–3	–2	–1	0, +1
Cervical consistency	Firm	Medium	Soft	
Cervical position	Posterior	Midposition	Anterior	

Assessing the fetal response to uterine activity includes an assessment of the variability and periodic and nonperiodic heart rate changes. It is important to remember that variability indicates how the fetus is able to tolerate stress; therefore, it is the most useful indicator of fetal status. There are several factors that attribute to the changes of variability of the fetal heart rate including fetal sleep patterns, maternal infection, gestational age, and the use of drugs such as narcotics, barbituates, or other drugs that depress the central nervous system.

Uterine blood flow is normally impeded with labor contractions. However, if a labor stimulant causes an increase in frequency, intensity, or duration of contractions, the uterine blood flow can be further impeded, resulting in a nonreassuring fetal heart rate pattern.

It is also important for the obstetrician to determine the maternal pelvic type because different pelvic types may have different effects on the progress of labor. The four pelvic types are gynecoid, android, anthropoid, and platypelloid. The gynecoid pelvis is present in 50% of all women. It is most favorable to normal labor due to its transversely round shape. The android pelvis is present in 23% of all women. Its heart shape contributes to the fetal head engaging in the transverse or posterior position, therefore increasing the need for forceps to rotate and deliver the fetus (Petrie & Williams, 1993). The anthropoid pelvis with its oval shape often causes the fetal head to present in the occiput posterior position. This pelvic type is present in 24% of all women. The platypelloid pelvis is present in 3% of all women and the fetus is usually delivered by cesarean section because of the flat and widely transverse appearance of the pelvis.

Baseline maternal vital signs should be obtained and assessed prior to induction of labor, along with baseline lab values such as a complete blood count and blood type and antibody screen. The initial assessment should also include an emotional assessment of the level of coping of the patient and significant others. From this information, a nursing diagnosis can be established and a plan of care formulated. The nurse determines if there are any knowledge deficits and answers all questions, explains all

procedures, and relieves fears and anxieties as appropriate. Many patients believe that induced labor causes stronger, more severe contractions. The patient should understand that spontaneous labor begins with irregular, mild contractions that slowly progress into active labor, allowing the patient to cope with the gradually increasing intensity of uterine contractions. However, with induced labor, the patient may go from absence of discomfort to strong, active labor in a relatively short period of time (Petrie & Williams, 1993). Any information given to the patient must be relayed on her level of understanding.

Risks and contraindications to labor induction or augmentation and/or vaginal delivery are also an important part of the assessment, and must be communicated as appropriate to the physician.

STAFFING

As recommended by the American College of Obstetricians and Gynecologists (ACOG), any hospital that provides labor and delivery services should be equipped to perform an emergency cesarean section within 30 minutes of the time the decision is made to operate. The facilities need to be readily available, as do the hospital personnel including nursing, anesthesia, a neonatal resuscitation team and an obstetrician (AAP & ACOG, 1988).

Display 10-2 illustrates the recommended nurse–patient ratios. Patient acuity, types of delivery, skill levels of staff, anesthetic choice, and other variables can alter the recommended ratios and are important to remember when making assignments.

PROTOCOLS RELATED TO PREPARATION AND ADMINISTRATION OF OXYTOCIN

The Association of Women's Health, Obstetric, and Neonatal Nurses (AWHONN) recommends that each institution have written policies, procedures, and protocols related to the preparation and administration of oxytocin. These are written by both nursing and medical staff incor-

DISPLAY 10-2

Staffing Ratio	Care Provided
1:1	Patients in second stage of labor
	Ill patients with complications
	Coverage of anesthesia
	Circulation for cesarean delivery
	Newborns requiring multisystem support
	Newborns needing intensive care
	Antepartum testing
1:2	Antepartum testing
	Laboring patients
	Oxytocin induction or augmentation of labor
	Postoperative recovery
	Newborns needing intensive care
1:3	Patients with complications but stable condition
	Mother–newborn care
	Newborns requiring intermediate care
1:3	Recently born infants and those needing close observation
	Newborns requiring intermediate care
1:6	Antepartum/postpartum patients without complications
	Newborns needing only routine care

porating the national standard of care, current nursing, and medical practice acts, and reflecting a reasonable practice for any given institution (AWHONN, 1993).

Written protocols should be in compliance with state nursing practice acts. They should include information reflecting indications, contraindications, potential complications, criteria for evaluating the patient, steps in preparing the infusion, starting dosages, dosing increments, time intervals between dose increments, monitoring parameters for both mother and fetus, and finally, physician and nursing responsibilities (Brodsky & Pelzar, 1991).

The initial dose of oxytocin varies and is different for induction or augmentation. Currently, the initial dose recommendation for induction is between 0.5 mU/min and 3 mU/min. For augmentation, the initial dose ranges from 0.5 mU/min to 6 mU/min (Owen & Hauth, 1992).

Dosing increments can be added (arithmetic), doubled (geometric), or a combination of both (Owen & Hauth, 1992). Dosing intervals are based on two theories. The first theory is related to the half-life of oxytocin, which is approximately 10 minutes. This is the basis for a dosing interval of 15 minutes. The second theory postulates that it takes approximately 40 minutes for oxytocin to reach a steady state of plasma concentration, therefore providing the basis for a 30–60 minute dosing interval (Seitchik, 1987). Based on several studies that have been conducted, the literature reports that the longer dosing interval theory comes closest to achieving the goal of minimizing side effects (fetal distress, uterine hyperstimulation), using the lowest dose possible, and maximizing the opportunity for a safe vaginal delivery in the shortest time (Lazor et al., 1993).

Uterine activity is assessed every 15 minutes for frequency, intensity, and duration of contractions along with uterine resting tone. Contractions that are less than 2 minutes apart and greater than 90 seconds in duration are considered hyperstimulation. A uterine resting tone of greater than 20 mmHg by an intrauterine pressure catheter is also considered hyperstimulation. In the event of hyperstimulation, the oxytocin infusion should be discontinued, the patient placed in a lateral position (left lateral position preferred), oxygen administered, and the obstetrician or certified nurse midwife notified. The oxytocin should be restarted at a lower dose only after reevaluation of the fetal heart rate pattern and uterine activity.

The potential for water intoxication exists, especially in those patients who undergo prolonged induction or in those patients who receive high doses of oxytocin. Signs and symptoms of water intoxication include headache, nausea, vomiting, mental confusion, decreased urinary output, hypotension, tachycardia, and cardiac arrhythmias. To prevent water intoxication the nurse should decrease the total amount of intravenous fluids used and prepare the oxytocin by double strengthening it in a balanced salt solution such as lactated Ringers or 0.9% sodium chloride.

NURSING CARE OF THE PATIENT UNDERGOING INDUCTION OR AUGMENTATION OF LABOR

The following is a checklist of key points to remember in caring for the patients undergoing induction or augmentation of labor.

1. Ensure that a physician who has privileges to perform a cesarean section is readily available (American Academy of Pediatrics & ACOG, 1992).
2. Assess cervical effacement and dilation before beginning the oxytocin infusion (may be performed by the qualified registered nurse or physician).
3. Assess the patient's and the support persons' (or persons') understanding of induction or augmentation, providing appropriate education and reassurance as needed.
4. Prepare oxytocin intravenous solution (usually 10 U/1,000 ml) using a physiologic electrolyte-containing solution.

5. Establish a primary line for infusion of a non-oxytocin-containing intravenous maintenance solution.
6. Connect secondary line with oxytocin solution into the proximal port of the primary intravenous line to avoid a bolus dose of oxytocin should the primary line's rate be increased.
7. Use an infusion pump to ensure accuracy of the oxytocin intravenous solution flow rate.
8. Position the patient to avoid vena-caval compression.
9. Monitor uterine contractions and fetal heart rate through continuous fetal monitoring. Prior to the start of induction, a 20-minute baseline fetal monitoring strip is usually recommended.
10. Follow policy, procedure, and protocol established by the institution. If the physician requests deviation from the institution's policy, procedure, or protocol, ensure that the physician writes the order.
11. Assess intake and output. Ensure documentation is accurate and clear.
12. At a minimum, assess uterine contractions, fetal heart rate, and maternal blood pressure before every dosage increase. Other factors such as stage of labor, maternal and fetal risk factors, and institution policy, procedure, and protocol also must be taken into consideration when determining frequency of assessments.

NURSING CARE OF THE PATIENT UNDERGOING RAPID AUGMENTATION

Rapid augmentation or active management of labor was first studied in Ireland and proposed as a strategy to decrease the cesarean births secondary to dystocia. The goal is to establish efficient labor and deliver the fetus within 12 hours of admission. Rapid augmentation differs from other augmentation options by a higher initial dosage of oxytocin. For a woman to be a candidate for rapid augmentation of labor, all of the following criteria must be met: nulliparity, gestation of 37 weeks or greater, a single fetus in no distress, and the diagnosis of spontaneous labor (AWHONN, 1993).

A patient is admitted to the hospital once a diagnosis of spontaneous labor is established. Spontaneous labor is defined as the presence of regular, painful contractions every 5 minutes associated with the complete effacement of the cervix or the spontaneous rupture of membranes (Lopez-Zeno et al., 1992). Amniotomy is performed 2 hours after admission if the membranes remain intact. If cervical dilation is less than 1 cm per hour, oxytocin augmentation may be considered. The dosing protocol for rapid augmentation involves starting the oxytocin at 6 mU/min. The dosing increment and interval would be 6 mU/min every 15 minutes until 7 contractions occur within a 15-minute period or an infusion rate of 36–40 mU/min is reached (AWHONN, 1993).

CASE EXAMPLES

Lawsuits that arise out of complications from use of pitocin almost always involve severely brain-damaged children and occasionally involve maternal death. Because these severely brain-damaged children have astronomic medical care needs both at birth and throughout their lives, these lawsuits consistently result in jury verdicts of several million dollars.

A 22-year-old primigravida was admitted to the labor suite at 39 weeks gestation with spontaneous rupture of membranes 18 hours prior to admission. The fetal heart rate was 136, vital signs were stable (afebrile), and the patient exhibited no signs of labor. The nurse began an elective induction after the patient's cervix was examined and found to be a fingertip dilated.

The physician ordered the oxytocin to be increased by 30 mU every 15 minutes. The nurse increased the oxytocin as ordered. Frequent contractions and an obvious decrease in the long-term variability of the fetal heart rate were noted 2 hours later. The staff continued to increase the oxytocin infusion every 15 minutes despite tetanic contractions. The oxytocin was doubled 5 hours after the start of the induction. A fetal scalp electrode was placed and the tocodynamometer was removed and never reapplied.

Within a 20-minute period the oxytocin was decreased, stopped, and restarted along with documentation showing several maternal position changes. The fetal scalp electrode showed diminished short-term variability.

A female neonate with Apgar scores of 2 and 5 was delivered 16 hours and 30 minutes after the oxytocin induction was started.

The expert's opinion found the nursing care to be far below the standard of care of an average obstetrical nurse for the following reasons:

a. failing to adequately monitor fetal status
b. failing to question oxytocin orders
c. administering oxytocin in excessive amounts
d. failing to recognize a side effect of oxytocin and utilize appropriate interventions
e. failing to follow protocols outlined by AWHONN.

The expert also stated that the nursing care was a proximate cause of the asphyxiation and the outcome was preventable.

An out-of-court settlement was reached in which the plaintiff was awarded a substantial amount of money to care for the severely handicapped child (McRae, 1993).

A second case involves a gravida 4 para 3. The woman was at a routine prenatal checkup 4 days prior to her due date, when upon examination, she complained of experiencing a decrease in fetal movement. A nonstress test was performed to evaluate the fetal status. The results were "questionably nonreactive" and the woman was admitted to the hospital for observation.

At 4:30 PM, the chief resident on duty concluded from examination that the patient was a candidate for Pitocin augmentation. He felt the patient to be in prodromal labor because she was experiencing contractions every five to six minutes and her cervix had already begun to efface and dilate. The chief resident presented his findings to the attending physician, and approval was obtained to begin the Pitocin infusion.

The intravenous infusion of Pitocin was started at 5:00 PM. The initial infusion was ordered to be 4 drops per minute. It was also ordered that the infusion be increased by 2 drops every 10 minutes until an adequate labor pattern was established.

The infusion was continued for 8½ hours until being discontinued at 1:30 AM when the patient's contractions had reached a frequency of one per minute. The hospital records fail to indicate the total amount of Pitocin the patient received, or whether the infusion was at all modified during the 8½-hour administration period. The records did show that at approximately 12:30 AM, the patient was uncooperative, restless, and screaming with contractions.

Within 15 minutes of discontinuing the Pitocin infusion, the patient's contractions resumed at a normal rate of 1 every 2–3 minutes. This pattern continued until the fetus experienced bradycardia at approximately 4:00 AM. Because of the unacceptably low level of the fetal heart rate, it was determined that a caesarean section was necessary.

As the patient was being prepped for surgery, she began to experience convulsions, followed by respiratory arrest. She began to hemorrhage, and suffered a heart attack. CPR was performed for two hours unsuccessfully, and the patient was pronounced dead at 6:00 AM.

The plaintiff's medical expert witness testified that Pitocin was contraindicated because the fetal head was unengaged and still floating in the patient's uterus when the Pitocin infusion was initiated. He also stated that Pitocin is a very potent drug that must be carefully monitored while in use. The records clearly indicated that the patient was not adequately monitored and as a result, received an excessive dosage of Pitocin. The records also show no indication of the patient's status between the hours of 12:30 and 1:30 AM, the time that her contractions became severe.

The jury found in favor of the plaintiff for a principal sum of $1.25 million ($400,000 for conscious pain and suffering and $850,000 for wrongful death).

STRATEGIES TO MINIMIZE RISK

Strategies to minimize liability risks of caring for a patient undergoing induction or augmentation of labor include attaining nursing competencies, utilizing appropriate and timely interventions, accurate documentation, and the proper use of the chain of command.

Competency is the professional standard of care required by an average member of that profession with a similar background under similar circumstances. It is determined and validated by preparation, orientation, and continuing education. Examples of this include being able to mix a solution appropriately, such as oxytocin, or being able to obtain an adequate nursing history. In addition to knowing the pharmacokinetics of oxytocin and its potential dose-related effects, the labor and delivery nurse should have a thorough knowledge base of the normal physiology of labor, its complications, and an established competency of fetal monitoring (Brodsky & Pelzar, 1991). The nurse has the responsibility to follow written protocols, question orders, and refuse to administer oxytocin if contraindications exist.

Risk management is identifying risks and establishing preventative practices to avoid the identified risks. Quality assurance is a form of risk management that reviews and evaluates client care to determine if it meets the standard of care. If standards are not met, policies and protocols should be reviewed and changes made to ensure that the care received by patients meets or exceeds the recommended standards (Harris, 1993). Peer review, chart review, and performance evaluations are all forms of quality assurance.

Risk management has three main goals. The primary goal is to reduce the number and severity of patient, employee, and visitor injuries. The second goal is to ensure adequate documentation of the care given to patients so that adequate defense can be obtained should a professional liability claim be initiated. The third goal of risk management is to protect the health care provider and institution against financial loss by ensuring availability of adequate liability insurance (Cohn, 1990).

It is also important to utilize appropriate and timely nursing interventions. For example, in the event of hyperstimulation, was the oxytocin infusion stopped, patient's position changed, oxygen administered, physician notified, and oxytocin restarted at the appropriate dose after reevaluation of the fetal heart rate and uterine activity?

In order for documentation to provide accurate communication among health care providers it must be accurate, objective, and comprehensive (Harris, 1993). To ensure accurate documentation one must remember that the fetal monitor tracing is considered a legal part of the medical record and therefore should contain the patient's identifying information and times and events related to ongoing patient care. It is also important to record any maternal and fetal response to all interventions. If oxytocin is administered, it needs to be documented on the medication record, the fetal monitoring strip, and in the nurse's notes.

Although the use of abbreviations in charting are generally not desirable, they have become a time-saving device. Staff needs to make sure they are conforming to hospital policy when using abbreviations and to avoid using obscure abbreviations (Cohn, 1990).

The hospital is responsible for providing a chain of command policy that is clear and allows the nurse to use it without fear or penalty. The chain of command works only if used. The nurse has a duty to be a patient advocate; therefore, assertiveness is required to use the chain of command. Most hospital chains of command indicate that the nurse should first speak with his or her own immediate supervisor, then the house nursing supervisor, then the director of nursing, then the physician head of the department. An example of when the nurse should initiate the chain of command would be when the nurse is providing care to a patient who is receiving oxytocin for augmentation/induction. The fetal monitor strip shows minimal long-term variability at best. The fetus develops late decelerations and the contraction pattern is showing contractions less than two minutes apart. Intrauterine resuscitation measures are initiated that include discontinuing the oxytocin. The physician is notified and arrives to view the strip. After reviewing the strip, the physician orders the nurse to restart the oxytocin. The nurse confers with the physician outside the patient's room and the physician insists the nurse restart the oxytocin. The chain of command should now be implemented.

Another example would be when the nurse is providing care to a patient whose fetal monitor strip is nonreassuring. The nurse notifies the physician of his or her interpretation of the strip and the physician does not come to assess the strip. The nurse has communicated with the physician several times via the telephone but the physician has not responded to the nurse's request to come view the strip. The nurse's next step is to implement the chain of command.

CONCLUSION

The induction/augmentation of labor is a practice that is being managed by registered nurses. The nurse performing the induction/augmentation must be proficient in performing the required skills and must have additional educational preparation in this area. Competency must be demonstrated and documented. The employing institution has an obligation to provide continuing education so that the nurse in this role keeps current with the rapidly changing medical practices and advances to ensure that safe and effective care is being given to patients.

REFERENCES

American College of Obstetrics and Gynecology (1995). Dynstocia and the augmentation of labor. (Technical Bulletin No. 218). Washington, DC: Author.

American College of Obstetrics and Gynecology (1995). Induction of labor. (Technical Bulletin No. 217). Washington, DC: Author.

Association of Women's Health, Obstetric, and Neonatal Nurses. (1993). AWHONN practice resource-cervical ripening and induction and augmentation of labor. Washington, DC: AWHONN.

Bobak, I. (1993). Essential factors and processes of labor. Maternity and gynecologic care: The nurses and the family (pp. 352–360). St. Louis, MO: Mosby.

Brodsky, P., & Pelzar, E. (1991, November/December). Rationale for the revision of oxytocin administration protocols. Journal of Obstetrical, Gynecological, and Neonatal Nursing, 440–444.

Cohn, S. D. (1990). Risk Prevention and management. Malpractice and liability in clinical obstetrical nursing (pp. 1–20). Rockville, Maryland: Aspen.

Gabbe, S. (1987). Amniotic fluid indices of maturity. Protocols for high risk pregnancies (pp. 54–60). NJ: Medical Economics Co.

Gilbert, E., & Harmon, J. (1993). Labor stimulation. <u>Manual of high risk pregnancy and delivery</u> (pp. 528–546). St. Louis, MO: Mosby.

Harris, C. (1997). Legal and ethical issues. In Lowdermilk et al., Maternity and Women's Health. St. Louis, MO: Mosby.

Hayshi, R., & Castillo, M. (1993). Bleeding in pregnancy. <u>High risk pregnancy: A team approach</u> (2nd ed., pp. 539–560). Philadelphia: W. B. Saunders.

Keller-Bronte, C. (1986). Normal and dysfunctional labor, <u>Nursing management of uncomplicated and complicated births</u> (pp. 1–43). East Hanover, NJ: Medical Media Associates.

Lazor, L. Z., Philipson, E. H., Ingardia, C. J., Kobetitsch, E. S. & Curry, S. L. (1993). A randomized comparison of 15- and 40-minute dosing protocols for labor augmentation and induction. <u>Obstetrics & Gynecology, 82,</u> 1009–1012.

Lopez-Zeno, J. A., Peaceman, A. M., Adashek, J. A., & Socol, M. L. (1992). A controlled trial of a program for the active management of labor. <u>The New England Journal of Medicine, 326,</u> 450–453.

Lowdermilk, D., Perry, S., & Bobak, I. (1997). Labor and birth at risk. Maternity and Women's Health (pp. 1046–1081). St. Louis, MO: Mosby.

Marshall, C. (1985, January/February). The art of induction/augmentation of labor. <u>Journal of Obstetrical, Gynecological, and Neonatal Nursing,</u> 22–26.

McRae, M. J. (1993). Litigation, electronic fetal monitoring, and the obstetric nurse. <u>Journal of Obstetric, Gynecologic, and Neonatal Nursing, 22,</u> 410–419.

Owen, J., & Hauth, J. C. (1992). Oxytocin for the induction or augmentation of labor. <u>Clinical Obstetrics and Gynecology, 35,</u> 464–475.

Petrie, R., & Williams, A. (1993). Induction of labor. <u>High risk pregnancy: A team approach</u> (pp. 303–315). Philadelphia: W. B. Saunders.

Sokol, R. (1987). Dysfunctional labor. <u>Protocols for high risk pregnancies</u> (pp. 360–365). Oradell, NJ: Medical Economics Co.

Sweeten, K., Graves, W., & Athanassiou, A. (1995). Spontaneous rupture of the unscarred uterus. <u>American Journal of Obstetrics and Gynecology,</u> June, 1851–1856.

Vogler, J. (1993). First stage of labor: Maternity and gynecologic care. <u>The nurse and the family</u> (pp. 422–465). St. Louis, MO: Mosby.

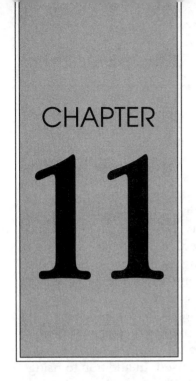

CHAPTER 11

Care of the Neonate: Nursery, Resuscitation, and Transfer Issues

Kimberly E. Carr

For most families, the birth of a newborn is one of the happiest times in their lives. Many days are spent in anticipation of the event and there are great expectations for the child. Whereas admitting a sick relative to the hospital may bring feelings of fear and uncertainty, families plan for an uncomplicated birth of a normal newborn with no surprises of unexpected outcomes. The expectation of a routine delivery and a healthy newborn intensifies the reaction to unforeseen events.

Cases involving children can be very expensive for a variety of reasons. Emotional ties cause parents to be very sensitive regarding actions that affect their children. Juries see infants and young children as being less able to care for themselves than adult patients, and children who suffer permanent disability are often awarded large settlements (Calfee, 1993). Because of their small size, newborns are at greater risk when medication or intravenous fluid errors are made than are adult patients whose body size may be able to tolerate a miscalculation. Nurses who care for newborns must be aware of the standards of care of this special population and how deviation from these standards place the nurse at risk for liability.

STANDARDS OF CARE

Standards of care can be broken down into two categories: internal and external. Internal standards of care are those written by the hospital and include the nurse's job description and the hospital's policies and procedures. External standards of care include those set by state boards of nursing, professional organizations, specialty nursing organizations, federal organizations, and federal guidelines (Guido, 1997). Standards of care specific to nursery practice have been published by the American Academy of Pediatrics; the American College of Obstetricians and Gynecologists; the Association of Women's Health, Obstetric, and Neonatal Nurses; and the National Association of Neonatal Nurses. Nurses are responsible for keeping up with changes that occur over time.

The Association of Women's Health, Obstetric, and Neonatal Nurses (or AWHONN, formerly The Nurse's Association of the American College of Obstetricians and Gynecologists or NAACOG) identifies three standards specifically related to neonatal care:

Standard I: Nursing Practice

Comprehensive neonatal nursing care focuses on helping newborns, families, and communities achieve their optimum health potential. This is best achieved within the framework of the nursing process.

This standard focuses on promoting the health of the newborn and family. Nursing interventions are aimed at supporting the newborn through transition to life and integration into the family unit. Health and social risks are anticipated and planned for. Alterations in physiological functions are assessed and managed.

Standard II: Health Education and Counseling

Health education for the newborn, family, and community is an integral part of comprehensive nursing care. It encourages participation and shared responsibility for health promotion, maintenance, and restoration.

Health education issues include newborn care, health promotion issues, signs of illness, adolescent parenting and family dynamics, perinatal loss, and information on follow-up care.

Standard III: Policies, Procedures, and Protocols

Written policies, procedures, and protocols clarify the scope of nursing practice and delineate the qualifications of personnel authorized to provide care to the newborn within the health-care setting.

A summary of suggested policies, procedures, and protocols for neonatal care is listed in Appendix 11-1 (NAACOG, 1991). AWHONN's publication *Standards for the Nursing Care of Women and Newborns* details nursing practices related to these standards, which serve as a reference for policy, procedure, and protocol development; educational programing; and short- and long-range planning.

LIABILITY IN THE NURSERY

Guido (1997) describes changes within hospitals in the last 30 years that require nurses to have increased accountability and responsibility. These changes as applied to the nursery nurse recognize the special training and skills needed to care for newborns at birth, during the transition to extrauterine life, and in the postnatal period. In an intensive care setting, the changes involve using advanced nursing knowledge, technology, and equipment. Failure to keep current, failure to adequately supervise and staff, and failure to communicate concerns and problems to the appropriate health care personnel place the nurse at risk for liability.

In the past 30 years nursing has evolved from a practice of step-by-step policies and procedures to a science of assessment, planning, intervention, and evaluation. Along with integrating thought and judgment into patient care, technological changes challenge today's nurses (Driscoll, 1993). The professional nurse is responsible for keeping up with changes in her field. For the nursery nurse, this may involve reading current specialty journals, attending conferences, attending inservices related to new technology, and being involved in specialty organizations. Staying abreast of current standards of practice reduces the risk of liability.

As the health care marketplace changes, hospitals are forced to examine the way in which nursing resources are used. In addition to using unlicensed personnel supervised by registered nurses, hospitals cross-train staff so that they can work in more than one area. These strategies can be very effective in saving money as well as being challenging and rewarding for nurses who want to increase their skills and have variety in their workplace. However, the hospital must provide adequate, competent staff. *Northern Trust Co. v. Weiss Memorial Hospital* (1986) illustrates the importance of providing appropriately trained, adequate staff.

On September 23, 1970, Donna Collins was born after a normal pregnancy and labor. At delivery the amniotic fluid was noted to contain copious meconium. Her Apgar scores were 7 at 1 minute and 10 at 5 minutes. However, her cry was noted as weak and her color slightly bluish. The physician ordered that she be placed in an isolette containing oxygen and transferred to the newborn nursery—a "well baby" nursery.

Over the next 18 hours Donna had worsening respiratory distress with a respiratory rate of up to 150, increased temperature, vomiting, and duskiness. Nurse A cared for Donna on the 11:00 PM to 7:00 AM shift. Nurse A did not notify the physician until 6:00 AM of Donna's worsening condition. The physician arrived at 8:15 AM to examine Donna and arrange for transport to a children's hospital. By this time Donna had already suffered brain damage from inadequate oxygen.

Nurse A recalled that she had approximately 5 weeks of training in nursing school related to newborn care. She had been employed at Weiss Hospital for approximately 3 months and had split her time between the nursery, postpartum, and labor and delivery areas. She had no choice of where she would work.

The jury returned a $1.5 million dollar verdict against the hospital for failure to provide an appropriately trained professional nurse to supervise the nursery, which led to the developmental disability of a newborn. The hospital appealed, claiming that its staffing failure did not cause the injury. However, the verdict was upheld (Calfee, 1993).

Nurse A may have protected herself from the risk of liability by recognizing that she did not have the proper training to care for this infant. This child was clearly a patient that was not in the scope of practice of a "well baby" nursery and needed more supervision than could be offered by Nurse A. Nurse A should have communicated these concerns to her supervisor both verbally and in writing. Further, Nurse A failed to communicate the worsening condition of the infant to the physician until approximately 7 hours had passed.

It is the nurse's responsibility to inform a supervisor if he or she does not feel adequately prepared to carry out an assignment (Northrop, 1987). Nurses who lack proper education, experience, or training to handle a particular patient population, volume of patients, or piece of equipment should notify their supervisor both orally and in writing. It then becomes the supervisor's responsibility to solve the problem. Soliciting the help of others or requesting additional resources when faced with an unfamiliar or overwhelming situation protects the nurse as well as the patient. A $125,000 settlement was reached in the wrongful death of a premature infant in *Clark v. University of Washington* (1984). A newborn was delivered at 30 weeks gestation and had respiratory difficulties. During the next four days the newborn had major spells of apnea that went untreated. This resulted in brain damage and eventually death. The plaintiff charged that the nurses were improperly trained and supervised and failed to medically manage the neonate and respond to his apnea (Northrop & Kelly, 1987).

In addition to communicating with a supervisor about concerns, the professional nurse is responsible for communicating with other hospital team members, physicians, and families. Pertinent observations and information about the plan of care must be passed from one nurse to the next to provide continuity of care. Physicians must be notified of abnormal vital signs, symptoms of disease, lab values, and other pertinent patient information. Families should be kept up to date about the plan of care for their newborn and given sufficient information to care for their newborn after discharge. Communication is both oral and written. Legible, clear records of observations, plans, interventions, and evaluations as well as records of oral conversations with other health care providers and patients is one of the best ways to reduce the nurse's liability.

The use of unlicensed personnel in the health care setting is increasing. Unlicensed personnel require supervision by a professional nurse. The responsible nurse must know each team member's capabilities and corroborate data gathered by the unlicensed person. The professional nurse, not the unlicensed caregiver, is responsible for planning and evaluation of interventions for patient care.

ASSESSMENT OF NURSING COMPETENCY

Certification

Licensure is governmental recognition that a person has the minimal skills and education to practice general nursing. Licensure is required by each state in order to practice as a professional nurse. Certification is recognition by a nongovernmental body that a person has advanced education, experience, and skills in a specific area. With a few exceptions, certification in a specific area of nursing is voluntary and not required by the institution in order to work in a specialty unit. The purpose of both licensure and certification is to protect the public from unsafe nursing care. Certification may allow the nurse to escape potential liability by demonstrating that the nurse has the expertise to make necessary decisions and care for patients in the nursery or intensive care nursery areas (Guido, 1997).

Certification for low-risk neonatal nurses is offered through the National Certification Corporation for the Obstetric, Gynecologic, and Neonatal Nursing Specialties (NCC). Both the NCC and the National Association of Critical Care (AACN) offer certification for intensive care neonatal nurses. Nurses applying to take the certification exam must present proof of state licensure, must have worked a required number of hours in the past few years in the specialty area, and must have had experiences caring for patients with a variety of diagnoses in that specialty area. Formal continuing education related to the specialty is required to maintain certification.

Additional Requirements

The American Academy of Pediatrics and the American Heart Association developed the *Neonatal Resuscitation Program,* an educational program for professionals who are responsible for the newborn at delivery. Many institutions have adopted completion of this program as a requirement for staff members that attend deliveries and require staff to renew their proof of competency every two years. The content is accepted as the standard of care for infant resuscitation across the nation. The Neonatal Resuscitation Program guidelines recommend at least one person trained in resuscitation be at every delivery (Bloom & Cropley, 1994). Nurses consistently attend deliveries although physicians and respiratory therapists may also be present. Nursery nurses who attend deliveries must know and follow the proper procedure to resuscitate a newborn in order to escape liability.

As nursing care has become more technologically focused, states have recognized the need to protect patients from unsafe care. States vary in their requirements, but most states have guidelines that must be followed regarding the practice of invasive procedures. These guidelines may include providing written policies and procedures, providing education and a practice lab, and providing supervised experiences. For the neonatal nurse practicing in an intensive care setting, these invasive procedures may include arterial puncture, placement of percutaneous catheters, placement and removal of umbilical catheters, removal of chest tubes, and needle thoracentesis. Renewal of the nurse's competency at a designated interval protects the patient and provides the nurse with documentation of her skills should those skills ever be questioned.

RISK AREAS

Assessment Factors

Assessment provides the basis for planning, implementing, and evaluating the newborn's plan of care. Although assessment is ongoing, there are three major assessments performed in the neonatal period: at birth, during the first few hours after birth, and prior to discharge (Endo & Nishioka, 1993). The first assessment evaluates the newborn's adaptation from intrauterine to extrauterine life.

The most accepted tool for assessing this transition is the Apgar scoring system. If used properly, the Apgar score assists the practitioner to quickly evaluate the newborn's status, guide the interventions that are necessary, and evaluate the response to the resuscitation. The newborn's heart rate, respiratory effort, color, muscle tone, and reflex response are given a score of 0, 1, or 2 points each for a maximum score of 10. This evaluation occurs at 1 and 5 minutes after birth. Additional scores may be assigned at 5-minute intervals depending on the newborn's response to resuscitation (Letko, 1996). The American Academy of Pediatrics (AAP) and the American College of Obstetricians and Gynecologists (ACOG) recommend obtaining scores until 20 minutes have passed or until two successive scores of 7 or greater are obtained (Freeman & Poland, 1992). A score of 0 represents a newborn with no heart rate or respiratory effort who is cyanotic, hypotonic, and unresponsive. A score of 10 represents a newborn with a good heart and respiratory rate, who is active and pink. Newborns that receive a score between 7 and 10 rarely need any resuscitation. Although scores of 0–3 at 10, 15, or 20 minutes after birth may be predictive of poor outcomes for the newborn, low Apgar scores alone cannot be used to substantiate a claim of birth asphyxia (Letko, 1996). Individual scores for each assessment category (heart rate, respiratory effort, color, muscle tone, and reflex response) and the total scores at 1 and 5 minutes should be documented on each newborn delivery record.

The next examination should be completed within the first 2 hours after birth (Freeman & Poland, 1992). This may take place in the mother's room or in the nursery. This assessment should include a thorough physical examination including color and condition of skin, respiratory status, heart and circulation, abdomen, head, eyes, mouth, nose, ears, neck, trunk, chest, back, anogenital area, and extremities. Reflexes are also checked. Newborns who are particularly small or large or are the newborn of a diabetic mother should have a blood glucose analysis. An evaluation of gestational age should also be completed. Information obtained from the gestational age assessment allows the nurse to anticipate problems in newborns who are evaluated and found to be premature regardless of weight or due date.

Families are often present during this assessment and should be encouraged to learn more about their newborn. If deformities are noted or the newborn's condition is deteriorating, the family should be reassured that the newborn will be thoroughly evaluated and treated. The nurse is responsible for keeping the family informed of the nursing plan of care and the necessary interventions. Families who remain involved and informed may be less likely to feel that the staff is hiding something and less likely to pursue legal action in the event of an unexpected outcome.

The last major assessment is just prior to discharge. An accurate weight should be obtained and a physical exam completed. The newborn's ability to breastfeed or bottle feed and bladder and bowel function are assessed. The family's ability to care for the newborn is also assessed. The information is recorded in the chart and verifies that the newborn was ready for discharge or identifies risk areas that may need referral to and follow-up by community practitioners.

In addition to these three major assessments, ongoing evaluation of the newborn's status is vital. The AAP and ACOG recommend that a newborn be monitored (temperature, heart and respiratory rates, skin color, adequacy of periph-

eral circulation, type of respiration, level of consciousness, tone, and activity) once every 30 minutes until stable for 2 hours. Once stable, the newborn must be monitored at the time interval set by the institutional policy. Documentation should include the data collected at each assessment and any special circumstances of problems noted. Interventions to correct the problems or the need for further assessment should also be documented. Newborns who are premature or admitted to an intensive care area will require more frequent monitoring.

Assessment data should be recorded in the chart in a standardized way. Using a systematic format will make documentation easier for the nurse and facilitate communication of the information to other practitioners. A standardized form may also remind nurses to record information that is required by hospital policies. For example, Hospital A has a policy that requires the IV site in an infant be checked every 2 hours. By creating a standardized form with a particular area for charting that information, compliance with the policy will be increased because the nurse will be reminded to enter the observation on the chart.

Problems that require immediate intervention must be communicated to the physician and this communication must be documented in the record. Failure to report assessment data that are abnormal or represent changes in condition not only places the patient at risk but also increases the liability of the nurse. If the physician fails to return the call or respond to the situation, the nurse should follow the chain of command to obtain assistance in caring for the newborn. In the case of *Harris v. Screech* (1985), physicians as well as nurses were found negligent in failing to observe increased head circumference and failure to recognize and treat signs and symptoms of intracranial bleeding. The newborn was delivered by forceps, which was contraindicated in this birth due to a family history of hemophilia. A bulging fontanelle, which may indicate intracranial hemorrhage, was noted on the initial exam. No treatment was given until three days later when the newborn was found seizing. He suffered mental retardation, partial blindness, deafness in the right ear, and intermittent seizures.

The settlement was $1.86 million (Northrop & Kelly, 1987).

Assessment/Intervention Errors

Interventions fall into three main categories: nursing interventions that do not require a physician's order (independent nursing functions), physician-ordered interventions (interdependent nursing functions), and emergency interventions. Hospital policy, state nurse practice acts, and general nursing practice usually dictate which actions fall into which category. The lack of appropriate interventions or inappropriate nursing interventions place the nurse at increased liability.

Nursing interventions may be directed at many areas of patient care including general nursing care (such as monitoring an IV and placing an extra blanket over a newborn who has a low temperature), safety (such as placing an identifying band on the newborn or making sure the sides of the warmer are raised), comfort (such as offering a pacifier or rocking), and education (such as teaching the family about bathing or breastfeeding). Nursing interventions are planned after assessment data are collected. Assessing the patient and planning nursing interventions are independent functions of nursing and require education, intelligence, and independent decision making. Nursery nurses are expected to individualize the plan of care and interventions to meet patient and family needs while following the standards of nursing practice.

Interventions can range from the complex task of starting an intravenous line to the simple task of communicating a lab result to the physician. There are many interventions that could be considered the ultimate responsibility of the physician but require communication from the nurse to be carried out. For example, the nurse cannot independently provide interventions such as administering dextrose to a newborn who has a low blood sugar. The nurse cannot prescribe an amount of dextrose so he or she must communicate observations to the physician and obtain the order. Then the nurse can complete the intervention by administering the medication. In *Butts v. Cummings* (1985), $2.3 million was awarded to the family of a child who suffered brain damage due to hyperbilirubinemia. At 5 days of age, the newborn had a bilirubin level over 34 mg/100 ml. Jaundice is clinically observable at levels over 10 mg/100 ml. The evidence showed that it would have taken a few days for the level to increase to 34 mg/100 ml and that the probability of brain damage increases as the levels rise. The court found that the nurses were negligent in failing to report the jaundice to the pediatrician (Northop & Kelly, 1987).

Nurses must identify when an intervention is necessary, be able to communicate that need, and decide when an intervention is inappropriate. A nurse can be held liable for carrying out an order that is not a part of usual procedure (Fiesta, 1994). In *Willis v. El Camino Hospital* (1985), a $4.35 million verdict was awarded on behalf of twin boys who were born 9 weeks premature and suffered permanent blindness due to oxygen administration. The boys were given oxygen and although they had abnormally high oxygen levels on the blood gas tests during the first 7 days of oxygen administration, the oxygen was not decreased appropriately. During the last 9 days of oxygen administration the blood gases were not monitored. The jury found that the nurses failed to adhere to protocols for monitoring oxygen levels, to advise the pediatrician that an excessive amount of oxygen was being administered, and to independently decrease the oxygen (Northrop & Kelly, 1987).

Management of emergency situations and neonatal complications must be outlined in hospital policies, procedures, and protocols. Interventions such as administering oxygen to a newborn who is rapidly deteriorating needs to be done in a timely fashion without wasting time by waiting for a physician's order. Many hospitals have standing orders for routine admissions to their nurseries. The AWHONN standards suggest that written procedures should also exist for emergencies such as cardiopulmonary distress and arrest, central nervous system alterations, drug/substance withdrawal, metabolic alterations, respiratory/oxygen therapy initiation, thermal alterations, transfer to an intensive care unit, and emergency diagnostic testing (NAACOG, 1991).

In *Williams v. St. Joseph's Hospital* (1984), Baby Williams was born at 29 weeks gestation and admitted to the nursery at St. Joseph's Hospital. He was treated with continuous oxygen for 38 days and 10 additional nights. Arterial blood gases were never drawn. The infant had severe retinopathy of prematurity thought to be secondary to the continuous oxygen therapy. The jury awarded $2.5 million against the nurses for negligence in continuing oxygen administration without any clinical signs or symptoms justifying its use. The pediatrician was also found negligent in failing to decrease the oxygen and wean the baby to room air (Northrop & Kelly, 1987).

This case demonstrates the necessity of having procedures for interventions such as giving oxygen. Oxygen can also be considered a medication and the nurses failed to recognize the indications for the oxygen and perform appropriate monitoring techniques. If the nurses recognized that the oxygen was being used inappropriately, the physician should have been notified and this notification should have been documented on the chart. Failure of the physician to act would have necessitated following the nursing chain of command to rectify the situation and protect the nurse from liability.

Requiring physicians to write their orders on the order sheet instead of giving them verbally helps to safeguard the nurse against being responsible for the order. Although having the physician present to write all orders is optimal, it is not practical in many instances. Verbal orders may be appropriate in emergency situations. If the physician is present, orders should be written by the physician instead of by the nurse. Repeating telephone orders back to the physician validates what was heard and provides an opportunity for the physician to correct errors. The Joint Commission on Accreditation of Health Care Organizations requires that verbal orders be cosigned by the physician within the time frame defined in the medical staff rules and regulations (JCAHO, 1996). State laws usually require that hospitals' orders be validated and checked for accuracy within 24 hours.

Medication Administration

One of the most frequent interdependent interventions that nurses practice is medication and intravenous fluid administration. Healthy term newborns receive very few medications. However, those newborns who exhibit signs of illness or are born prematurely may be given medications that are lifesaving when administered properly. Because of the newborn's small size, drug dosages that are not accurately calculated can be more harmful than in an adult patient. (See Display 11-1.)

The concept of the "five rights" in drug administration is taught in most basic nursing curriculums. These five rights include the right patient, drug, dose, route, and time. These "rights" are applicable to any patient including the neonate. Each newborn should have an armband attached to a limb that is checked prior to medication administration. In the intensive care setting, armbands are often removed due to IV insertion and to maintain the integrity of the fragile skin in a very premature newborn. The armbands for these newborns should be attached to the warmer or isolette holding the newborn until the newborn is large enough and well enough to have it placed on the arm or leg.

DISPLAY 11-1

Practices to Decrease Neonatal Dosage Errors

Identify the newborn using armband

Verify the drug name

Know the purpose of the drug

Know the proper dose of medication

Verify dose by using a reference book

Double-check the volume and dose with a second nurse prior to administration

Double-check any dose volume over 1.0–1.5 ccs

Know the appropriate route

Give medications in a timely manner

Monitor blood drug levels

Report all medication errors

Nurses should pay special attention to newborns who are products of multiple births or who share common last names. Identifying numbers instead of names can prevent the patient from receiving medications meant for another newborn.

The name of the drug should be read from the vial or label. There are many drugs that are packaged similarly. Grabbing a vial with a purple top does not always ensure that you are getting the drug you intended. Pharmacies may supply the same drug in different packaging. It is the responsibility of the nurse administering the drug to verify that the label reflects the drug that was ordered. The nurse is also responsible for knowing why the drug is being administered and what to monitor after administration. Knowing the purpose for administration of a particular drug can help prevent errors. For example, an order is written for pentobarbital for a term newborn who has been seizing for 10 minutes. The nurse who is familiar with pentobarbital would know that it is a sedative and that the physician probably meant to order phenobarbital. If the pentobarbital had been given, the nurse as well as the physician could have been liable for any harm to the newborn. Although nurses are expected to follow orders, nurses have a duty to question and refuse to follow inappropriate orders.

Neonates come in different sizes ranging from 1½ pounds up to 10 or 12 pounds. Drug dosages are calculated in milligrams of drug per kilogram of body weight to ensure that newborns receive the proper amount. The most common math error made is incorrect positioning of the decimal point so that the child could end up with ten times the desired dose or one tenth of what is needed. Unfortunately, it is more common to give too much than too little. There are several practices that can decrease the chance of making a dosage error. First, the nurse should know the proper dose of the medication that is being given. There are many excellent reference books that give quick, concise information, such as the *Neofax—A Manual of Drugs Used in Neonatal Care* (Young & Mangum, 1996). Next, each drug dosage should be verified by using an accepted reference when the initial order is received. A good time to do this is when the drug is transcribed from the order sheet to the medication administration record. Checking the dose prior to transcribing it will reduce the chance of a wrong dose being given on the assumption that the person who transcribed the order verified the proper dose.

Having two nurses check the medication to make sure the proper dose is drawn up in the syringe is a third safeguard. Neonatal medications often do not come in unit doses from the pharmacy and must be obtained from an ampule, vial, or multidose bottle. In the nursery or intensive care setting another person is usually available who can check the dose and volume calculations. Most neonatal medications are given in volumes of less than 1.0–1.5 cc. A few drugs are exceptions, but any volume that is calculated to be larger than 1.0–1.5 ccs should be double-checked.

Neonatal drugs are given in a variety of ways such as through an endotracheal tube, orally, by oral or nasogastric tube, intravenously, intramuscularly, topically, rectally, and, infrequently, intraarterially. Knowing the appropriate route is a nursing responsibility. Perhaps the most critical time is during resuscitation. Many drugs can be given via the endotracheal tube instead of waiting for an IV insertion. Some drugs such as epinephrine cannot be given intramuscularly because the absorption is too slow to help a compromised newborn and because it causes tissue damage in the muscle. Orders of inappropriate routes should be questioned.

The last of the "five rights" is time. The frequency of the drug administration is ordered by the physician. However, nurses usually determine the actual hour that drugs are administered. Orders should be carried out in a timely fashion and the scheduled time of the drug administration should be adhered to. Occasionally, there is a delay in giving a drug such as when an IV must be restarted. The reason for these delays should be documented.

Some drugs require blood level monitoring. Blood levels of antibiotics, caffeine, aminophylline, digoxin, and anticonvulsants are usually ordered by the physician. It is the nurse's responsibility to see that the blood is drawn at the appropriate time to obtain the appropriate level: peak, trough, or random. The nurse is also responsible for communicating abnormal levels to the physician.

Hospitals have policies for reporting drug errors. The practice of reporting these incidents is not intended to be disciplinary but rather to collect facts surrounding the error while knowledge of what happened is fresh in mind. Following drug errors can provide important data about procedures that may need to be changed in order to prevent future errors. Keeping these reports can also provide factual information during litigation.

Rooming-In

The Interprofessional Task Force on Health Care of Women and Children supports the practice of family-centered newborn care. The Task Force was formed by the American College of Obstetricians and Gynecologists, the American College of Nurse-Midwives, the Association of Women's Health, Obstetric, and Neonatal Nurses, the American Academy of Pediatrics, and the American Nurses' Association. The definition of family-centered care emphasizes giving safe maternity and newborn care while fostering family unity (Phillips, 1996). One model of maternity nursing that promotes family-centered care is "rooming-in." The optimal policy allows 24-hour family/newborn contact with the option of returning newborns to the nursery as needed by the mother. Such a policy allows families to spend time getting to know their newborn but provides a safe place for the newborn if the mother has received sedation, needs to take a shower, or is sick and cannot care for the newborn. Even a febrile postpartum mother may handle and feed her newborn after washing her hands and placing a gown over her clothing if she feels well enough. An exception to rooming-in should be made if the mother has a communicable disease that may be transmitted to the newborn. In this case the mother should be separated from the newborn until the threat of infection is gone (Freeman & Poland, 1992).

Assessment of the newborn is still required even though the newborn may not be in the nursery. The family's observation does not replace the assessment and observation of a professional nurse. This model may provide a challenge to the nursing staff if the physical layout of the unit or the staffing pattern was not planned for rooming-in. The same assessments and procedures required of nurses caring for newborns in the traditional nursery are required for newborns who remain with their family. The advantage of this model is that it provides the nurse with the opportunity to complete patient teaching while the routine work is done. For example, a bath demonstration can be done with the family instead of bathing the newborn in the nursery. Rooming-in also allows the nurse to assess the family/newborn interaction. Education and psychosocial needs can be added to the plan of care.

Educational needs should be met prior to discharge. Areas that only are allowed 24-hour postdelivery stays by insurance companies must be very creative in meeting these needs during such a short stay. Prenatal classes regarding newborn care and breastfeeding may help to fill this need. Families should not be discharged if they have not received basic newborn care instruction including feeding, bathing, diapering, use of the bulb syringe, positioning, and signs of illness. The JCAHO requires that newborns and their families be provided with appropriate education to learn skills and behaviors to promote optimal health (Cahill, 1996).

For the neonate that was born premature, sick, or has complicated health or family problems, more complex discharge planning is required. Patients are being discharged at lower weights and with more involved health care needs than ever before. Discharge planning provides continuity of care and decreases waste and delays in treatment (Dammed, 1991). A discharge plan begun well in advance of the discharge date will protect the nurse and hospital from the liability of sending an unprepared family home to care for a medically fragile newborn. Topics to be included in discharge teaching are listed in Display 11-2 (NAACOG, 1991).

All patient teaching and written materials that are given to the family should be documented in the chart. There should also be documentation that families who must learn skills such as suctioning and ventilator management have

DISPLAY 11-2

Discharge and Home Care Education for the Low-Risk and High-Risk Newborn

Newborn care

Newborn nutrition and feeding practices

Newborn protection and safety

Parenting skills

Infant responses and interaction with others

Family dynamics

Hospital, community, and other resources

Pediatric health promotion and maintenance

Newborn growth and development

Immunizations

Use and maintenance of necessary equipment

Medication administration

Perinatal loss and bereavement

Signs of illness

demonstrated these skills. The most protective documentation of teaching and skill demonstration requires the parent's signature.

Kidnapping

Although rooming-in provides family-centered nursing care and promotes a good teaching environment, it challenges newborn security. Traditional nurseries allow for a nurse to have visual contact with the newborns. Mothers and families with newborns rooming-in are often not familiar with legitimate hospital staff members. Impostors with hospital clothing and name badges may easily be able to take the baby from an unsuspecting family.

Between 1970 and 1980 only one hospital kidnapping was reported. However, between 1983 and 1991, 68 kidnappings were reported. Each year approximately 12 to 18 newborns are abducted from hospitals (Beachy & Deacon, 1992). This is probably a conservative estimate because many attempts at kidnapping are probably not reported. Fortunately, 95% of all newborns who were abducted from hospitals are usually located safely and returned within a few days (Rabun & Lincoln, 1994).

By studying people who have kidnapped newborns in the past, a description of the typical abductor has emerged. Characteristics for nurses to be aware of are set forth in Display 11-3.

John Rabun (1993) of the National Center for Missing and Exploited Children promotes a comprehensive program of hospital policy; teamwork by staff, parents, and security; and electronic security devices. A hospital policy should provide a plan for educating staff and a plan for immediate response to any missing newborn. Staff should be given the profile of the typical abductor, be instructed to report any suspicious people, and be knowledgeable about the procedure to follow in the event that a newborn is missing. Each newborn and parent should be banded with a bracelet identifying that they belong together. Parents need to be instructed to never leave their newborn unattended, even in their room. They also need to be told not to give their newborn to anyone who is not wearing an identification badge. Some hospitals go one step further and mark the identification badges of nursery/maternity staff with a special symbol or color. Parents are told about the special marking and limited hospital employees are permitted access to newborns. Electronic alarms and surveillance equipment are more costly and difficult to implement but may be effective in documenting and deterring abductions. However, the most effective preventative measure is the awareness of staff and parents that there is a potential problem.

Resuscitation

Neonates are more likely than any other age group to require resuscitation (Bloom & Cropley, 1994). One study found that approximately 6% of all neonates require resuscitation (Byrne, Tyebkhan, & Laing, 1995). Of the 30,000 newborns born each year weighing less than

**Characteristics of an
Infant Abductor**

Female

Age 14–48

Often overweight

Frequently unable to conceive or has lost a newborn

Usually is married or living with someone; the significant other's desire to have a child may be a motivating factor

Lives in the community where the abduction occurs

Is a frequent visitor to the nursery and maternity area; may ask questions about procedures and gets information on layout, stairways

Plans the abduction but does not target a specific newborn; takes advantage of whatever opportunity is presented

Impersonates a nurse or other hospital staff member

Is familiar with the hospital staff and maybe even the newborn's parents

Can provide good care for the newborn once she has kidnapped the child

Source: Rabun & Lincoln (1994).

1,500 grams, 80% will require resuscitation. An unknown number of newborns who weigh more than this will also need intervention at birth. The quality of care given during the first few minutes after birth can affect the rest of the newborn's life (Bloom & Cropley, 1994). Necessary equipment and a person skilled in resuscitation must be present at every delivery. A $9 million judgment was awarded against the hospital in *Mather v. Griffin Hospital* (1988) due to the unavailability of appropriate resuscitation equipment and negligence of a nurse employee. The newborn needed intubation and suctioning for respiratory distress at approximately 3 minutes of age. The nurse failed to respond to the physician's request for an appropriate size suction catheter, which led to the need to reintubate the child. When the physician requested a larger endotracheal tube, the same size tube was provided, which led to another intubation. When the newborn was intubated and suctioned, the physician requested an ambu bag but was unable to remove the mask from the bag in order to connect it to the endotracheal tube. The nurse was also unable to remove the mask or provide another ambu bag. By this time the child was very cyanotic and the physician provided respiratory support by blowing air from his mouth into the newborn via the endotracheal tube. During the next few hours the child suffered seizures and was left with developmental delays and cerebral palsy secondary to neonatal asphyxia. At the trial, the nurse testified that it was the responsibility of nurses to make sure that appropriate equipment is available at deliveries (Calfee, 1993).

In term neonates and most prematures over 26 weeks gestation, there is no question of whether or not to resuscitate. However, in the very-low-birth-weight neonate under 26 weeks gestation, there are many legal and ethical questions and concerns about when to act. The main question deals with whether resuscitation would be futile. In other words, does the burden of treatment outweigh the benefits? What will the quality of life be? Will the treatment be effective? Is death imminent? (Rushton & Hogue, 1993). The decision of whether or not to treat the newborn is made between the health care team, primarily the physician, and the parents. The constitution, case law, and many individual state laws protect an individual's right to make decisions about health care. Many parents make these decisions for their children based on religious, cultural, and personal preferences (Fry-Revere, 1994). For some parents the decision is an easy one, whereas for others it is very difficult.

The nurse who is part of the team struggling with the decision of resuscitation of the very-low-birth-weight newborn should document interactions between the family and health care workers that involve discussions about treatment. The nurse should give support and factual information but refrain from offering a personal opinion. Discrepancies between the physician's plan of care and the family's wishes should be brought to the attention of the supervisor. The decision-making process for impending deliveries must be started as early as possible. A last-minute attempt to discuss the best option for a particular newborn and family cannot yield the best decision.

Transport

Transporting neonates between hospitals is often essential in perinatal care today. All parties involved (referring hospital, receiving hospital, ambulance company, and transport team) assume responsibility in the process. The referring physician and hospital are responsible for providing resuscitation and adequate stabilization, making the referral, explaining why the newborn should be transferred, obtaining consent, and caring for the newborn until care is transferred to the transport team (Reimer-Brady, 1996). The hospital that employs the team assumes responsibility for the team. The official point of transfer of responsibility from the referring physician to the transport may be considered to be the point when the team leaves the referring facility. At this point, most receiving hospitals consider patients who are in route to their center as their responsibility (Freeman & Poland, 1992). However, some institutions believe that once the transport team arrives, receives the report, and begins to give care, the transport team assumes the responsibility. A written agreement between hospitals can clarify this matter (Task Force on Inter-hospital Transport, 1993).

The Task Force on Inter-hospital Transport of the American Academy of Pediatrics first published *Guidelines for Air and Ground Transports of Pediatric Patients* in 1986. The document was intended to provide guidelines for safe, effective, and skilled care needed for each individual child. More specific guidelines can be found in *Guidelines for Perinatal Care* published by the American Academy of Pediatrics and the American College of Obstetrics and Gynecology. The National Association of Neonatal Nurses (NANN) has also published *Neonatal Transport Standards and Guidelines*. NANN addresses education and competency of the transport team members, quality of care, support of parent's communication, quality improvement, safety, and medicolegal issues and regulations (NANN, 1992).

Transport team personnel should have the combined skills to care for any newborn that they will be transporting. The level of care given should be equal to the level of care the newborn will receive at the referral center. Medication and equipment should be available for general care and emergencies. The team must be able to communicate with the physician in charge at all times. Team members should work within their scope of practice, using the physician in charge as needed (Reimer-Brady, 1996). In addition to providing a high level of physical care, the team must provide care to the family. Family members should be informed of the plan of care and the receiving hospital's phone number and location. All questions should be answered to the best of the team's abilities. The family should be allowed to see and touch the newborn. Consent to transport and consent to treat in route should be obtained by the team if not done by the referring physician (Reimer-Brady, 1996).

Supervision

Of all the risk areas, the one area that places the individual nurse at greatest liability is lack of knowledge on how to respond when in a hazardous situation. This situation might be one caused by his or her action, the action of another, or events beyond his or her control. Every hospital should have a written policy regarding notification of one's supervisor when faced with a difficult situation. If the immediate supervisor is unavailable or the action of the supervisor is not acceptable to the nurse, he or she should follow the chain of command in notifying the next level of management. The chain of command should be a part of the notification policy. Chains of command apply not only to nurses, and there should be a policy outlining the management tiers for other health professionals—even physicians.

STRATEGIES TO DECREASE RISK

Policies and Procedures

Policies and procedures can be used for a variety of purposes. They are used to teach new nurses how things are done. They serve as a reference for procedures that are done infrequently. They set the standard of care for an institution. And they are used in court to judge whether a particular standard of care was breached. Moniz (1992) suggests the following when writing protocols:

1. Develop protocols that consist of simple steps that are always applicable.
2. The protocols should represent the minimum needed for safe care instead of the maximum needed for ideal care.
3. The information should be updated as scientific knowledge develops.
4. They should be realistic for the practice setting.
5. Once approved, the standards and protocols should be carried out as written. Any deviation from what is written should be documented in the chart.

Using these guidelines may save the nurse from being held liable for a breach in the standard of care set forth by the nurse's own institution. In *Parker v. Southwest Louisiana Hospital Association* (1989), the hospital was found liable for failure to adhere to its own written policy. Approximately 24 hours after birth, a newborn had a cardiac and respiratory arrest in the nursery. Resuscitation was begun immediately but the infant suffered brain damage and died nine months later. The hospital policy required visualization of newborns every 10–15 minutes, much more frequently than the AAP 30-minute standard. The staff's failure to follow the written policy resulted in the hospital's liability (Aiken & Catalano, 1994).

The Association of Women's Health, Obstetric, and Neonatal Nurses in *Standards for the Nursing Care of Women and Newborns* details policies, procedures, and protocols necessary for the care of low-risk/healthy newborns, high-risk or neonatal intensive care, and neonatal complications and emergencies. Institutions safeguard themselves against potential liability by having these documents in place, educating their staff, and monitoring compliance with the policies.

Risk Management

Anticipating risks and working to prevent them is the best risk management for newborn nurses. Preventative strategies have been discussed previously in this chapter: knowing the policies and procedures and following them, keeping families and other team members informed, and documenting all aspects of care. Quality assurance programs provide identification of risk areas, assurance of consistent quality patient outcomes, promotion of professional nursing practice, and education of staff (NAACOG, 1991). For the newborn area, the quality assurance monitoring should include measuring standards that affect the aspects of care. For example, chart reviews can reveal babies admitted without Apgar scores, babies who did not get their vitamin K within the specified time frame, and other patient care-related data. Family interviews can yield information regarding the quality of discharge teaching. Each institution and nursery area will have areas that can be improved. Identification of the problem, formulation of a plan to solve the problem, education of staff, and follow-up will decrease the risk of failing to follow the standard of care.

Many nurses view incident reports as a punitive exercise. When a nurse is involved in any questionable situation, an incident report may be very beneficial should any lawsuit occur. Incident reports record factual information at the time an event occurs. The information is confidential and is generally only available to the nursing supervisor, risk management department, and the institution's insurance carrier. Most lawsuits take months or even years to process. The information recorded at the time of the event will supplement the chart and allow for better recollection of what happened. In addition to monitoring risky situations for the hospital, attention paid to trends noted by the risk management department can lead to changes in nursing practice that may lower the risk of liability for nurses in the future.

Documentation

The most used tool in any lawsuit is probably the patient's medical record. It is reviewed by people involved in the case as well as by expert witnesses who will give an opinion. Many people follow the philosophy that if you did not write it in the chart, you did not do it. Handwriting should be legible and information should be recorded in the appropriate part of the chart. Careful documentation of assessment, planning, intervention, and evaluation will be the nurse's evidence that he or she followed the standard of care.

Regarding newborns, documentation must include all assessment data and any deviations from normal. Apgar scores, admission assessments, and nursing care during the transition to extrauterine life and during the first few hours must also be recorded. Reassessment, teaching, and any communication with other health team members documents the continued care of the newborn. All medications, lab work, and other tests provide a record of how the orders were carried out. Discharge teaching, follow-up needs, and concerns that should be addressed should also be documented.

CONCLUSION

The neonatal nurse encounters families in a state of transition. Most families welcome their newborn into life and leave the hospital after having a happy experience. Nurses who work in the newborn setting must have special training and skills to meet the increased accountability and responsibility demanded by hospitals and the public. They must be familiar with the standards of care for the newborn population and adhere to those standards. Liability issues such as keeping up with new technology and advances in care, appropriate staffing for neonatal areas, and communicating with the health care team and family must be a concern for each nurse. Being aware of risk areas such as required assessments, planning and carrying out interventions, giving medications, assisting the family who chooses rooming-in, safeguarding newborns from kidnapping, resuscitation of the baby, appropriate transfer of babies not within the scope of care for particular institutions, and supervision of staff will assist the nurse in maintaining the required standard of practice and alert the nurse to risky situations. The risk of liability can be decreased if the nurse follows the policies and procedures of the institution, participates in risk management activities, and carefully documents all aspects of care.

REFERENCES

Aiken, T. D., & Catalano, J. D. (1994). Legal, ethical, and political issues in nursing. Philadelphia: F. A. Davis.

Beachy, P., & Deacon, J. (1992). Preventing neonatal kidnaping. Journal of Obstetrical, Gynecological, and Neonatal Nursing, 21(1), 12–16.

Bloom, R., & Cropley, C. (1994). Textbook of neonatal resuscitation, (pp. ix and O-1) Elk Grove, IL: American Heart Association and American Academy of Pediatrics..

Byrne, R., Tyebkhan, J., & Laing, L. (1995). Ethical decision-making and neonatal resuscitation. Seminars in Perinatology, 18(1), 36–41.

Cahill, M. (Ed.). (1996). Nurse's legal handbook. Springhouse, PA: Springhouse Corporation.

Calfee, B. E. (1993). Nurses in the courtroom: Cases and commentary for concerned professionals. Cleveland: ARC Publishing.

Dammed, E. (1991). Discharge planning from the neonatal intensive care unit. Journal of Perinatology and Neonatal Nursing, 5(1), 43–53.

Driscoll, K. (1993). Legal aspects of perinatal care. In C. Kenner, A. Breuggemeyer, & L. P. Gunderson (Eds.). Comprehensive neonatal nursing (pp. 36–51). Philadelphia: Saunders.

Endo, A. S., & Nishioka, E. (1993). Neonatal assessment. In C. Kenner, A. Brueggemeyer, & L. P. Gunderson (Eds.). Comprehensive neonatal nursing (pp. 265–293). Philadelphia: Saunders.

Fiesta, J. (1994, July). Failing to act like a professional. Nursing Management, 15–17.

Fiesta, J. (1988). The law and liability (2nd ed.). New York: John Wiley and Sons.

Freeman, R. K., & Poland, R. L. (1992). Guidelines for perinatal care (3rd ed.). Elk Grove Village, IL: American Academy of Pediatrics and American College of Obstetricians and Gynecologists.

Fry-Revere, S. (1994). Ethics consultation: An update on accountability issues. Pediatric Nursing, 20(1), 95–98.

Guido, G. W. (1997). Legal issues in nursing (2nd. ed.). Norwalk, CT: Appleton & Lange.

Joint Commission on Accreditation of Health Care Organizations. (1996). Accreditation manual for hospitals. Oakbrook Terrace, IL: JCAHO.

Letko, M. D. (1996). Understanding Apgar score. Journal of Obstetrical, Gynecological, and Neonatal Nursing, 25(4), 299–303.

Moniz, D. M. (1992, September). The legal danger of written protocols and standards of practice. Nurse Practitioner, 58–60.

NAACOG. (1992). Standards for the nursing care of women and newborns (4th ed.). Washington, DC: NAACOG.

Northrop, C. E. (1987, June). Adequate staffing . . . whose problem is it? Nursing, 87, 43.

Northrop, C. E., & Kelly, M. E. (1987). Legal issues in nursing. St. Louis, MO: Mosby.

Phillips, C. R. (1996). Family-centered maternity and newborn care. St. Louis, MO: Mosby.

Rabun, J. B. (1993, January/February). Preventing neonatal kidnaping. Journal of Obstetrical, Gynecological, and Neonatal Nursing, 15–16.

Rabun, J. B., & Lincoln, J. (1994). Preventing infant abductions from health care facilities. Neonatal Network, 13(8), 61–63.

Reimer-Brady, J. M. (1996). Legal issues related to stabilization and transport of the critically ill neonate. The Journal of Perinatal and Neonatal Nursing, 10(3), 59–69.

Rushton, C. H., & Hogue, E. E. (1993). When parents demand "everything." Pediatric Nursing, 19(2), 180–183.

Task Force on Inter-hospital Transport (1993). Guidelines for air and ground transport of neonatal and pediatric patients. Elk Grove Village, IL: American Academy of Pediatrics.

Young, T. E., & Mangum, O. B. (1996). Neofax: A manual of drugs used in neonatal care (9th ed.). Raleigh, NC: Acorn Publishing.

CASE CITATIONS

Butts v. Cummings, 28 ATLA L. Rep. 182 (May 1985).

Clark v. University of Washington, 27 ATLA L. Rep. 42 (February 1984).

Harris v. Screech, 28 ATLA L. Rep. 420 (November 1985).

Mather v. Griffin Hospital, 540 A.2d 666 (Conn. 1988).

Northern Trust Co. v. Weiss Memorial Hospital, 493 N.E.2d 6 (Illinois 1986).

Parker v. Southwest Louisiana Hospital Association, 540 So.2d 1970 (La. App. 3d Cir. 1989).

Williams v. St. Joseph's Hospital, 27 ATLA L. Rep. 42 (February 1984).

Willis v. El Camino Hospital, 28 ATLA L. Rep. 227 (June 1985)

APPENDIX 11-1. Neonatal Policies, Procedures, and Protocols

Low-Risk/Healthy Newborn
Admission criteria
Physical assessment parameters
Transitional care
Routine care (eye and cord care, vitamin K administration)
Vital signs
Length, weight, and head circumference
Identification of the newborn
Indication for, and initiation of, diagnostic assessments
Newborn nutrition
Medication administration
Circumcision, including assistance with procedure and follow-up care
Bathing
Heelstick for capillary blood assessment
Venipuncture for obtaining blood specimens
Oral/nasal suctioning
Phototherapy
Management of intravenous lines
Metabolic screening, including genetic screening
Use of pulse oximetry
Care of physiologic alterations in the newborn including
    cardiac murmurs
    respiratory distress
    feeding intolerance
    hypothermia
    hypoglycemia
    anemia
    polycythemia
    hyperbilirubinemia
    congenital hip dysplasia
    circumcision complications
    congenital anomalies
    alterations in skin integrity
    drug/substance withdrawal
    unusual physical findings
Screening test, including hearing
Preparation for transport
Scope of practice of health care providers

Organizational structure of the unit
Functional responsibilities of nursing, medical, and ancillary personnel
Nursing orders and institutional standards of care
Patient admission, transfer, discharge, and readmission
Rooming-in
Nurse's role in research
Infection surveillance, hand washing, universal precautions, isolation, and traffic control
Visitation
Setting up, calibrating, and trouble-shooting biomedical equipment
Documentation and record-keeping requirements
Lines of authority and responsibility
Hazardous materials
Relinquishment
Identification of parenting problems
Identification of consultation and referral resources and the referral process
Use and maintenance of department equipment and supplies

High-Risk Newborn
Admission assessment
Administration of blood and blood products
Vital signs and hemodynamic monitoring assessment
Measurement of length, weight, and abdominal and head circumference
Administration of medications and parenteral therapy
Administration of oxygen and respiratory therapy
Assistance with technical procedures
Cardiopulmonary distress and arrest
Care of central arterial and venous lines
Care of chest tubes
Collection of specimens
Endotracheal intubation and care of intubated infants
Assisting with eye examination
Hearing screening

Hyperalimentation

Setting up, applying, and trouble-shooting biomedical equipment

Infant demise

Assistance with insertion and care of peripheral and central lines

Maintenance of tracheostomy tubes

Metabolic alterations

Care of physiologic alterations in the newborn including

craniosynostosis

intraventricular hemorrhage

periventricular leukomalacia

seizures

anomalies and syndromes

congenital heart disease

drug/substance withdrawal

respiratory problems including persistent pulmonary hypertension, diaphragmatic hernia, hyaline membrane disease, bronchopulmonary dysplasia, pulmonary air leaks, meconium aspiration, and pneumonia

necrotizing enterocolitis

acute renal failure/acute tubular necrosis

esophageal atresia with or without tracheal esophageal fistulae

metabolic problems

hematologic problems

hypothermia/hyperthermia

retinopathy of prematurity

Phototherapy

Pulse oximetry

Perioperative care

Bathing

Suctioning/chest physiotherapy

Ostomy care

Thermoregulation

Immunizations

Admission, transfer, discharge, and readmission of patients

Designation of responsible individuals for attendance at deliveries and resuscitation team

Documentation and record-keeping requirements

Organizational structure of the unit

Infection surveillance, handwashing, isolation, universal precautions, and traffic control

Hazardous materials

Nurse's role in research

Nurse's role regarding patient consent

Nursing orders and standards of care

Scope of practice of health care providers

Transport procedures, including roles and responsibilities of the transport team

Use and maintenance of department equipment and supplies

Discharge planning and home care

Identification procedures for the newborn

Identification of consultations, referrals, resources, and processes

Parent health education

Perinatal loss

Spiritual care of the family

Complications and Emergencies of the Newborn

Cardiopulmonary distress and arrest

Central nervous system alterations

Drug/substance withdrawal

Metabolic alterations

Respiratory/oxygen therapy initiation

Thermal alterations

Transfer to an intensive care unit

X-ray, ultrasound, and other diagnostic testing

Source: NAACOG. (1992). Standard for the nursing care of women and newborns (4th ed.). Washington, DC: NAACOG.

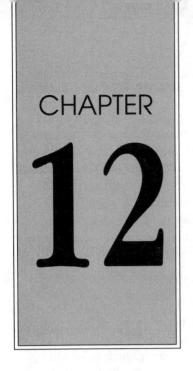

CHAPTER 12

Telephone Triage and the Office Nurse

Rebecca F. Cady

With the advent of managed care resulting in more perinatal patients being treated on an outpatient basis, perinatal office nurses have an increasing responsibility to provide care to perinatal patients who previously would have been hospitalized. The area of the perinatal office nurse's practice that presents the greatest risk for liability is that of telephone triage. The term "telephone triage" has been officially recognized only recently in the medical literature. Briggs (1997) describes telephone triage as a "systematic process that screens a caller's symptoms for urgency and advises the caller when to seek medical attention based on the severity of the problem described. The process also helps to direct callers to the most appropriate health care setting or advises home care" (pp. 1–2).

Wheeler and Siebelt (1997) estimate that about 35 million Americans now have access to telephone triage lines, compared to fewer than 2 million in 1990. The literature recognizes that telephone triage remains a controversial practice with undefined legal parameters (Wheeler, 1993). The Emergency Nurses Association (ENA) has noted the many pitfalls of telephone triage practice: "The caller may or may not accurately perceive or evaluate the urgency of the situation or condition that prompted the call. Often times the nurse may be asked to provide an opinion regarding potential medical or nursing diagnoses. When addressing medical diagnosis, the nurse may be in violation of state nurse practice acts and may be practicing beyond the scope of nursing practice. Whether addressing medical or nursing diagnoses, the . . . nurse providing advice over the telephone can be liable for that advice" (ENA, 1991). This chapter focuses on risk management strategies for telephone triage by the perinatal office nurse, and provides recommended protocols for dealing with various obstetric triage issues.

COMPETENCIES FOR PERINATAL TELEPHONE TRIAGE

The first risk management strategy for perinatal telephone triage is to ensure that the personnel providing this service meet minimal levels of competency. There is a great deal of confusion about what are considered safe telephone triage practices for medical personnel, and which personnel should be practicing telephone triage. The American College of Emergency Physicians (ACEP) recommends that no substantial diagnosis or treatment recommendations be made by telephone, and that when any doubt exists, the patient should be instructed to go to the emergency room. ACEP also recommends that telephone advice should give first aid information and recommendations on how to access medical care. ACEP recommends that telephone advice be given only by qualified medical professionals who know the limitations and ramifications of providing this service, and that the quality of telephone advice be ensured through the use of policies and protocols, documentation, and quality assurance programs to monitor outcomes (ACEP, 1988).

At a minimum, the person providing perinatal telephone triage should be a registered nurse with experience in an acute care obstetric setting, who has demonstrated clinical competence in the following areas: knowledge of protocols, decision-making and problem-solving skills, triage skills, resource identification, patient teaching and communication, health assessment and history taking, communication with physicians, and documentation.

Registered Nurse

The registered nurse or CNM is the most appropriate person to perform telephone triage for several reasons: The nurse is more cost effective than a physician, the nurse has the ability and is licensed to perform nursing assessment of the patient, and the nurse is customarily a gatekeeper between the patient and the physician in an office setting. The physician employer is obviously liable for his nurse-employee's actions, but the nurse would be independently liable for her own actions as well. It would be ill advised from a risk management standpoint to permit an unlicensed and lesser trained person such as a medical assistant to perform this function, due to the pitfalls previously outlined.

Acute Care Obstetric Experience

It is important for the nurse doing perinatal telephone triage to have acute care obstetric experience because of the potential complexity of the clinical issues likely to arise in this setting. The possession of acute care experience will allow the nurse to more accurately assess the patient by asking the appropriate questions, and will allow the nurse to more accurately assess the severity and urgency of the patient's complaints.

Clinical Competencies

Decision Making/Problem Solving

Triage is a function performed by the nurse independently, with the use of standard proto-

cols. The nurse is responsible for identifying which protocol is applicable to a given patient complaint. Even the most complete protocol cannot possibly account for every eventuality, thus the nurse may be faced with the need to make independent nursing decisions. Because of the independent nature of this task, the nurse must possess demonstrated skill in decision making and problem solving.

Knowledge of Protocols

Because triage must be performed in accordance with written standard protocols, the triage nurse must be intimately familiar with the protocols of the office. The triage desk must always have a copy of all protocols available, and the nurse must refer to the applicable protocol while speaking with a patient.

Triage

Triage is the act of determining the urgency and severity of a patient's complaints. Ideally, the nurse performing office telephone triage should have attended educational preparation such as seminars available via the hospital staff office or the physician's professional liability insurance carrier. Previous experience in obstetric triage in the acute care setting is also preferable.

Resource Identification

Because triage involves recommendations on how to access medical care, the triage nurse must be familiar with community perinatal resources, such as tertiary centers, teratogen registries, and public assistance.

Patient Teaching and Communication

Because perinatal patients in need of telephone triage services may be anxious and afraid, the importance of the nurse's skill in this area cannot be overemphasized. It is imperative that the nurse accurately communicate instructions to the patient and provide reasonable reassurance regarding the patient's complaint. It is likewise important that the nurse accurately receive complete information about the patient's condition. The nurse must be a careful listener, and must be sure that instructions given to the patient are based upon the patient's history and complaints.

Health Assessment and History Taking

Paramount to the selection of the proper triage protocol is a thorough health assessment and history taking by the triage nurse. Unless the nurse has a complete picture of what is going on with the patient, the nurse cannot make decisions about protocols or recommendations within the standard of care. It is especially important that the triage nurse not give a patient instructions without paying careful attention to the patient's history and complaints.

Communication with Physicians

The triage nurse must be able to identify which situations require immediate consultation with a physician. In the office setting, there should always be a physician available should the triage nurse need to consult with a physician regarding a caller. The nurse must be able to quickly and accurately communicate with the physician regarding the nature of the problem, and must be able to promptly carry out the physician's recommendations.

Documentation

The triage nurse must carefully document each triage conversation. The use of preprinted telephone contact forms can make this duty easier, but the nurse must be sure not to leave any blank spaces. The nurse should make notes during the call, and should record all content of the conversation, including the patient's name, the date and time of call, the length of the call, the primary physician, the complaints and history of the patient, the protocol used, the advice given, and the name of the nurse. There should be some method for ensuring that the physician periodically reviews these notes during the day. Carbonless copy logs may be useful in that a copy can be placed in the patient's chart, and a copy can be retained at the triage desk for future reference if the patient makes repeat calls.

DEVELOPMENT OF PROTOCOLS

The second risk management strategy is to develop and use protocols for dealing with telephone calls from patients. Protocols must be developed and used in the provision of telephone triage services to ensure accurate, complete, and consistent advice and to reduce exposure to claims of professional liability. Protocols may be requested by the plaintiff's attorney in a medical/nursing malpractice case to determine whether the facility's own standard of care was followed in a given situation. Protocols should be developed collaboratively by the nurses and physicians who will be utilizing them, and must be in line with the state nurse practice act. The physician must sign off on each individual protocol prior to its implementation. Wheeler (1993) suggests outlining the data collection portion of the protocol to identify the patient symptoms and associated symptoms; characteristics and course; history of symptoms; onset; location; aggravating factors; and relieving factors. Other information that must be gathered in the perinatal setting is the caller's estimated date of confinement (EDC), number and complications of previous pregnancies, allergies, current medications, complications of the current pregnancy, contraction status, status of membranes (ruptured or not), amount and nature of any vaginal discharge, fetal movement status, and current and chronic health problems. The nature of the patient's responses to these questions will guide the nurse in asking follow-up questions. The nurse should always seek to err on the side of caution by making an appointment for the patient or having the patient report to labor and delivery, if there is any doubt about the severity of the patient's condition or any unusual presentation of her symptoms. The nurse should never refuse to make an appointment for a patient who requests one. The nurse should consult immediately with the physician while the patient remains on the line if the nurse believes the protocol does not completely address the patient's situation, or for any other reason the nurse believes necessary.

All protocols must provide for a time frame for the patient to reevaluate her condition, and should include instructions to the patient that if the symptoms are not relieved within the appropriate time frame, she should either call the nurse back, go to the emergency room, or go to labor and delivery. The nurse must emphasize to the patient that the patient is responsible for calling back or seeking further care if circumstances worsen or fail to improve.

It is important that written protocols are backed up with policies and procedures regarding telephone triage. These policies should establish hours for telephone calls to be taken and the time within which all calls must be returned, as well as location of documentation, and a means for follow-up with the patient as needed.

Last, in order to have a quality telephone triage service, policies and procedures should provide for a means of evaluating the quality of telephone contacts and patient outcomes. This can occur via regular chart review and follow-up calls to patients who have used the service.

Kelley and Mashburn (1990) found that telephone triage calls from pregnant patients encompassed the following subjects in order of prevalence: systems complaints, calls requiring counseling (such as about test/procedure information, medications, activity level, early pregnancy questions, and disease exposure), test result requests, pregnancy problems, medication and pain, labor, gynecologic problems, and medication side effects. Calls related to pregnancy problems most commonly involved questions about preterm labor, followed by questions on vaginal bleeding and altered fetal movement. These patterns of calls from pregnant patients should be kept in mind when developing protocols and procedures.

SAMPLE PROTOCOLS

In general, the nurse performing telephone triage has four responsibilities: assess the severity and urgency of the problem, implement the appropriate action, evaluate the patient's understanding of the instructions given, and document all aspects of the contact.

The severity of the patient's problem will be classified in one of three ways: emergent, urgent, and nonurgent. Obviously, the patient with an emergent condition must be instructed to go to labor and delivery immediately. The patient with an urgent condition must be given an appointment with the physician for that day, or if outside of office hours, sent to labor and delivery within a few hours. The nonurgent problem

can usually be managed with home care and telephone follow-up, and/or follow-up at the next regularly scheduled prenatal visit.

In implementing the appropriate action, the nurse must first correctly identify the correct protocol. The nurse must then identify appropriate resources, and provide advice as indicated in the protocol. The nurse must then provide a thorough explanation and instruction to the patient regarding resource utilization, home care measures, and follow-up.

In evaluating the patient's understanding of instructions, the nurse should ask the patient to repeat the instructions given. The nurse should also encourage the patient to take written notes regarding advice given if necessary. The policies and procedures should provide criteria for evaluation of patient understanding of instructions, and the nurse must document that these criteria are met.

Last, as discussed earlier, the nurse must completely document the call including all signs and symptoms, advice given, and affirmation that the patient verbalized understanding.

Wheeler (1994) identifies the following pitfalls to avoid when performing telephone triage:

1. asking leading questions
2. using medical jargon
3. collecting inadequate data
4. inadequate length of conversation
5. stereotyping callers or problems
6. failing to talk directly with the patient
7. accepting a caller's self-diagnosis
8. second-guessing the caller
9. devaluing reassurance calls
10. overreacting, underreacting, and fatigue

Examples of questions and advice for specific protocols are given here as a starting point for the development of protocols for a physician office setting. To be effective, protocols must be tailored for the patient population and the health care providers involved in a particular clinical setting (protocol information adapted from Briggs, 1997, pp. 312–314).

Bleeding in Pregnancy

Information to be obtained from the patient should include EDC, time of onset of bleeding, amount, any clots or other tissue present, any recent trauma or illness, any medications or chronic health problems, primary obstetrician's name, any prior history of bleeding or miscarriage, DES exposure, history of infertility treatments resulting in this pregnancy, multiple gestation, and associated symptoms of pain.

If the patient is under 12 weeks gestation and is not bleeding heavily, offer an ultrasound appointment to determine origin of bleeding within 24 hours, instructing the patient to call back if bleeding worsens prior to the appointment. If the patient is 12–24 weeks gestation, offer a physician appointment within 2 hours or refer to labor and delivery if the patient prefers or if an appointment is not available. If the patient is 24–40 weeks, is passing large clots, or has pain or recent trauma, refer the patient to labor and delivery immediately, via ambulance if necessary.

Rule Out Labor

Information to be obtained from the patient should include onset, nature, and duration of contractions, cramping, onset, nature and amount of vaginal discharge, gravity, parity, last office visit, distance from the hospital, any recent trips to labor and delivery regarding possible labor, EDC, and primary obstetrician.

If delivery appears imminent, the patient should call an ambulance immediately. If she has regular contractions or her water is broken she should report to labor and delivery as soon as possible (within 2 hours).

Abdominal Pain

Information to be obtained from the patient should include history of recent trauma, any associated gastrointestinal problems, nausea, vomiting, diarrhea, bloody stools, EDC, primary obstetrician, vaginal discharge, or history of hypertension/diagnosed preeclampsia.

If she has had recent trauma, she should call an ambulance or go to the emergency room. If she has no associated symptoms, make appointment within 2 hours or send her to the emergency room if the patient prefers or an appointment is not available. If she has associated gastrointestinal symptoms, make an appointment within 24 hours.

Headache

Information to be obtained from the patient should include EDC, diagnosed preeclampsia, history of hypertension, other associated symptoms, trauma, visual disturbances, epigastric pain, abdominal pain, bleeding, dizziness, irritability, disorientation, swelling of face, hands, lower back, and medications taken/nature of relief provided.

If severe headache, double or blurred vision, disorientation, dizziness, or irritability are present, the patient should call an ambulance or report to the emergency room immediately. If she has diagnosed preeclampsia with new onset of headache, or associated swelling or visual disturbances, give an appointment within 2 hours or send her to the emergency room if the patient prefers or an appointment is not available. If she has a persistent headache not responding to pain relievers without any of the mentioned associated symptoms, make an appointment within 24 hours.

Fetal Activity

Information to be obtained from the patient should include EDC; primary obstetrician; nature, pattern, and frequency of fetal movement; other symptoms; kick count results; and complications of this pregnancy and previous pregnancies.

If there are fewer than 10 movements an hour, consult the physician immediately. If there are more than 10 movements an hour, reassure the patient, instruct her on the method for kick counts, and arrange for the patient to reassess movement several times over the next 24 hours and call back if anything changes.

Nausea and Vomiting

Information to be obtained from the patient should include EDC; onset, character, and amount of vomiting; associated pain; other GI symptoms; fever; recent travel; and name of primary obstetrician.

If the patient is in her first trimester and there are no associated symptoms, she should call back if there is no improvement, and follow home care instructions: Eat dry crackers before

DISPLAY 12-1

Safeguards against Legal Problems Resulting from Telephone Triage

- Use medically approved protocols to establish a standard of care. Do not deviate from the protocols unless changes are in writing and approved by the appropriate medical authority.
- Document the call and advice provided. For example, if a suit is filed three years later claiming the nurse did not advise the mother appropriately, the nurse's position is much more defensible if the documentation shows that protocols were followed and appropriate advice was given. Documentation may include a log, a note in the patient's chart, or a recording of the call.
- Provide callers with an option to seek medical attention sooner if they do not agree with the advice or the condition persists or worsens.
- Develop a mechanism to regularly review documentation and advice for consistency, accuracy, and quality.
- Orient and train staff in telephone triage protocols, policies and procedures, phone encounter techniques, dealing with difficult calls, and documentation.
- Measure outcomes. Conduct regular consumer satisfaction surveys. Follow up promptly on problems and quality issues.
- Establish a positive helping relationship at the outset of the call. The average call lasts approximately six minutes. The effectiveness of this short encounter is often dependent upon skillful communication. The initial contact can often make or break the caller's confidence and satisfaction with the telephone interaction.
- Encourage the caller to briefly describe the problem and its duration, onset, and location; past medical history; medications; and allergies. Be sure to obtain the age of the person with the problem.
- Use terminology the caller can understand. Avoid medical jargon as much as possible.
- Listen carefully to the caller and avoid jumping to conclusions. Callers may mask their real concern for fear of embarrassment, particularly regarding sensitive issues such as sexually transmitted diseases or mental health problems.
- Try to talk to the person with the problem directly if possible. Direct communication is usually more reliable and inclusive than secondhand information.
- Thoroughly assess the problem before determining an action plan. The caller may underplay the symptoms and want reassurance that the problem is insignificant.
- Pay attention to the degree of anxiety and concern expressed by the caller. Remember, the telephone nurse is at a disadvantage and cannot see or touch the person. If the caller is emphatic that the person is ill even though protocols may recommend home care measures or observation while waiting for an appointment, encourage the caller to seek medical attention sooner. It is better to be overly cautious than to miss a serious condition.
- Always provide the caller with the option to call back or seek medical attention if the condition persists or worsens or new symptoms develop.
- Attend conferences, workshops, and continuing education offerings to establish competency in communication skills, assessment, and telephone triage to reduce the risk of medical-legal problems.

From Briggs, Julie K. (1997). *Telephone triage protocols for nurses* (pp. 3–4). Philadelphia: Lippincott. Used with permission.

getting out of bed in the morning, get up slowly, eat frequent small meals, drink ginger ale between meals, and avoid fatty and spicy foods. If persistent vomiting or abdominal pain is present or associated GI symptoms are present, make an appointment within 24 hours.

Vaginal Discharge

Information to be obtained from the patient should include the nature, amount, and onset of vaginal discharge; EDC; associated cramping or contractions; any douching or recent yeast infection diagnosis; and associated urinary difficulties.

If there is any question as to whether the membranes have ruptured, have the patient either come to the office or report to labor and delivery within 2 hours. If there is bleeding, follow the bleeding protocol. If the discharge is other than clear fluid or bleeding, schedule an appointment within 24 hours.

Breast Complaints

Information to be obtained from the patient should include nature, location, and onset of problem; history of breast cancer; EDC; last mammogram or breast exam; any other symptoms; and name of primary obstetrician.

If this is a new lump, make an appointment within 24 hours. If an old lump has enlarged, make an appointment within 24 hours. If there is bleeding from the nipples, make an appointment within 24 hours.

CONCLUSION

The strategies of proper selection of personnel, and development and use of protocols are part of a risk management strategy for perinatal office nurses performing telephone triage. Display 12-1 lists safeguards against legal problems resulting from telephone triage. By heeding these safeguards, perinatal office nurses can work to ensure their patients get optimum care while at the same time minimizing their own risk of liability.

REFERENCES

American College of Emergency Physicians. (1988). Statement on emergency telephone advice.

Briggs, Julie K. (1997). Telephone triage protocols for nurses. Philadelphia: Lippincott.

Emergency Nurses Association. (1991). Emergency Nurses Association position statement: Telephone advice, 17(5), 52A.

Kelley, M., & Mashburn, J. (1990). Telephone triage in the office setting. Journal of Nurse Midwifery, 35(4), 245–251.

Wheeler, S. Q. (1993). Telephone triage: Theory, practice & protocol development. Albany, NY: Delmar.

Wheeler, S. Q. (1994). Telephone triage: Sidestepping the pitfalls. Nursing, 24(5), 32LL–32OO.

Wheeler, S. Q., & Siebelt, B. (1997). Calling all nurses: How to perform telephone triage. Nursing, 27(7), 36–41.

Home Health and Ambulatory Nursing Liabilities

Diana C. Ballard

H ome health care services utilization is on the increase and is proving to be cost effective, and in many cases significantly less costly than traditional inpatient care.

Advances in technology, growth in managed care, and market-driven health service delivery innovations are coming together in a way that is placing home care at the front of the continuum of care—as a means of cutting back acute care costs while providing the high-quality outcomes associated with inpatient care. In fact, the Congressional Budget Office predicts that home care spending will quadruple between 1993 and 2000 (Lumsdon, 1994).

Where the right clinical criteria exist, even highly specialized areas of service, such as high-risk maternity and neonatal care, can be managed at home; in some instances for less than half the cost of comparable inpatient care (Lumsdon, 1994).

TRENDS, USES, AND THE INFLUENCE OF MANAGED CARE

The managed care environment is leading a shift in health care that fundamentally affects not only the way in which health professionals practice, but also the location in which patient care services are delivered.

Home health care is one area so affected. Utilization of home care services is growing at annual rates of 20–40%, due in large part to the early hospital discharge initiatives (Lumsdon, 1994). Some of the most dramatic changes in home care utilization have occurred in high-risk maternity care and neonatal care. In fact, publicity surrounding initiatives attributed to managed care organizations that "rush" new mothers and newborns out the doors of hospitals has prompted the introduction of legislation at both the state and federal levels aimed at setting minimum limits for maternity stays. These "mandated benefits" bills are controversial, prompting concerns from some about the inability to contain and reduce health care costs, whereas some see such cost management measures affecting the quality of health care services.

Insurers and health maintenance organizations argue they are not responsible for such medical decisions, but the so-called drive-through delivery dilemma has struck a chord of frustration and dissatisfaction among consumers that could jeopardize the great strides in acceptance that managed care has made. Resolving the issue and similar issues in the future could prove complicated from both cost and quality perspectives.

These trends in limiting benefits are likely to continue as are the efforts to assert more regulatory constraints directed at the managed care industry. The cost-saving element of managed care is so irrefutable that today, one out of every five Americans, or some 50 million people, are enrolled in some type of managed care organization (Lumsdon, 1994).

MOVING AWAY FROM INSTITUTIONS: HOME CARE AND OTHER AMBULATORY SETTINGS

Characteristics of the Environment and Legal Implications

As nurses practice in less institutional settings such as offices, ambulatory centers, and clinics, or in fully noninstitutional settings such as in the home of the patient, they face certain conditions that require specialized legal analysis. This chapter is intended to include offices and clinic type settings, and where specific reference is made in that regard such will be noted. However, because the patient's home is at the far end of the noninstitutional continuum and the characteristics analyzed are more emphasized in the home care context, the reader will note that the discussion most frequently addresses directly the home setting.

Home Health Care and the Services Continuum

Home health services present a cost-effective alternative to inpatient care. Many home-based services are now directed at younger managed care populations. Physicians, using such tools as care maps and clinical pathways, will direct certain patients into home care rather than hospital care. Home care is now becoming a "front-end substitution" for hospital care, a change from the traditional "after hospital separate site business" (Lumsdon, 1994, quoting Kevin O'Donnell).

The beneficiaries of home care, then, are in many instances clients who would have been hospitalized, and their home care in these cases constitutes a substitute for the hospital. Their physical condition can therefore be expected to be more acute, even though they qualify medically for home-based services.

Degree of Autonomy and Responsibility

The more distant the practicing nurse is, clinically speaking, from the traditional institutional setting, the more likely it is that decision making and application of judgment must and will occur autonomously. The reasons for this are apparent in light of the following factors.

1. The home care setting lacks the *stability and control* of the institutional setting. The residence of the patient is under the control of the patient and family. The nurse will be subject to whatever conditions exist in that setting in providing care to the patient. This is indeed a most dramatic change from the hospital setting.

2. The availability of *immediate backup and support* for actions taken in response to situations that occur in the home are not present as in the institution. Although support may be available in a reasonably timely manner, the nurses are usually alone or in the company of family caregivers. They do not have the ability to push a "panic button" to summon immediate skilled assistance when needed.

3. The nurse practicing in the home may be *relying on untrained or less prepared persons,* such as family caregivers or unlicensed home health staff, for follow-up care and observations. The professional nurse must educate, communicate with, and supervise these other persons. However, this environment is without the actual physical presence of this type of support for more hours of the day than is the case in the institutional setting. In addition, the nurses must know their duties and which ones can properly be delegated to other categories of personnel (Sullivan, 1994).

4. The *degree and constancy of supervision* such as exists in the institutional setting is not usually possible or practical in the

home setting. Consequently, the potential for ascertaining compliance with the plan of care and response to treatment may be compromised. The nurse will at appropriate periods assess the response of the patient and the level of care provided by others, but at home there is no constant presence for ensuring such compliance.

5. *Reimbursement for services is likely to be very precisely defined and limited,* presenting the potential that the nurse may face the dilemma of having to balance the ability to terminate or limit services with the possible continuing needs of the patient. The nurse should know what the reimbursement limits are in advance so that planning can be carried out in order to avoid such problems.

These factors present a complicated paradox. The utilization of home care services is growing dramatically. The traditional users of home care services have been Medicare patients receiving a fairly basic range of services for more stable and chronic conditions (Lumsdon, 1994). Yet, the growth in home care services as they are currently being used in many cases is a substitute for hospitalization. Furthermore, many of the patients served are the most vulnerable (new mothers and infants), and often their care involves the use of high-technology equipment such as home isolette care, infant phototherapy, and maternal uterine contraction monitors.

More will be presented about these issues later in this chapter. For now, though, one can see why the home care environment, and indeed the other less institutional settings, may present some of the most interesting and compelling legal challenges that nurses practicing in this important area face.

IMPORTANT GENERAL APPROACHES

Care Planning and Communication

Providing care in the home may involve the services of a number of organizations and agencies. Although consolidation is occurring in this segment of the health care system, there are still many small home care agencies and other agencies specializing in specific in-home care, such as infusion therapy. This can result in fragmentation that makes it difficult to coordinate the care of the patient. Verbal feedback and written reports may come from many sources. Caregivers may experience difficulty communicating effectively with one another, and all may be communicating separately with the attending physicians(s).

In addition, the family must be included in the process of care planning. Involvement of the family is required by professional standards of practice, by law, and regulations. (See, for example, *American Nurses Association Standards for Professional Practice for the Perinatal Nurse Specialist, Standard III.*)

Observation and Evaluation of the Environment

As has been noted herein, the home setting is more frequently being used as a substitute for hospitalization. Accordingly, the home care setting must be evaluated in terms of the services to be provided to the patient and the needs of the caregiver in order to provide the needed care. The level of equipment, back-up personnel, and second opinions, such as are available in the hospital, will not be present in the home (Abbott, 1996).

In addition the nurse must assess the ability of the family and/or other home caretakers to follow through on the necessary aspects of the care plan. This should involve their ability to understand the patient and family education provided, and the identification of any cultural or language barriers that may interfere with their ability or willingness to participate (Abbott, 1996).

Unique Nursing Skills Required

Home- and ambulatory-based perinatal nursing care requires unique skills of the nurse, such as the need to be comfortable in a highly autonomous setting, the ability to responsibly depend on others for observation and follow-up, and the application of high-technology equipment in the home setting.

In addition, since the movement into the less institutional setting has so dramatically encompassed the care of mothers and infants in the perinatal context, the specialized services available within this nursing specialty must now be adapted for safe and responsible management in the home and/or noninstitutional setting. Given that the managed care movement is proceeding with vigor, this trend will most certainly continue.

PERINATAL HOME HEALTH CARE INITIATIVES: CLINICAL APPLICATIONS

In this section, some of the contemporary home health care programs in perinatal nursing are discussed. This information is not intended to be an exhaustive presentation of clinical expertise. Rather, it is provided to review those areas currently discussed in the literature as amenable to home health care management and to point out some of the clinical factors and vital characteristics that will guide the nurse in ascertaining the appropriate standard of care.

Nurses working in these areas should be familiar with the scientific principles and standards of clinical care as may be in effect at any time and from time to time. Nursing practice should be carried out in such a way as to address the key clinical principles appropriate with the particular services being delivered.

In reviewing the adequacy of care in the legal context, the performance of the nurse will be measured against the relevant and applicable standards of care. More discussion on standards and their development can be found in Chapter 3.

Specialized Home Health Care Services

Many communities have home health services specializing in prenatal care. Nurses from these services provide specialized care for pregnant patients at home, including evaluation of

- weight
- urine analysis
- blood pressure
- blood glucose levels
- bed rest compliance
- psychological status
- uterine contractions
- fetal heart tones using a fetoscope

Home services also include medication therapy as prescribed by a physician. Gestational diabetes and preterm labor are two serious medical conditions that cause expectant parents much concern and worry. High costs of hospitalization and the rate of illness and death in newborns are factors promoting the increased use of home monitoring for women who have high-risk pregnancies due to these conditions. Educating expectant mothers to get early prenatal care, eat nutritionally sound diets, stop smoking, practice stress reduction, and detect signs of preterm labor can go a long way toward lowering the incidence of infant mortality and illness.

Early Discharge Program

The growth in managed health care and increased utilization of cost-containing short-stay programs have resulted in earlier hospital discharge for a growing population of newborns. The following report of a coordinated early discharge program offers valuable insights into certain key elements of the program that helped the program to be effective and provided benefits to the patients. These factors are important when considering the elements of an early discharge program that will measure up to a reasonable standard of care.

Case Study of an Early Discharge Program: A Coordinated Approach

An early discharge program, with a stated goal of discharge by 24 hours of life for all vaginal deliveries, was initiated in response to community pressures to reduce length of stay. Coordination of postnatal services was a central element of the program. Nurses from a hospital-based, care-coordinating unit visited the mother before discharge to verify the location for a first home visit and were also responsible for coordination of home visits and postdischarge use of other services.

Timing of the home visit was planned in consultation with the nursery physicians caring for the infant, and a follow-up appointment with the primary care pediatrician at 2 weeks of age was made before discharge. All appointments at the study hospital's primary care clinic were made with a particular resident physician or nurse practitioner.

The name of the physician or nurse practitioner was documented on the discharge instruction sheet. During the visit, the home health nurse, previously screened for experience with newborns, assessed the mother and infant including infant weight, provided education about parenting issues and recognizing signs of illness, and verified follow-up with the primary care provider. Information on special needs of particular infants was communicated to the home health agency before discharge.

Adjustments in follow-up, including the need for subsequent home visits, were made with the care-coordinating nurses linking home health nurses and primary care physicians. Reports on visits were made available within 24 hours of the visit, or sooner as indicated (Cooper et al., 1996).

The study concluded that a coordinated early discharge with home nursing visits for inner-city infants may result in earlier use of primary care services. Furthermore, there was a significant decrease in use of the emergency department during the first 3 months of life, and no increase in re-hospitalization.

The information gained from this study could indeed be very persuasive to a court if they were asked to determine whether a particular early discharge program had been conducted in a manner that provided for the safety of the clients.

Metabolic Prescreening

Through early detection and treatment, neonatal screening programs have prevented the serious sequelae of metabolic and congenital disorders such as congenital hypothyroidism, phenylketonuria, and congenital adrenal hyperplasia. Screening of the newborn has traditionally been performed at the time of discharge on the infant's second or third day of life. However, cost-containment measures have recently resulted in earlier hospital discharges.

Accordingly, early discharge programs should include coordination of time-appropriate metabolic screening in order to prevent the inadvertent loss of these important screening tools, and to ensure compliance with appropriate standards of care.

Home Monitoring for Preterm Labor Risk

Clinical studies suggest that in conjunction with patient education, home uterine activity monitoring (HUAM) may reduce the incidence of preterm births for women at high risk for preterm labor (United States Preventive Services Task Force, 1993). Home monitoring for signs of preterm labor may help reduce costs and continue to provide a safe and satisfactory means of monitoring pregnancy.

The Food and Drug Administration (FDA) has approved certain systems to monitor uterine activity in women past their 24th week of pregnancy who have histories of previous preterm births. The purpose of such monitoring is the early detection of uterine activity, which can cause cervical dilation and preterm birth.

Wearing an elastic belt around her waist, the woman places a transducer attached to the belt on her abdomen. The transducer is a small, flat, pressure-sensitive recorder that looks like a small "beeper" and detects uterine contractions. A computer program transfers the data reporting the uterine activity over the telephone lines to communication centers such as the obstetrician's office, the home health service office, or a hospital relay station.

Consequently, the role of the nurse involves, in addition to familiarity with the technology itself, the education of the patient and assistance to the physician in observing and interpreting the monitored results, whether via personal visits or telephone contact. Documentation should include determination of data reporting intervals, notes on the interpretation and communication of the monitored results, and the plan for follow-up based on those results.

Breastfeeding

Short stay programs should be accompanied by a program of home health care for routine follow-up to prevent hypernatremic dehydration in breastfed newborns. Clinical reports stress the importance of early systematic medical follow-up for breastfed babies (Cooper et al., 1996).

In a study of infants with severe breastfeeding malnutrition and resulting profound hypernatremia, factors identified as possibly contributing to the increased incidence of breastfeeding malnutrition included minimized opportunities postpartum for teaching about early recognition of problems with breastfeeding and lack of timely newborn medical follow-up. The mothers of the infants, although well prepared prenatally, had no previous breastfeeding experience (Cooper et al., 1995).

Although the infants in the cases included in that study were discharged later than many infants enrolled in cost-saving early discharge programs, it is likely that a confluence of factors related to education about breastfeeding technique and early signs of breastfeeding failure, along with a delay in presentation to a physician, contributed to these problems.

Of further note in the study was the finding that none of the families supplemented the breastfeeding more than once between discharge and readmission. It was not clear whether the avoidance of supplementation was prompted by health care provider concerns or family concerns, but a stringent approach by both parents and health care providers to avoiding supplementation in attempts to establish breastfeeding might have exacerbated the problem (Cooper et al., 1995).

Although these families had varying levels of contact with health care providers during the first week of life, no infant was weighed or examined by a pediatrician.

Clearly, breastfeeding malnutrition and dehydration is a serious newborn health issue. This study suggests that the incidence and severity of breastfeeding malnutrition and hypernatremia may be increasing, and that the needs of many breastfed infants are not currently being met. In view of early discharge programs where home care follow-up by nurses constitutes an essential element of the program, assessment of the newborn's nutritional and hydration status is paramount in evaluating whether the standard of care has been met.

The optimal time for infant follow-up has not been determined. However, a follow-up visit in the first week of life for breastfed infants might have prevented some of the problems seen in this group of infants.

If there is a link between the shorter length of initial hospital stay for newborns, inadequate strategies for follow-up, and worsening breastfeeding malnutrition, then the current system of follow-up must be adjusted for changes in the health care system.

Jaundice or Hyperbilirubinemia

For many decades, newborn babies with jaundice were treated under bright lights in the hospital. Jaundice, or hyperbilirubinemia, appears in infants born with underdeveloped livers that are unable to process bilirubin, a natural molecule of the red blood cells released when the blood cells break down. When the immature liver fails to break down the bilirubin, it builds up in the fat tissues, turning the skin yellow.

Although usually harmless, neonatal jaundice, can become toxic and cause brain damage. Bright light on the skin breaks down the bilirubin, which is then naturally excreted by the baby.

In the traditional hospital treatment for this condition, the infant is placed under a bank of overhead fluorescent lights that shine down on the child. The infant is typically unclothed in order to derive the therapeutic benefits from the exposure of light on the skin, and wears eye shields to protect the eyes from the light source. During this form of treatment, the infant's temperature must be closely monitored. In addition, treatment in this manner poses restrictions on the holding of the infant by its parents.

The introduction of portable fluorescent systems and innovative fiberoptic pad units for jaundice treatment gave pediatricians the option, in appropriate situations, of sending infants home for the therapy.

Home phototherapy for jaundice is less stressful for the parents and infant, reduces medical costs, and allows the parent–child bonding process to continue uninterrupted.

There are different types of phototherapy units. One consists of a soft fiberoptic pad connected to an illuminator box, which contains a halogen light bulb, the source of the therapeutic light. The pad, which slips into a disposable cover, transmits a unified blue light through woven plastic fibers. The baby lies down with his or her back or chest on the pad or secured by a vest, so that the infant can be held without interrupting treatment.

The home health caregiver, clinic, or office nurse must be familiar with this equipment and the selected method of treatment. Parents will need reinforcement with regard to issues such as the duration of treatment and the manufacturer's specifications and recommendations with respect to use and application of the equipment. For example, some equipment may permit light settings to be adjusted. The baby's eyes may need shielding, depending on how or whether the eyes are exposed to the light source. The nurse should determine whether there is a need for temperature monitoring or any other nursing intervention. Parents may also need advice on issues of heat exposure or exposure to electricity.

Puerperal Infection

Postpartum or puerperal fever is a common obstetric complication. Often it results from endometritis but it can also be caused by urinary tract infection, wound infection, or phlebitis (Hamadeh, Dedmon, & Mozley, 1995). Postpartum fever is a complication in 2–4% of vaginal deliveries and in 29–95% of cesarean deliveries. The rate of endometritis is at least 10 times higher in patients who have a cesarean delivery, compared with patients who have a vaginal delivery.

Treatment options for patients include administration of antibiotics with specific activity against anaerobic bacteria.

Additional diagnostic modalities, such as computed tomography, ultrasonography, heparin administration, and surgical exploration, should be employed when the patient fails to respond to antibiotic therapy.

Risk factors for each of the described postpartum febrile complications have been identified. It is important to note that if invasive procedures are performed on a patient in labor who has other risk factors, a higher risk exists for a febrile complication. This is particularly true in the case of endometritis, in which the risk for a febrile complication increases from less than 4% in an uncomplicated vaginal delivery to as much as 85% in an indigent patient with membranes ruptured for more than 6 hours and multiple pelvic examinations followed by a cesarean section.

The identification of these risk factors provides essential information for the nurse who is monitoring the postpartum care of the client. The assessment process should include analysis of these factors including socioeconomic conditions, and they should be considered in the development of the plan of care.

AREAS OF RISK

Alternate Site Providers

Alternative care delivery sites must be appropriate to the condition and needs of the patient. The failure to provide the proper standard of care in this regard can lead to a finding of negligence.

A failure to equip and staff a medical facility to handle high-risk pregnancies resulted in an award of $2.8 million to a plaintiff for past and future pain and suffering and future loss of earnings. In *Diamond v. Friendly Hills Medical Group* (1994), repeated ultrasound tests had found a distended fetal bladder in the plaintiff. The patient's record noted that she was high risk, but the defendant medical group did not transfer her to a hospital. Further, when another ultrasound determined an absence of amniotic fluid, timely induction of labor or a caesarean section was not performed. The infant was born with complete renal failure.

This case points out the need to constantly assess the appropriateness of patients to the setting in which they are receiving care, to employ appropriate clinical judgment, and to follow the proper standard of care. This is particularly important in light of changes in the patient's condition.

DUTIES OF THE HOME HEALTH CARE AGENCY OR OTHER ORGANIZATION

Agency/Organization Licensing

Most states require the licensing of home health agencies. (See, for example, Connecticut General Statutes Section 19a-490; McKinney's Consolidated Laws of New York, Public Health Law, §3600-3620 and §3614a; Florida Statutes 1989, §§400.461 to 400.505; General Statutes of North Carolina, §§131E-135 to 131E-142.) The majority of licensing requirements apply to any private organization that provides home health services. (See, however, California Deering's Health and Safety Code, §1727, which applies the requirements of licensing to public and private organizations who provide skilled nursing services to persons in their "temporary or permanent place of residence.") Further, most jurisdictions require that a home health agency provide nursing services and at least one other home health service as defined in the specific statute. Additional home health services may typically be provided directly by the licensed agency or pursuant to a contract with another duly qualified provider.

The definition of home health services may vary by jurisdiction. The statutes typically require that home health care is defined as part time or intermittent nursing care provided by or under the supervision of a registered nurse; additional services may include physical, speech, or occupational therapy; medical social services; and home health aide services. There may be additional requirements of law with respect to the provision of certain drugs, biologicals, uses of medical appliances, and other therapeutic services.

Usual licensing provisions also include the requirement for a plan of treatment for each patient; the maintenance of a clinical record; supervision of licensed and unlicensed personnel by a registered nurse or a licensed therapist for services within their scope of professional practice; establishment of policies regarding the delivery and supervision of care; and the provision that all requirements of laws and regulations that are in effect at the time are complied with.

Given the variation and complexity of the state and federal laws and regulations affecting the delivery of health care services, it is important for nurses working for a home health agency to be familiar with the statutes that govern their agency. This advice also applies to nurses working in offices, clinics, and ambulatory center settings, because governing laws vary and the nurse needs to know what specific practices may be required, prohibited, or in any other way affected by the applicable law.

Nurses should request a copy of the relevant statutes and regulations and be familiar with their jurisdiction's definition of home health or other ambulatory services.

In some states an agency furnishing only specific services, such as home dialysis services, supplies, or equipment may not fall under the state's licensing laws. (See, for example, Florida Statues 1993, §400.462.)

Individual Home Health Care Provider

Hiring

QUALIFICATIONS. In the autonomous and independent setting of home based health care, there can be no substitute for an appropriately qualified practitioner. As has been noted, there may be no readily available back up person who can be summoned in on a moment's notice. The environment is not a clinical and controlled environment, set up to accommodate the performance of nursing services. The uniqueness of the environment must be recognized: It should not be assumed that even a well-qualified hospital nurse without home heath care experience or training can effectively practice in this setting.

Further, patients in need of perinatal nursing being managed in the home often require the use of specialized technology. The nurse must not only be familiar with the use of the equipment, but also must be able to instruct and supervise the patient in the use of the equipment.

Nurses working in this setting should prepare carefully to ensure effective and safe practice, and their qualifications should be verified by the employer. In addition, local statutes and regulation should be reviewed to see whether there are any specific legal requirements that apply with respect to the specific acts that the nurse is undertaking.

BACKGROUND SCREENING. State laws vary greatly as to what criminal and/or professional screening is required of new employees for home health care agencies and other health providers. In some instances state statutes are specific, indicating whether criminal background checks or verification with other state licensing authorities must be carried out by the prospective employer. (See, for example, Florida General Statutes sections 400.512, and 943.053, 943.0585, and 943.059.) In addition some states have particular requirements as to experiential and educational qualifications for staff positions and for administrative posts. In some states, there may not be any requirements for preemployment screening.

Even where there are no such requirements, employers may still be well advised to develop reasonable company policies to ensure the suitability of their employees. This is especially true in the home health care setting, where workers may be alone with the patient and without direct supervision at all times. In these settings, the employer's actions in selecting and screening employees must provide a reasonable level of assurance that the worker will perform according to the requirements of the position and, even more importantly, will not cause harm to the patient.

The civil liability of employers that is associated with not conducting thorough criminal and professional background checks is increasing every day.

In developing appropriate and reasonable policies, employers should consider out-of-state licensing or registry checks for licensed, certified, or otherwise listed employees. Often an employer does not do this unless it is specifically required by statute. Most states do not require health care providers to conduct criminal and out-of-state licensing checks; consequently it is not often done. However, failure to do such checks may be considered a failure to take reasonable steps in hiring new employees if it turns out that the person should not have been hired and causes harm to a patient.

The fact that such checks may not be legally required does not necessarily relieve an employer of potential liability for damages resulting from negligent hiring practices.

Employers should consider the legal ramifications of a civil action for negligent hiring. This is becoming a more frequently seen cause of action, and results when an employer does not take all reasonable actions to verify a prospective employee's suitability for a position. In such cases, the employer may be liable for damages suffered as a result of that employee's actions, or inactions, while on the job.

For example, in a California case, home health care workers used their employment status to obtain information from patient files. Later, when they were no longer employed by the agency, they robbed and assaulted elderly patients. The court records showed that they had been hired without adequate checks for either qualifications or background. The agency was found liable for negligent hiring in connection with the harm done to the plaintiff (*Morett v. Kimberly Services, Inc.,* 1996).

The courts have found that checking a prospective employee's background for a criminal record, especially those employed in health care positions, is a reasonable action (Debatto, 1995). Not doing so may leave the employer liable for damages if an incident occurs causing injury or abuse. This could include not checking for a criminal record and professional license verification, both in-state as well as in other states where the employee is known to have worked.

ORIENTATION AND TRAINING. No direct care staff should begin work for an agency or in a patient's home before completing an orientation program. In addition to general orientation, all current staff should attend special training on identification of patient abuse, including proper reporting procedures and prevention. All training should be documented and such records placed in the employee's permanent file.

Failure to properly orient and train new employees can also lead to agency liability. In *Fink v. Kimberly Services, Inc.* (1993), a patient was injured when dropped by a home health aide. Liability was assessed against the agency when it was shown that the injury occurred because the aide had not been properly trained and supervised.

Clarity of Scope of Practice: Potential for Performance of Medical Acts

The practice of nursing is defined by the Nurse Practice Act, which is in effect in every state. Nurses must be familiar with the definition of nursing practice in their state. In many jurisdictions, the Nurse Practice Act has been expanded to define the practice of the advanced practice nurse.

The acts governing the practice of nursing define the scope of nursing practice. Specifically, this means that the particular range of responsibilities of the nurse within the defining act is spelled out. Adherence to the mandates of these acts is vital to avoid allegations of infringement into areas of practice that are reserved for other professionals, such as the practice of medicine (Brent, 1994).

The likelihood of exceeding the scope of practice is greater when the nurse is practicing in an expanded role (Brent, 1994). The autonomous nature of the nurse practicing in the home health or similar setting may, therefore, expose him or her to a greater likelihood of exceeding the scope of practice as defined by the governing act. This exposure can also extend to the practice of other home health team members who provide care to the clients.

Further, this exposure may occur when the definition of nursing practice for the registered nurse or advanced practice nurse allows for nontraditional patient care responsibilities, such as diagnosis and prescription of medications and treatments, even when done according to the use of physician-based treatment and prescriptive protocols (Hadley, 1989).

A thorough understanding of the act and its interpretive and administrative regulations is essential if the home health care nurse and the agency wish to avoid the prospect of alleged violations of the practice law (Brent, 1996). For example, it is important to know whether the act provides the authority for the home health care nurse to prescribe medications, and what basis may be used for a finding of violation of the act by a nurse. The act will also identify other obligations the nurse may have, such as reporting of suspected child or patient abuse or neglect. The act and its interpretations will also determine the best way for an agency to delegate responsibilities to other agency staff. Home health care nursing requires the legal authority to provide nursing care consistent with the demands of this specialty, and both the agency and the nurse must ascertain the existence of such authority or modify their practice accordingly (Brent, 1996).

PERSONNEL SAFETY RISKS

OSHA Advisory on Workplace Violence

The Occupational Safety and Health Administration (OSHA) is the administrative agency charged with promulgating and enforcing workplace safety and health standards. Because of the increasing safety concerns and hazards posed by assaults on health care workers, OSHA issued advisory violence prevention guidelines to reduce this risk (OSHA, 1996). Although these standards are not mandatory, the guidelines are provided for consideration and voluntary use by employers. Based on OSHA and Bureau of Labor Standards data, more assaults occur in health care and social services than in any other industry (OSHA, 1996, paragraph 15,060). Almost two thirds of the nonfatal assaults occurred in nursing homes, hospitals, and establishments providing residential care and other social services.

Reasons cited for the increased risk of violence include the prevalence of handguns and other weapons among patients, their families, and friends; working alone in remote high-crime locations without adequate means to summon assistance if needed; and lack of staff training to recognize and respond appropriately to escalating hostile behavior.

OSHA has identified the four main components of a safety program:

1. Management commitment and employee involvement. These factors might be reflected through assigning organizational responsibility for the safety and prevention program; allocation of authority and company resources; providing counseling and debriefing for employees when needed; using employee suggestion/complaint procedures to provide for prompt and accurate reporting of violent incidents; and training and education.

2. Worksite analysis. A threat assessment team should be established to analyze the workplace for "potential hazards" that might lead to violence. The team would include representatives from senior management, operations, employee assistance, security, safety and health, legal, and human resources.

3. Hazard prevention and control. This aspect of the program would serve to evaluate where engineering measures, or administrative or work practices might be employed to prevent hazards.

4. Safety and health training. All staff should receive education regarding workplace violence, including training about preventing or diffusing volatile situations, a policy for reporting incidents, and a policy for obtaining assistance after a violent incident.

What are the employer's liabilities when a worker is injured due to workplace violence? The law regarding workplace violence does not provide clear, comprehensive guidance for employers (Yohay & Peppe, 1996).

Worker's compensation statutes have a significant effect upon an employer's liability for injuries caused by violence in the workplace, and provide parameters for the employer's liability to the injured employee. Such statutes are state-specific and vary greatly.

In general, an injured employee who is covered by worker's compensation cannot sue the employer directly because the worker's compensation statute identifies worker's compensation as the employee's exclusive remedy for injuries and illnesses that occur within the scope of the individual's employment.

In the majority of jurisdictions, if an assault occurs during work and resulted from a work-related situation, it is covered under worker's compensation. Every situation must, however, be analyzed on a case-by-case basis. The determination of what constitutes a "work-related situation" can require considerable legal analysis.

As more employers acknowledge the threat of workplace violence and implement programs to address it, their potential liability for the injuries caused by such violence may be clearer, as it may become more difficult for cited employers to assert that the hazard is not a recognized and foreseeable one.

Illegal Activities

Every state has laws that protect vulnerable populations from all manner of abuse. Children, the elderly, and the mentally or emotionally challenged may be included in such laws.

A health care professional should be alert to signs of illegal abuse or to other signs indicating that illegal activity may be occurring. The patient's home is an environment not controlled by the health professional. When signs of illegal activity of any sort are present, company policy should dictate the proper action to be taken, so that it is clear to whom and in what manner such reporting is done. Remember, certain types of reporting, such as child abuse, must be reported by health care professionals upon a reasonable belief that such abuse may exist, and failure to do so can lead to various legally imposed sanctions. The nurse does not have to verify or ascertain that abuse has occurred. Most statutes require reporting based upon a reasonable suspicion, even if it later turns out that the nurse was mistaken.

DOCUMENTATION

Communication in the delivery of health services is fundamental to continuity and effective delivery of patient care. The medical record should tell the story of a client's course of care. If any essential information is not included, then the story will be incomplete.

Primary Means of Communication to Other Caregivers

In home health care and noninstitutional settings where services may be delivered by numerous providers at varying times, the challenge to communicate effectively on behalf of the patient is greater indeed.

In a study of records where hospital patients were referred for posthospital home-based services, only about 58% of the necessary data were found to be transmitted in the referral form. This usually consisted of background and medical data, some nursing care instructions, and very little psychosocial data. More data were transferred when standardized written forms were used, when smaller hospitals provided the information, and when the home health agency was affiliated with the hospital (Anderson, 1993). In another case, the failure of an emergency room nurse to produce the medical record of an infant's previous emergency room visit, which had occurred one month earlier, was alleged to be negligence and a contributing factor in the death of the infant from sudden infant death syndrome (SIDS) (*Butterfield v. Holy Cross Jordan Valley Hospital*, 1992).

In that case, an expert testified that the nurse's failure to produce this record contributed to one of two physicians allegedly faulty diagnosis of the infant's condition. This type of situation is an example of failure to have available the necessary information for management of the patient. The patient record must be completely written and it must be available to the physicians and health professionals when needed.

Computerized Patient Records

More and more patient records are being computerized. There are important public policy reasons for this shift: Patient records can be readily available wherever and whenever needed, and large volumes of medical data are available to benefit health care research.

However, along with the storage of massive amounts of individually identifiable medical data come concerns about medical privacy and security of records.

There is no national or uniform law that governs the privacy of medical information contained in computerized databases (Ballard & Cohen, 1995). However, at this point it is clear that whoever is responsible as the custodian of such records must take reasonable steps to ensure the security of the information contained in the records.

Nurses working with computerized medical record systems should remember that their password, which enables their access to the system, is in fact their signature and its security should be treated accordingly. That would include not sharing the password with any other person, and changing it regularly.

Reimbursement for Services

In this managed care era there is tremendous emphasis on the cost of care. Reimbursement from governmental payment sources, such as Medicaid and Medicare, requires compliance with certain specific conditions, such as medical necessity, in order to qualify for payment of benefits. In addition, fraud in the health care payment system is a major focus of government efforts to eliminate such abuse and the resulting misuse of funds.

The patient record, properly written, will provide information that can verify the need for services and help to justify the payment for services.

Continuation of Care/ Duration of Payment

Documentation of the patient's continuing needs and the communication of those needs to the physician and to the managed care entity are essential. The record should also show the risks to the patient if home care or other services are not continued, as this may become crucial if services must be terminated due to lack of payment source.

A source of concern for home health services is the exposure to charges of abandonment if services are discontinued. Services may be discontinued when there is no longer a source of payment or when the environment is unsafe for the caregivers. In such instances, careful documentation of the specific facts and circumstances is essential.

Such documentation should include the steps taken to provide notice to the patient and physician, and also of the alternative means taken to prevent the patient from being endangered due to the termination of services. Careful attention to these facts will help to safeguard the patient as well as protect the rights of the caregiver and provider.

Evidence in Legal Proceedings

Guardianship, Child Neglect, and Custody Proceedings

Nursing records can provide important evidence in cases involving the abuse or neglect of children. Courts will examine the observations and recording of nurses to help in determining whether a child has been mistreated.

In *Re: Willie A. III* (1991), a cocaine-addicted mother was permitted to take her newborn home with referrals to the local visiting nurse. Court records show that the nurse's observations on more than one occasion indicated that the infant was being neglected. The notes documented unsanitary conditions in the home, inadequate feeding of the child, and a spreading diaper rash. In specifically making note of these observations, the judge in this case found a basis for termination of parental rights.

Nurses should also note that in most states, statutes require that any basis for a reasonable belief that a child is being neglected or abused must be reported. These are called mandatory reporting requirements, and sanctions may exist for failure to report as required by statute. Agencies and health centers should be sure that their policies and procedures include the specific steps that must be taken in order to comply with such mandates.

However, in another interesting case, it was held that the physicians, the home health agency, and the nurse employees of the agency could be held liable for conspiracy, if adjudication of the facts supported an allegation that they acted in concert with state officials in depriving a child's father of his constitutional rights. In *Bendiburg v. Dempsey* (1990), facts were alleged that if proven could show that the home health agency, its nurse employees, and physicians might have intentionally exaggerated the emergency nature of the minor child's medical problems in order to supply state officials with the facts needed to obtain temporary custody of the minor.

TELEMEDICINE

Telemedicine involves the use of communication systems by medical experts to collaborate on a patient's diagnosis and treatment (Pendrak & Ericson, 1996).

The home health care setting is an environment actively pursuing utilization of these techniques. In fact, the potential of telemedicine is generating excitement in almost every health care setting. Health systems have been quick to recognize that new technologies can allow physicians in isolated and rural areas to directly access a full range of specialists and cutting-edge treatment options traditionally available only at large, urban medical centers (Pendrak & Ericson, 1996).

Telemedicine systems depend on advanced telecommunications technologies to exchange health information and provide health care services. The impact of these new technologies on professional liability cannot yet be determined. A lack of professional guidelines and clear legal opinions makes it difficult to predict the effects on practitioner liability.

The legal analysis surrounding the application of telemedicine involves many complicated legal issues concerning licensing, credentialing, professional standards of care, and even assessment of telemedicine technology systems.

Currently malpractice analysis centers on the existence of a duty owed to the patient by the practitioner and whether or not that duty was violated by a failure to perform according to the appropriate standard of care. Malpractice analysis will likely continue to focus on these issues. However, the existence of a duty may be less clear in telemedicine cases, and only a handful of professional associations thus far have developed specific telemedicine standards.

Another key issue is whether a practitioner's license in one state permits that person to provide telemedicine consultation in another state. Currently, most jurisdictions view telemedicine practice as practicing in the state in which the patient is located. Unless this is modified, practitioners will have to be licensed in the state in which the patient is located to provide telemedicine services.

Current steps that can be taken to limit potential liability for practitioners and health systems include keeping detailed records of telemedicine consultations and activities—even videotaping such activities—and ensuring the security and accessibility to computerized medical records necessary to ensure uninterrupted care (Pendrak & Ericson, 1996).

CONCLUSION

The focus of health care is changing. In an effort to control costs and conserve resources, health care is now provided in many different venues including ambulatory and home care settings. High-risk maternity patients and neonates are now often managed at home. Perinatal nurses should actively participate in research to determine the best methods for delivery of home and ambulatory care. The nurse providing home health care must be familiar with principles and standards of clinical practice to avoid liability and deliver safe, effective nursing care to perinatal and neonatal patients.

REFERENCES

American Nurses Association. (19). American Nurses Association standards of professional practice for the perinatal nurse specialist, Standard III. Kansas City: ANA.

Anderson, Mary Ann, & Helms, Lelia. (1993, Winter: ANA. Hospital & Health Services Administration, 38(4), 537.

Ballard, Diana, & Cohen, Joshua. (1995). Confidentiality of patient records in the computer age. Journal of Nursing Law, 2(4), 49–61.

Brent, Nancy J. (1994). Risk management and legal issues in home care: The utilization of nursing staff, Journal of GNN, 23(8), 659–666.

Brent, Nancy J. (1996). The home healthcare nurse and the state nurse practice act: Gaining familiarity is as easy as 1-2-3. Home Healthcare Nurse, 14(10), 788–789.

Cooper, William O., Kotagal, Uma R., Atherton, Harry D., Lippert, Carrie A., Bragg, Elizabeth, Donovan, Edward F., & Perlstein, Paul H. (1996, October). Use of health care services by inner-city infants in an early discharge program. Pediatrics, 98(4), 686.

Debatto, David. (1995). Criminal care. Nursing Homes, 44(2), 28.

Occupational Safety and Health Administration. (1996, March 14). Guidelines for preventing workplace violence for health care and social workers. Washington, DC: U.S. Department of Labor.

Hadley, E. H. (1989). Nurses and prescriptive authority. A legal and economic analysis. American Journal of Law & Medicine, 14(2 & 3), 245–299.

Hamadeh, Ghassan, Dedmon, Cindy, & Mozley, Paul D. (1995). Postpartum fever: American Family Physician, 52(2), 531.

Lumsdon, Kevin. (1994). No place like home? Market sings show that home care may eclipse hospital care. Hospitals & Health Networks, 68(19), 44–46, 48, 50–52.

Pendrak, Robert F., & Ericson, R. Peter. (1996, September 30). Telemedicine may spawn long-distance lawsuits. National Underwriter Property & Casualty-Risk & Benefits Management, 40, 17.

Sullivan, Gayle H. (1994.) Home care: More autonomy, more legal risks. (Legally Speaking, Column), RN, 57(5), 63.

United States Preventive Services Task Force. (1993). Home uterine activity monitoring for preterm labor. <u>Journal of the American Medical Association, 270,</u> 371–376.

Yohay, Stephen C., & Peppe, Melissa L. (1996). Workplace violence: Employer responsibilities and liabilities. <u>Occupational Hazards, 58</u>(7), 21.

Case Citations

Bendiburg v. Dempsey, (1990) 909I2d463 (11th Cir; cert. den.).

Butterfield v. Holy Cross Jordan Valley Hospital, 831 P2d97 (1992).

Fink v. Kimberly Services, Inc., No. 91-11794; FJVR Ref. No. 93:12 70 (1993).

Morett v. Kimberly Services, No. 127096; Verdictum Juris No. 10 Mar. (1996) 127068.

Re: Willie A. III, Ct. Sup. 4945, CSCR, Sup. Ct., Juvenile Matter, Judicial District of Hartford-New Britain at Hartford (June 28, 1991).

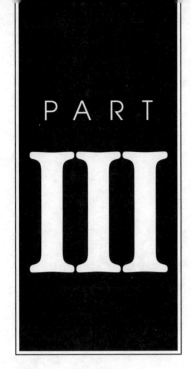

PART

III

Miscellaneous Liability Issues

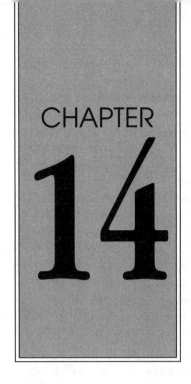

CHAPTER
14

Patient Rights

Mary Catherine Rubert

This chapter concerns the rights of the individual patient. These rights extend to all patients, regardless of their medical condition. Some rights are a result of state legislation, and others are a result of federal legislation. Some rights have developed through guidelines established by the Joint Commission on Accreditation of Healthcare Organizations, a nonprofit organization that reviews and evaluates health care facilities.

Perinatal patients present certain patient-rights problems. Most patient-rights problems develop when there is an issue concerning treatment or the refusal or rejection of treatment. They also develop when the patient is unable to decide for herself what treatment protocol should be used. Problems may develop if the baby is born with a severe illness or birth defect that is not curable. Parents do not have an unqualified right to have medical care withheld for an infant. Under state and federal laws, depending on the age of the fetus, the rights of the fetus may exceed those of the mother.

This chapter includes information about advance directives for health care decision making, and how they evolved. It also covers the durable health care power of attorney. Also included is information concerning the Joint Commission on the Accreditation of Healthcare Organizations, information about the OBRA or antidumping legislation, and information about

the National Practitioner Data Bank. These documents and entities are designed to protect the rights of the patient.

ADVANCE DIRECTIVES

In 1991, the federal Patient Self-Determination Act (PSDA) went into effect. Those health care facilities that participate in Medicare and Medicaid reimbursement programs must comply with the PSDA regulations. Failure to comply prohibits reimbursement for treatment rendered. The PSDA gives patients the right to make advance directives and decisions concerning their health care.

Advance directives are written instruments or legal documents that provide a means of communicating a person's wishes concerning his or her future medical treatment if he or she is unable to personally make the decision. With a few exceptions almost every state and the District of Columbia have some form of legislation covering advance directives.

As long as a patient is competent and able to communicate, she can make treatment decisions for herself. A patient can choose to have treatment started, modified, or stopped. If the patient chooses to discontinue treatment, and health care providers ignore that decision and continue the treatment, the health care providers are potentially liable for an intentional tort and lawsuit. In

Schloendorff v. The Society of the New York Hospital (1914), the plaintiff patient came to the hospital in January 1908 complaining of a stomach disorder. After several weeks in the hospital, it was determined that she needed an examination under ether. She consented to the examination, but told the doctor that there must be no operation. Ether was administered and while the patient was unconscious, the doctor removed a tumor. It was alleged that because of the surgery, the patient developed gangrene in her left arm and some of her fingers had to be amputated. Schloendorff sued the hospital. Although this case involved additional issues, it held that the wrong complained was of trespass and not merely negligence.

The case held that "Every human being of adult years and sound mind has a right to determine what shall be done with his own body; and a surgeon who performs an operation without his patient's consent, commits an assault for which he is liable in damages" (*Schloendorff v. The Society of the New York Hospital,* 1914).

The Incompetent Patient

Black's Law Dictionary defines "incompetency" as "lack of ability, legal qualification, or fitness to discharge the required duty" (*Black's Law Dictionary,* 1968, p. 906).

A court at the request of a family member, friend, attorney, or other interested party may be called upon to determine and declare whether a person is incompetent and then to appoint a guardian to make decisions, including health care decisions, for that person.

Legislation providing for advance directives was enacted to respond to various cases nationwide that involved the courts in health care decision making for those patients who were unable to make decisions for themselves. The patients in many of those cases were determined to be incompetent due to severe mental retardation, or because they were in persistent vegetative states due to disease or severe head trauma.

In *Matter of Quinlan,* one night in April 1975, Karen Quinlan ceased breathing for at least two 15-minute periods. Mouth-to-mouth resuscitation was ineffectual. Quinlan eventually was in a per-

sistent vegetative state. Her father sought to be appointed guardian of her person and property. The father also sought the express power of authorizing the discontinuance of all extraordinary procedures for sustaining Karen's vital processes.

The Supreme Court of New Jersey held that a decision by the patient to permit a noncognitive, vegetative existence to terminate by natural forces was a valuable incident of her right to privacy that could be asserted by her guardian. However, the court also held that there was a need to have a concurrence of agreement of guardian and family, and if the attending doctors concluded that there was no reasonable possibility of the patient emerging from her comatose state and that the life support equipment should be discontinued, then the physicians should consult with the hospital ethics committee, and if the committee agreed with the doctors' prognosis, then the life support systems could be withdrawn and there would be no civil or criminal liability on the part of any participants.

In another case, Nancy Cruzan, a young woman, was injured in a motor vehicle accident. She suffered severe injuries that rendered her unable and incompetent to make health care decisions for herself. Her parents, as guardians, sought a court order directing the withdrawal of Nancy's artificial feeding and hydration equipment after it was determined that she had virtually no chance of recovering her cognitive faculties.

The Supreme Court of Missouri held that there was no clear and convincing evidence of Nancy Cruzan's desire to have life-sustaining treatment withdrawn under such circumstances. Her parents did not have authority to effect such a request.

The case reached the United States Supreme Court. In the underlying case there was testimony by a former housemate that Nancy would not have wished to continue to live unless she could live at least halfway normally. The United States Supreme Court held that Missouri could apply a clear and convincing evidence standard. Missouri had a State Living Will statute that embodied a state policy strongly favoring the preservation of life, and the law required clear and convincing evidence. The housemate's testimony did not meet that criteria (*Cruzan v. Missouri Dept. of Health,* 1990).

Types of Advance Directives

The main types of advance directives are the living will and the durable health care power of attorney, also known as a health care proxy.

The Living Will

A living will is a legal document in which a competent person lists and describes the type of treatment or lack of treatment that the person wishes to receive in the event that he or she becomes incompetent and is unable to make health care decisions for him- or herself. A living will provides guidelines for the health care providers concerning treatment, nutrition, and hydration, and the withdrawal of life-support measures. When the directives are followed, it provides protection of the patient's rights as well as legal protection for the health care provider.

Living wills are not valid in every state. For example, New York has a health care proxy statute (see N.Y. Public Health Law, §29-C), but it does not have legislation that requires a living will to be honored, although there is case law that permits it to be considered.

Durable Health Care Power of Attorney

The durable health care power of attorney or health care proxy is a written legal document wherein the principal designates a health care agent to make health care decisions for the principal when he or she is unable to make such decisions for him- or herself. The person executing the proxy should have discussed his or her wishes concerning health care with the agent, so that the agent can make decisions based on the person's desires. For example, in New York State, if the principal has not discussed the issues of administration of artificial nutrition and hydration, the agent cannot make decisions concerning those issues. (See N.Y. Public Health Law, 29-C.)

If there are statutory provisions in place for a durable health care power of attorney, the provider of the health care is usually protected by an immunity against civil or criminal liability as long as the provider acts in good faith and honors the agent's health care decision. As a health care provider, the perinatal nurse needs to become acquainted with the laws of the state or governmental entity in which the nurse practices.

HEALTH CARE AGENT. In general, anyone who has reached the age of majority can be appointed the health care agent. However, there are some exceptions, which may vary from one governmental entity to another. In New York State, for example, administrators, operators, or employees of a hospital in which the principal is a patient or who has applied for admission to that facility may not be appointed as a health care agent, unless the individual is related to the principal by blood, marriage, or adoption. A physician may be appointed as an agent provided that he or she does not act as the principal's physician after the appointment. There may be additional restrictions on physicians practicing in mental health facilities, unless the physician is related to the patient (N.Y. Public Health Law, §29-C).

Connecticut extends the limitation on agents to include an administrator or employee of a government agency which is financially responsible for a person's medical care. (Ct. Public Health & Well-Being, 19a-576.)

A statute may limit the appointment of an agent if that person is already a designated agent for a specified number of people.

REVOCATION OF AUTHORITY. The principal may designate in the proxy that it expires on a date certain or upon the occurrence of a specific event. If there is no such date or occurrence specified, then the proxy will remain in effect until it is specifically revoked by the principal. See Display 14-1 for a sample of a health care proxy.

All patients, including perinatal patients, should be concerned about advance health care directives, whether they are a living will, a durable health care power of attorney, or a do-not-resuscitate order. Although the expectant mother may not see herself as a patient, there is the possibility that complications could occur that would prevent the perinatal patient from being able to make a decision concerning her health and/or the health of the fetus.

JOINT COMMISSION ON ACCREDITATION OF HEALTHCARE ORGANIZATIONS

The Joint Commission on Accreditation of Healthcare Organizations (JCAHO) is an independent, not-for-profit organization. Established in 1951, its members include the American College of Physicians, the American College of Surgeons, the American Dental Association, the American Hospital Association, and the American Medical Association. The main activities of the JCAHO are to develop organizational standards for health care facilities, to make accreditation decisions, and to provide educational and consultation services to health care organizations.

After meeting eligibility requirements, any hospital or other defined health care organization may apply for an accreditation survey. After completing the required paperwork and paying the appropriate fee for costs, surveyors from the JCAHO are sent to the facility. The survey includes on-site observations as well as document review and other information-gathering techniques. A decision is rendered and the facil-

DISPLAY 14-1

Sample Health Care Proxy

I, JANE DOE, hereby appoint JOHN DOE of 1234 Main Street, Anytown, New York 00000, (000)000-0000, as my health care agent to make any and all health care decisions for me. In the event that JOHN DOE is unable, unwilling, or unavailable to act as my health care agent, I hereby appoint MARY DOE, of 789 Smith Street, Anytown, New York (000)000-0000, as my successor health care agent.

In the event that I become unable to make my own health care decisions, this health care proxy shall take effect, and I hereby authorize my health care agent or my successor health care agent, as the case may be, to make any and all health care decisions for me, without exception.

I declare that I have discussed with my agent my wishes regarding artificial nutrition and hydration, and it is my intention that my agent shall have authority to make all decisions concerning these measures as fully as I could if I were able.

I have discussed health care decision-making matters with my agent and with my successor agent. However, should there be any doubt, I ask that their decisions be followed. I also direct that if it appears that due to injury or illness, I become extremely disabled and it appears that there is no reasonable expectation of my recovery, or that I will regain a meaningful quality of life, I direct that no medical treatment be initiated. If at that time medical treatment has already commenced, I direct that such treatment be discontinued.

I retain the power to revoke this proxy at any time and for any reason. I understand, unless I revoke it, this proxy will remain in effect indefinitely.

Date: _____

Witness: _____

_____

Signature
1234 Main Street
Anytown, New York 00000

Witness: _____

_____

ity is accredited, conditionally accredited, or denied accreditation. Accreditation is for a three-year period of time. There is an appeal process if the institution is denied accreditation.

Ramifications of Not Being Accredited by the JCAHO

Patients may be less likely to want to be treated at a facility that does not meet minimal standards. If a facility is not accredited, it will be unable to attract highly qualified physicians and staff. The facility may not be able to obtain grants and other types of funding if it fails to meet the JCAHO's standards.

The mission of the JCAHO is "to improve the quality of care provided to the public" (see JCAHO, 1996, at P.I.). As part of this mission, the JCAHO sets forth its standards in a manual that can be used by the health care facility to assess itself. In addition to the more technical aspects of the health care facility, the JCAHO also has set standards for patient rights.

The JCAHO reviews the health care organization's policies and procedures. The JCAHO has set standards concerning the right of the patient to have the facility respond in a reasonable way to the patient's requests and needs for treatment, as well as the patient's right to considerate and respectful care, which includes attention to the professional and spiritual as well as the cultural variables that affect the patient.

The JCAHO reviews the facility's policies and procedures concerning the right of the dying patient to have optimal comfort and dignity throughout the dying process. This includes the policies addressed to pain management and treatment of symptoms that respond to treatment, all of which should be based on the decision by the competent patient or the agent of the incompetent patient.

In addition, standards are set and policies reviewed that pertain to the patient's right to accept to refuse treatment, and the right to be informed of the consequences of her decision.

There are standards for protecting the right of the patient to appoint an agent to make health care decisions and for the patient to make advance directives if she desires. The JCAHO looks to see if the facility has a procedure to determine if the patient has advance directives and if there is a policy in place to assist the patient in the preparation of advance directives when the patient is admitted to the facility. The standards are such that the JCAHO looks for policies that indicate if the facility will provide care whether or not the patient has advance directives and whether it limits care if there are no advance directives.

The review also looks to whether there is a provision for the advance directives to be a part of the patient's medical records and provisions for a periodic review of those directives with the patient or the agent.

The JCAHO also has standards that address the patient's rights to participate in the consideration of ethical issues that could arise during the course of treatment; the right to be informed if there is any human experimentation or other research that would affect his or her care; the right to privacy and confidentiality; the right of the patient, at the time of admission to the facility, to be informed of the facility's patient-rights policies and the procedure for resolving the patient's complaints concerning his or her quality of care.

Furthermore, the JCAHO reviews the facility-wide policies concerning the withholding of resuscitative procedures and use or withdrawing of life-sustaining treatment.

The JCAHO survey looks at what steps the facility has taken concerning partitioning in patients' rooms, curtains in the emergency room, spacing of stretchers and exam areas to give auditory privacy, interviewing patients out of hearing range of other patients, and providing locked storage areas for patients' personal items. Other issues surveyed are whether translators are available, what communication facilities there are for hearing impaired patients, whether there are educational materials available, and how the hospital supports the patient's right to access protective services.

In addition to the patient rights set forth by the JCAHO, individual states may have enacted or promulgated various statutes, rules, or regulations that broaden the rights of the patient.

The standards as set forth by the JCAHO should be considered as materially significant if a practitioner becomes involved in litigation.

They are often cited by attorneys as evidence of the appropriate standard of care. A good argument could be made to have the JCAHO standards admitted into evidence if the case alleges that the patient's rights were violated. Nurses should be familiar with the JCAHO standards, because they are used in various lawsuits as evidence of the standard of care and they can be used to show that the nurse has deviated from that standard.

The JCAHO sets the standards for health care facilities. If the facility is accredited by the JCAHO there is some comfort to the patient that the institution is meeting the minimal standards and is protecting the rights of the patient.

ANTIDUMPING LEGISLATION

All patients have certain rights. There has been legislation to prevent the transfer of patients from one facility to another solely for financial reasons. Under other legislation similar protection has been extended to perinatal patients. In 1986, as part of the Omnibus Budget Reconciliation Act, Congress passed the Emergency Medical Treatment and Active Labor Act (EMTALA) (see 42 U.S.C.A. §1395dd). This legislation was created to prevent hospitals from refusing to treat and then dumping patients onto the street who came to the Emergency Room for treatment. For the most part these patients were poor and uninsured, and they drained the finances and services of the hospitals.

Protected Persons

If a hospital has an emergency department and a patient comes to the facility and requests either an examination or treatment for a medical condition, the hospital must provide an appropriate medical screening exam to determine if an emergency medical condition exists.

Emergency Room Patients

If a patient has an emergency medical condition as defined by the statute, that patient is protected and the hospital cannot refuse to treat the patient. The statute defines "emergency medical condition" as follows:

(A) a medical condition manifesting itself by acute symptoms of sufficient severity (including severe pain) such that the absence of immediate medical attention could reasonably be expected to result in

(I) placing the health of the individual (or, with respect to a pregnant woman, the health of the woman or her unborn child) in serious jeopardy,

(ii) serious impairment to bodily functions, or

(iii) serious dysfunction of any bodily organ or part;

(See 42 U.S.C.A. §1395dd (e) (A) (I), (ii), & (iii).) Therefore, any patient presenting with any of these conditions is protected and a hospital cannot refuse to treat the patient. The hospital *must* treat the patient.

Women in Active Labor

The statute extends the definition of "emergency medical condition" with respect to women who are having labor contractions to include

(I) that there is inadequate time to effect a safe transfer to another hospital for delivery, or

(ii) that transfer may pose a threat to the health or safety of the woman or the unborn child.

(See 42 U.S.C.A. §1395dd (e) (B) (I) & (ii).)

Requirements for Transfer to Another Facility

The hospital may undertake an "appropriate transfer" of a patient to another medical facility if the transferring hospital has provided the necessary treatment within its means, which minimizes the risks to the patient's health and the health of the unborn child. In addition, the receiving hospital must have the space and the qualified personnel to provide the necessary treatment, and it agrees to accept the transfer and to provide the necessary treatment. Also, the transferring facility must provide copies of their medical records related to the emergency condition. Furthermore, the transfer must be done by qualified personnel and transportation equipment including the provision for life support measures if that is required.

If the patient's emergency medical condition is not stabilized, the hospital may not transfer the patient unless the patient has been informed of the hospital's obligations and of the risk of transfer and then, in writing, requests a transfer. The transfer may be completed if a physician—or in the absence of a physician, another qualified medical person—has certified that the medical benefits that are expected to be received at the other facility outweigh the increased risks of the patient if she is not transferred. In addition the transfer must be an "appropriate transfer" as previously described.

Penalties

If a hospital violates the rules as set out in this statute, it is subject to civil penalties. Also any physician who is responsible for the examination, treatment, or transfer of a patient, and who negligently violates the statute, is subject to civil penalties for each violation. If the violation is gross and flagrant and is repeated, the physician may be excluded from participation in the reimbursement program.

The statute provides for civil enforcement for any patient who is harmed by the hospital's violation. In addition, any hospital that suffers a financial loss due to a participating hospital's violation of the law may seek and obtain those damages from the violating hospital.

The statute provides protection to any qualified medical person or physician who refuses to authorize a transfer of a patient who has not been stabilized. It also provides protection to any hospital employee who reports a violation of any of the requirements of the statute.

On December 5, 1986, Rosa Rivera went to the Emergency Room at DeTar Hospital in Victoria, Texas. She was pregnant and in labor with her sixth child. She was having one minute, moderate contractions every 3 minutes, and her membranes had ruptured. She was examined by two obstetrical nurses who found her to be in labor as well as having extremely high blood pressure. Mrs. Rivera had had no prenatal treatment, nor did she have a regular doctor nor means to pay for her treatment.

Michael L. Burditt was the doctor on call. After receiving the patient's history, he told the calling nurse that he did not want to take care of the patient. The nurse was asked to prepare the patient to be transferred to another hospital located 170 miles away.

The nurses advised their supervisor and the hospital administrator that they believed it would not be safe to transfer the patient. When Dr. Burditt called back, he was advised that the administrator understood that under the hospital regulations and federal law Dr. Burditt would have to examine the patient and then personally arrange to have her transferred.

Burditt came to the hospital and examined the patient. Her blood pressure was 210/130. He assumed that she had been hypertensive throughout her pregnancy. Burditt was an experienced head of the hospital's OB/GYN department. Burditt knew that the patient's condition could cause complications that could result in the death of the patient and her baby. Burditt obtained acceptance from the other hospital, which was better equipped to care for underweight infants.

The nursing supervisor showed Dr. Burditt the hospital's guidelines regarding EMTALA, but he refused to read them. Burditt told the supervisor that Mrs. Rivera represented more of a malpractice risk than he was willing to accept. He was told that he had to sign a form authorizing the transfer. Although the form provided a space for a reason for transferring the patient, he did not complete it. The patient was not transferred until approximately 1½ hours after Burditt first examined her. He remained in the hospital during that time period, but he never reexamined her. He did not order any medications or life support equipment for the patient during the transfer.

During the transfer, an OB nurse who was accompanying the patient delivered the baby when the ambulance was approximately 40 miles from DeTar Hospital. The nurse directed the ambulance to a nearby hospital and then called Burditt. He ordered that she continue to the distant hospital. However, the patient wanted to return to DeTar. Upon arrival, Burditt refused to see the patient. Burditt ordered the patient to be discharged if she was stable and not bleeding excessively. However, the hospital intervened and another doctor saw and treated

Mrs. Rivera for three days after which she was discharged in good health.

The Inspector General of the United States Department of Health and Human Services demanded a $25,000.00 civil penalty from Dr. Burditt for violating EMTALA. There was an appeal to the Departmental Appeals Board (DAB). Upon losing there, he appealed the final decision to the United States Court of Appeals, Fifth Circuit, which upheld the violation of EMTALA (*Burditt v. U.S. Department of Health and Human Services,* 1991).

Although the EMTALA statute limits civil actions of violations of EMTALA to hospitals, there are still some Federal District Courts allowing civil actions against physicians. Federal Circuit Courts have held that EMTALA does not authorize a private right of action against a physician. A recent Third Department case in New York agrees with the Federal Circuit Courts and recently dismissed an EMTALA violation cause of action against a physician (*Almond v. Town of Massena et al. & Jhaveri,* 1998).

NATIONAL PRACTITIONER DATA BANK

In 1986, President Ronald Reagan signed into law the Health Care Quality Improvement Act (HCQIA, 1986). This legislation resulted from a congressional finding that there had been an increase in medical malpractice cases and that there was a need to improve the quality of medical care, and that such issues needed to be dealt with at a national level. In addition, Congress found that there was a need to restrict the mobility of incompetent physicians and to prevent them from moving from state to state without any disclosure of the physicians' prior damaging or incompetent treatment and activities.

Congress decided that a professional peer review program was needed, and that protection was needed for physicians who engage in effective professional peer review. In general, the legislation pertains to professional review actions that began on or after October 14, 1989.

The legislation does not affect the rights and remedies of any patient to seek compensation for any damage or injury that may have resulted from negligent treatment by any physician, health care provider, or health care facility.

The National Practitioner Data Bank is a product of this legislation. The data bank is used to collect and release information concerning the competence and conduct of physicians and health care practitioners.

Reporting Requirements
Mandatory Reporting

Any entity that makes a payment to settle or to partially settle or to satisfy a judgment in a medical malpractice action or claim is required to report this information to the National Practitioner Data Bank. The statute defines a medical malpractice action or claim as a "written claim or demand for payment based on a health care provider's furnishing (or failure to furnish) health care services and includes the filing of a cause of action, based on the law of tort, brought in any court of any State or the United States seeking monetary damages" (U.S.C.A., title 42, §11151 (7)).

Physicians are subject to the reporting requirements as are other health care practitioners. Health care practitioners are those licensed, registered, or certified (depending on the jurisdiction) health care providers other than physicians. This includes nurses, midwives, and nurse practitioners.

The specific information to be reported to the National Practitioner Data Bank includes

1. name of physician or licensed health care practitioner who benefited from the payment that was made for the claim or the judgment;
2. amount of payment;
3. if known, the name of the hospital with whom the individual is affiliated;
4. a description of the acts or omissions and injuries or illnesses upon which the action or claim was based. (See Display 14-2.)

In addition, if a Board of Medical Examiners revokes or suspends a physician's license or censures, reprimands, or places a physician on probation for reasons that go to the physician's professional competence or conduct, that board must report such information to the Data Bank.

DISPLAY 14-2

Specific Information to be Reported to the NPDB for Settlement of a Claim

1. Name of physician/practitioner on whose behalf the claim/judgment was paid
2. Amount of payment
3. Name of hospital with whom affiliated
4. Description of acts/omissions
5. Injuries and/or illnesses

If an entity fails to report that a payment was made, the entity could be subject to a civil money penalty of up to $10,000.00 for each payment not reported. If a Board of Medical Examiners fails to report, and certain procedural steps to correct the error of failing to report have not been taken, then another entity may be appointed to do the reporting.

Elective Reporting

With regards to physicians, a health care entity *shall* (emphasis added) report to the Board of Medical Examiners information concerning the following:

> (1) If the entity takes a professional review action that adversely affects the clinical privileges of a physician for a period of more than thirty (30) days. Or if the entity accepts the surrender of clinical privileges of a physician while the physician is under investigation relating to possible incompetence or in return for not conducting such an investigation. (2) If the entity is a professional society and it takes a professional review action that adversely affects the physician's membership in the society.

However, if the above-mentioned activities related to a licensed health care practitioner who is not a physician, then the health care entity *may* (emphasis added) report the required information (USCA, title 42, §11133).

What does all of the legalese mean? Mandatory reporting is required of all of the previously mentioned activities for all physicians. If a payment is made on behalf of a health care practitioner named in a medical malpractice action, that information must be reported. The entity may report, but is not required to report, to the Data Bank if it takes action that adversely affects clinical privileges for more than a 30-day period or accepts the surrender of clinical privileges while the licensed health care professional is under investigation for professional incompetence or improper professional conduct, or if the entity accepts the surrender of the licensed health care professional's privileges in return for the entity's not conducting an investigation. In addition, if a professional society takes action that adversely affects the membership of the licensed health care professional in that society, the society may report the information. (See Display 14-3.)

Responsibility to Inquire

A hospital has the duty to request information from the National Practitioner Data Bank when the physician or licensed health care professional applies to be on the medical staff or when he or she applies for clinical privileges. In addition, the hospital must request information every two years for all physicians or practitioners who are on the medical staff or who have been granted clinical privileges at the hospital. The hospital may request information at other times.

Who May Access Information

Access to information is limited to state licensing boards, hospitals, and to other health care entities that have entered or may be entering into employment or an affiliation relationship with a physician or health care practitioner or to which the health care professional has applied for clinical privileges or appointment to the medical staff. Access is not available to individuals, attorneys, or insurance companies.

Due to the required reporting, physicians and health care practitioners named in a lawsuit are often reluctant to have a case settled, because

DISPLAY 14-3

Types of Information to be Reported to the NPDB

Mandatory Reporting for a Physician

1. Payment information to settle claim.
2. Actions taken by Board of Medical Examiners that adversely affect professional license.
3. Professional review action that adversely affects clinical privileges for over 30 days.
4. Surrender of license while under investigation relating to possible incompetence.
5. Surrender of license in return for entity not conducting investigation.
6. Professional society taking a professional review action that adversely affects the physician's membership in the society.

Reporting by a Health Care Practitioner

1. Mandatory.
2. Discretionary.
3. Discretionary.
4. Discretionary.
5. Discretionary.
6. Discretionary.

their names will be sent to the Data Bank. The reported information will be available if that person decides to relocate to another state. This could cause difficulty in obtaining a license and employment.

SUMMARY

In recent years, the rights of the patient have received a great deal of attention. There has been appellate litigation in various jurisdictions. This has led to statutory legislation that defines and specifically sets out the patient's rights and the procedures to protect those rights. The health care practitioner must be aware of these rights and proceed accordingly when caring for the patient. If the law is followed, there is protection for the practitioner from civil and criminal liability. If the law is ignored, then the practitioner may be liable for malpractice, civil penalties, criminal charges, and license suspension or revocation.

REFERENCES

Black's Law Dictionary. (1968). (Rev. 4th Ed.). St. Paul, MN: West Publishing.

Connecticut Public Health & Well-Being, 19a-576.

Health Care Quality Improvement Act, Pub. L. 99-660, Title IV, 402, Nov. 14, 1986, 100 Stat. 3784.

Joint Commission on Accreditation of Healthcare Organizations (1996). The joint commission 1996 accreditation manual for hospitals, Vol. I, Standards. Oakbrook Terrace, IL: Joint Commission on Accreditation of Healthcare Organizations.

Krugh, Timothy D. (1990). Is COBRA poised to strike? A critical analysis of medical COBRA. Journal of Health and Hospital Law, 23(6).

Naclerio, Gregory J., Conneely, Brian S., Rubert, Mary C., & Goodman, Richard S. (1992). New York state health care agents and proxies law: The last right? Journal of the Suffolk Academy of Law, 8.

New York Public Health Law, §29-C.

Paridy, N. (1993, Summer). Complying with the patient self-determination act: Legal, ethical and practical challenges for hospitals. Hospital and Health Services Administration 38, 287–296.

Pozgar, George D. (1996). Legal aspects of health care administration (6th ed.). Rockville, MD: Aspen.

Richards, Edward, P., III, & Rather, Katherine C. (1983). Medical risk management. Rockville, MD: Aspen Systems.

Sanbar, S. Sandy, Gibofsky, Allan, Firestone, Marvin H., LeBlang, Theodore R. (1995). Legal medicine. St. Louis, MO: Mosby-Year Book.

42 U.S.C.A., Title 42, §1395dd.

42 U.S.C.A., Title 42, §11151.

CASE CITATIONS

Almond v. Town of Massena et al. & Jhaveri, N.Y. App. Div., Third Department (1-8-98).

Burditt v. U.S. Department of Health and Human Services, Ct. of Appeals, 5th Cir., 934 F.2d 1362 (1991).

Superintendent of Belchertown v. Saikowitz, 370 N.E.2d 417 (1977).

Nancy Cruzan, by her parents and co-guardians Lester L. & Joyce Cruzan v. Director, Missouri Department of Health, 497 U.S. 261 (1990).

Matter of Quinlan, 137 N.J. Super. 227, 348 A.2d 801 (1975), modified, 70 N.J. 10, 355 A.2d 647, cert. denied sub nom. *Garger v. New Jersey,* 429 U.S. 922 (1976).

Schloendorff v. Society of New York Hospital, 211 N.Y. 125, 105 N.E. 92 (1914).

Informed Consent

*Carolyn Harris, Carolyn Curtis,
and Pamela Copeland*

This chapter addresses the doctrine of informed consent and its application in the perinatal period. The concepts that underlie this doctrine may be applicable in any phase of the perinatal period and should be implemented with due diligence where appropriate. The nurse provider should note that the information contained in this chapter is presented to assist with critical thinking when confronted with certain clinical issues or circumstances. It is not intended to replace policies, rules, or other authority under which the provider practices. It remains the nurse's responsibility to become familiar with the case law, statutory law, and nurse practice acts that govern a particular jurisdiction.

DEVELOPMENT OF THE DOCTRINE OF INFORMED CONSENT

The doctrine of informed consent is derived from both the legal and ethical disciplines (Lichtman & Papera, 1990). Since the early 1900s courts in common law have recognized that providers of health care treatments have a duty to obtain the client's (consumers of health care) consent for that treatment. This duty was articulated by Justice Cardoza in *Schloendorff v. Society of N.Y. Hospital* (1914), where he stated "that every human being of adult years and

sound mind has a right to determine what shall be done with his own body . . ." (Rozovsky, 1990). The courts initially upheld liability in tort on a theory of battery. Battery in most jurisdictions is an intentional tort requiring an unauthorized or "offensive" touching of another. The client had to establish that the provider, usually a physician, had failed to obtain the requisite permission for treatment, and that the treatment was the proximate cause of the client's injury (Northrop & Kelly, 1987). However, as clients have become increasingly more aware of their rights, liability in tort has shifted from a battery action to liability in negligence.

The informed consent doctrine reflects the belief that an individual has a right to be free from nonconsensual interference with his or her person, and a basic moral principle that it is wrong to force or encourage another to act against his or her will (Blanpain, 1993). Precedence for the modern-day doctrine was established in 1972 in the case of *Canterbury v. Spence* (1972). The issue in *Canterbury* was whether a 1% chance of paralysis caused by a laminectomy was sufficient to require disclosure of this "very slight" possibility (Goldworth, Silverman, Stevenson, Young, & Rivers, 1995). The neurosurgeon failed to discuss this particular risk with the client, who underwent a laminectomy and subsequently suffered a partial paralysis from the waist down.

The court held that the neurosurgeon had a duty to inform the client, and that the scope of the disclosure (what information must be provided to obtain informed consent) in this instance was shaped by the client's right of self-decision. This case helped to establish the client's right to self-determination and gave rise to the "reasonable patient" standard. This standard takes into consideration what the reasonable client deems important instead of what the practitioner considers important when determining what risks should be disclosed (Northrop & Kelly, 1987). However, this standard is subjective. It permits clients to testify retrospectively about what they would have done if information about the complication that has already been experienced had been known at the time of the procedure (Cohn, 1990).

The standard of disclosure may vary by jurisdiction, but increasingly the "reasonable person" or objective standard of disclosure is used (Cohn, 1990). In the reasonable person jurisdiction the provider is required to give the client, a rational agent, enough information for him or her to determine what information is material (Goldworth et al., 1995). Other jurisdictions may use the "professional" disclosure standard (Cohn, 1990). This measures the duty to disclose by looking at what a provider with similar training, education, and experience would have done under the same or similar circumstances (Blanpain, 1993).

The test for determining whether a particular peril must be disclosed is determined by its materiality to the client's decision. Blanpain (1993) cites *Shinn v. James Mercy Hospital* (1987) to illustrate that courts often hold that remote risks can be omitted. Likewise, *Kissenger v. Lofgren* (1988) also notes that risks commonly known by clients can be omitted.

During the unpredictable perinatal period, the expecting family may be required to make planned and/or unplanned decisions about treatments or interventions relating to the pregnancy, and to provide or refuse authorization for those treatments or interventions. In the absence of emergency circumstances or lack of decision-making capacity, the pregnant woman and her significant others should always be given sufficient information about proposed interventions. Additionally, she will need adequate time to discuss the information with the health care provider in order to render informed consent to or informed refusal of treatments.

INFORMED CONSENT PROCESS

Informed consent is an outcome of a deliberate decision-making process, not a form or a document. It involves

- *conversation* about a proposed intervention (that is, diagnostic, surgical, medical, or research),
- *negotiation,*
- *reflection,* and
- *debate* between the client and the provider.

Consultants and significant others may also have a need to participate in the process (Younger & Conner, 1987; King, 1994). The informed consent process promotes empowerment of the client and provides opportunities for autonomous decision making.

Rozovsky (1990) iterates that informed consent is a decision-making process that contains a number of important elements. These elements include

- illness or injury (also disease prevention and health promotion),
- development of a treatment relationship,
- history taking and examination,
- treatment or test recommendation,
- disclosure of pertinent information,
- exchange of questions and answers, and
- agreement on what should be done.

Staff nurses, whether in an outpatient, inpatient, or community setting, have a responsibility to educate clients about certain aspects of their treatment as it relates to the nursing care plan, specifically the diagnoses and interventions. Advanced practice nurse providers (nurse practitioners, nurse midwives, and nurse anesthetists) also have diagnostic and prescriptive responsibilities, and are required to obtain informed consent for all interventions that fall within their areas of authority. Consequently, advanced practice nurses also have a duty to disclose, educate, and ensure that the client understands the risks and benefits of a treatment or intervention to the best of their ability. Put another way, all providers should try diligently to ensure that clients understand the facts presented, believe the facts, and have reasonable decision-making capacity (Loewy, 1996).

The level and the scope of disclosure responsibility for the primary providers, consultants, and specialists are circumscribed by such variables as employment policies, educational preparation, certifications, and professional practice standards.

Rhodes and Miller (1984) state that nurses may have disclosure responsibility in four types of situations:

- procedures offered by nurses in independent practice roles;
- nursing procedures not directly related to medical procedures, such as starting an IV;
- nursing aspects of medical procedures where the primary procedure is being provided by another practitioner, such as wound management after surgical intervention; and
- medical procedures being provided by another practitioner.

DISCLOSURE REQUIREMENTS

The nurse has a duty to assist the client in making an informed decision about a given intervention. When the physician, nurse-midwife, or nurse practitioner fails to disclose pertinent information or material issues that may impact the client's decision to submit to or refrain from having a particular intervention, the provider may be legally liable if the client has a less than desirable outcome from the intervention. The nurse should ensure that the client has an understanding of the following in an effort to optimize client satisfaction and minimize the possibility of a lawsuit:

(a) the diagnosis (the client's condition or problem);

(b) the nature and purpose of the proposed treatment/intervention;

(c) the probable outcome of the treatment/intervention;

(d) the likely benefits of the intervention;

(e) what the diagnostic, medical, or surgical procedure will involve including any probable complications, temporary discomfort, disability, or discomfort;

(f) disclosure of risks and consequences of the proposed interventions that are reasonably foreseeable at the time consent is obtained, including an explanation of any permanent results of a medical or surgical procedure such as a scar or alteration in body functions and the required care;

(g) any remote risks that are material for the particular client;

(h) feasible treatment alternatives; and

(i) the prognosis if the proposed treatment is not given (Younger & Conner, 1987; Rozovsky, 1990).

During the client-teaching process the nurse provider should be aware that clients often do not remember much of what they have been told, and that clients tend to have their lowest level of knowledge about two of the most important aspects of treatment: alternatives and risks (Younger & Conner, 1987). The provider is only required to discuss the risks or alternative forms of care that are recognized at the time the consent is obtained. Should the client sustain an injury or insult that was not reasonably foreseeable at the time consent was obtained, then the provider cannot be held liable on that issue (Rozovsky, 1990).

Preconception Period

In the preconception period, informed consent is especially significant in the area of birth control where generally healthy people decide to use chemicals, hormones, and/or devices for family planning purposes. However, prior to the use of one of these methods, the client must be provided with all the necessary information required to make an informed decision about contraceptive choices. If the practitioner conscientiously provides the requisite information articulated in the following guidelines, he or she should be legally protected for and ethically secure in services rendered (Lichtman & Papera, 1990).

Informed consent for family planning encompasses the following:

(a) a description of the proposed method, how it works, what it does;

(b) the benefits of the proposed method, its effectiveness in preventing pregnancy, and other advantages;

(c) the disadvantages of the proposed method, including its risks;

(d) the cost of the proposed method, immediate and over time, including the need for provider follow-up and ongoing care;

(e) a full discussion of alternative methods, covering, for each method, a description, how it works, its benefits, effectiveness, advantages, disadvantages, risks, and cost. In family planning, alternative methods include all contraceptive choices, natural family planning, male or female sterilization, and abortion;

(f) a discussion of the benefits, advantages, effectiveness, disadvantages, risks, and cost of using no method of family planning;

(g) assurance of the right to ask (and have answered) questions at any time;

(h) the right to withdraw consent at any time; and

(i) a full disclosure of the experimental nature of any method when appropriate (Lichtman & Papera, 1990).

It is incumbent upon the practitioner to raise all of the informed consent issues with each client. A considerable number of lawsuits are filed in the area of injuries related to birth control. The salient issue in these cases is the provider's duty to disclose material information during the consent process. According to Rozovsky (1990) plaintiffs usually allege that their consent to using a birth control medication or a device was defective because they were not fully informed of the risks.

In *Klink v. G. D. Searle & Co.* (1980), a married, 19-year-old woman suffered a bilateral stroke after taking Ovulen-21, a birth control pill, for 17 months for amenorrhea. During the neg-

ligence suit against her private physician, the plaintiff stated in testimony that the physician had not told her that her underlying amenorrhea condition could be a sign of infertility, or that contraception was not a treatment for her condition. The plaintiff also stated that had she been so informed and had she been given other information relating to her condition, she would not have consented to taking the pill.

On appeal the defendant tried to establish that he had not been given the opportunity in presenting his defense, to show what other physicians disclosed in similar situations. The court concluded that the evidence did nothing to establish a defense justifying the defendant's failure to disclose certain facts to the client.

Health care practitioners including nurse providers at all levels are encouraged to actively minimize their vulnerability to potential lawsuits. Providers should remain current on developments involving family planning interventions; identify those women for whom birth control or devices are medically contraindicated; encourage clients to contact the health care provider immediately if a problem arises; monitor the time limits on prescriptions so that clients must come back for checkups and reassessment of continued use; use instruction sheets that describe the intended therapeutic effect of the medication or device, possible side effects, instruction for seeking immediate medical attention; and obtain signatures of the client and/or witness (Rozovsky, 1990).

The Antenatal Period

The antenatal period is filled with numerous decision-making opportunities for the pregnant woman and her family. This can be an ideal time for the nurse provider to implement teaching strategies that will enhance the woman's understanding of what is happening to her with this pregnancy. It should be a time when the pregnant woman and her family can make autonomous, uncoerced, and informed decisions about such things as antenatal tests and screens, and procedures or treatments for managing less than optimal results related to testing and screening.

Some of the most challenging issues in antenatal testing will be discussed in detail because of their impact on the informed consent process. However, there are other aspects of management in the antenatal period that must also be addressed and discussed with the client that will allow her to make an informed decision about the things that have a bearing on her pregnancy. These other aspects may include but are not limited to choice of provider, for example a certified nurse midwife or physician; fetal surveillance tests such as the nonstress test, biophysical profile test, and contraction stress test; and place of birth (home, hospital, or freestanding birth center). Each of these areas needs to be addressed in relationship to material disclosure and the client's philosophical, religious, ethical, and moral tenets, so that the client is empowered to render true, informed consent.

Often a woman's decision regarding a treatment modality or management plan may differ from that of the provider, the institution, or community. Speidel and Suarez (1995) caution the provider to remember that the client has the right of refusal and may decide to refuse treatment at any point during the pregnancy. This right of refusal is extended to the competent client because the client's autonomy and right to self-determination are also expressed in the refusal of treatment (King, 1994).

Antenatal Screening and Diagnosis

The substantive informed consent process includes a minimum of nine key elements. However, Speidel and Suarez (1995) state that the pregnant client should also be informed about the following aspects of management/treatment interventions:

(a) the probability of success of a particular intervention, and also what the provider means by success;

(b) the major problems anticipated in recuperation and the time period in which the client may be able to resume activities;

(c) how the procedure will be carried out;

(d) when test results will be available;

(e) how test results will be disclosed;

(f) the meaning of positive and negative test results; and

(g) any other information that is generally provided to women by other qualified providers.

The purpose of antenatal screening and diagnostic testing is to obtain information about the status of the pregnancy. This status information may provide an opportunity for parental reassurance of fetal well-being and reducing anxiety associated with reproduction; fetal therapy; parental preparation for birth of an affected child; abortion of an affected fetus; management options for delivery; and parents to ask questions within their particular social or religious framework. Clark and Devor (1989) state that the ultimate goal of prenatal diagnosis is to treat or prevent all prenatally diagnosed anomalies.

There are numerous tests that may be performed during the antenatal period. Screening tests include maternal serum alpha fetoprotein (MSAFP) and the triple test. Diagnostic antenatal tests include chorionic villus sampling (CVS), amniocentesis, ultrasound examination, the nonstress test, the contraction stress test, and the biophysical profile test. The nurse provider is required to have a working knowledge of these tests as part of managing women throughout their pregnancy. The provider also has a duty to disclose and review material aspects of screens or diagnostic tests.

The guidelines for disclosure should embrace the points previously articulated by Speidel and Suarez (1995). It is critical that women and their families are informed that when they enter the arena of prenatal screening and diagnostic testing, the decision-making process for informed consent is a tiered one. It is possible that they will face unexpected and unwanted information about the status of their pregnancy at some point in time during the pregnancy. Consequently, they may be faced with difficult ethical and personally moral decisions regarding the outcome of the pregnancy. Additional burdensome variables that the nurse provider must bear in mind is that antenatal testing has false positive and false negative occurrences. As a result of a false positive or false negative outcome, it is possible that a pregnancy decision can be adversely affected. It is also possible to lose a normal pregnancy related to complications of diagnostic procedures such as amniocentesis and chorionic villus sampling (Williams, 1992; Hepburn, 1996).

The antenatal client may have to make two major decisions: deciding to undergo antenatal testing, and for those receiving a positive result, deciding whether to continue the pregnancy. Because of the biopsychosocial, emotional, and spiritual impact these decisions may have on the client, it is imperative that women and their families know that at any point along the tier of antenatal testing, they have the right to exercise the right of refusal as a means of exercising their autonomy and self-determination.

Serum Antenatal Screening Tests

MATERNAL SERUM ALPHA FETOPROTEIN. Maternal serum alpha fetoprotein (MSAFP) screens for neural tube defects and is done between 15 and 18 weeks of pregnancy. MSAFP has a 90% sensitivity for anencephaly and an 80–85% specificity for spina bifida. The usual time for obtaining test results is one week, and results are reported as the median of the man (MOM). Elevated values include (a) MOM > 2.5 for the general pregnant population; (b) MOM > 2.0 for an insulin-dependent diabetic; and (c) MOM > 4.5–5.0 for twin gestation. Eighty to 90% of fetuses with neural tube defect will have values >2.5 MOM. Elevated values may also be indicative of other complications such as prematurity, premature rupture of the membranes (PROM), intrauterine growth retardation (IUGR), placental abruption, or ventral wall defect (Zamorski, 1996).

Accurate dating is required to interpret a low MSAFP value. Follow-up testing for values between >2.5–2.9 MOM and gestational age less than 18 weeks generally will require the MSAFP test to be repeated. An ultrasound may be done to ascertain correct dating, rule out multiple gestation, fetal demise, anencephaly, and missed abortion. An amniocentesis will be required if the reason for an abnormal value cannot be determined from the ultrasound. One in 15 women having an unexplained elevated MSAFP value will have an infant with a neural tube defect. Although a low MSAFP value may be an indication of Down's syndrome, the MSAFP test

does not screen for Down's syndrome (Gabbe, Niebyl, & Simpson, 1991).

TRIPLE SCREEN. The triple screen test is performed in the same manner and time frame as the MSAFP test. This test screens for Down's syndrome (Trisomy 21), Trisomy 18, as well as neural tube defects. It has a 95% specificity with a 5% false positive rate. The screen measures the maternal serum alpha fetoprotein for neural tube defects, estriol for Trisomy 21, and HcG for Trisomy 18 (Zamorski, 1995). Elevated results necessitate an amniocentesis to assess for the presence of congenital anomalies (Gabbe, Niebyl, & Simpson, 1991).

Antenatal Diagnostic Tests

CHORIONIC VILLUS SAMPLING. Chorionic villus sampling (CVS), an invasive procedure, may be performed as early as the fifth week of pregnancy, but is commonly done between 9 and 12 weeks gestation (Pillitteri, 1995). This test is used to detect genetic abnormalities. A catheter or needle is inserted into the uterine cavity to obtain a sampling of chorionic cells for analysis. If a multiple pregnancy is present with two or more separate placentas, then a sampling must be obtained from each placenta. Failure to do so may result in a missed opportunity to detect a genetic defect in a timely manner. Should termination be elected, it can be done early in pregnancy, thereby decreasing the risk of maternal morbidity and mortality associated with abortions later in pregnancy. An earlier termination also minimizes the time the woman and her family have to bond to the pregnancy.

Risks associated with CVS include infection (.1% or 1:1,000), ambiguous results secondary to maternal cell contamination, a 2–4% rate of associated labor contractions and excessive bleeding, and limb deformities (1.4:10,000–7.4:10,000). Spontaneous abortion occurs in approximately .5–1% (1:200–1:100) cases (Morbidity and Mortality Weekly Report, 1995). Although CVS is diagnostic of genetic anomalies, it cannot diagnose neural tube defects. The alternative procedure for CVS is amniocentesis.

AMNIOCENTESIS. Amniocentesis is also a diagnostic test for genetic anomalies as well as neural tube defects. This procedure is done between

15 and 18 weeks gestation and requires the removal of amniotic fluid from the uterine cavity. The fluid contains fetal cells that have been shed from the fetal skin, bladder, GI tract, and amnion. Because the test is not conducted until the second trimester, decisions regarding termination are delayed, which may result in increased maternal morbidity and mortality. The infection rate following amniocentesis is 0.1%, and rate of spontaneous abortion is .5–1% (1:200–1:00). Although CVS is the alternative to amniocentesis, it does not diagnose neural tube defects (MMWR, 1995).

Ultrasonography

Ultrasound has become an integral part of prenatal care for almost all women in the United States. Sonography is a diagnostic tool that is helpful in assessing a fetus for general size and structural defect of the spine and limbs. This procedure may be done concurrently with amniocentesis because it causes no apparent risk to the fetus (Pillitteri, 1995).

Several ethical issues associated with ultrasound emerge: The pregnant family knows the potential for confronting the unanticipated possibility of termination should an anomaly be detected; the results of ultrasound tests must be disclosed even when they are uncertain or incomplete; and bonding often occurs when the woman sees her infant during the procedure. The bonding may complicate the decisions related to abortion or benefit the decision to carry the baby to term (Chevernak & McCullough, 1992).

The Intrapartal Period

The same principles of informed consent apply during the intrapartal period. In the best-case scenario, the labor and delivery processes, possible related complications, and the general management of maternal/fetal complications were disclosed and discussed prior to the onset of labor. Due to the uncertainty of so many aspects of the intrapartal period, it is not practical for the certified nurse midwife or obstetrician to address every single possible development.

It is incumbent upon the practitioner to discuss methods of delivery and to obtain sig-natures on the appropriate consent forms. Depending on the setting, the nurse, student nurse, or another designee may be responsible for ensuring that a signed consent form is on the chart. In *Sinclair by Sinclair v. Block* (1991), the parents alleged among other things that the obstetrician failed to obtain informed consent specific to the use of forceps during the delivery of their newborn. During delivery, the newborn exhibited decelerations and was observed to be malpositioned in the birth canal. The obstetrician unsuccessfully attempted to correct the baby's position with the use of forceps and the newborn was subsequently delivered via cesarean section. After her birth, the newborn was observed to have areas of swelling on her scalp and a faint mark on her forehead, which were thought to be forceps marks. The parents contested that the use of forceps was a surgical procedure that required application of the informed consent doctrine.

On this issue the court determined that it was unnecessary for the practitioner to obtain the parents' specific consent to the use of forceps in delivery because the use of forceps is not a surgical operative procedure that requires application of the informed consent doctrine. At the trial the child's mother testified that the delivery procedures had been discussed and she had given authorization for the obstetrician or his partners to perform any procedure necessary to deliver her child.

The outcome in such cases is never predictable. Northrop and Kelly (1987) cite *Campbell v. Pitt County Memorial Hospital* (1985), where a jury verdict of $6.5 million was awarded against a hospital for negligence of its employee nurse. The nurse failed to ensure that the parents had given informed consent to a vaginal delivery under circumstances that warranted a cesarean delivery. Several hours after delivery, the nurse obtained the father's signature on the consent form.

The hospital was sued in its own capacity for failing to ensure that clients in labor had given informed consent for the method of delivery. The attending obstetrician had previously settled out of court for $1.5 million.

Postnatal Issues

There are numerous times in the postnatal period where the mother/family of a newborn may need to make decisions and authorize treatment for the neonate. Most states have laws that mandate neonatal immunizations, prophylactic eye treatments, and screening interventions. Parents need education and information about these interventions so they can make an informed decision.

Hepatitis B vaccine may be administered to the neonate 1–2 days after birth if the mother has a negative HBsAg status at the time of delivery. If the maternal status is HBsAg positive, the infant may receive the hepatitis immunization as early as 0–12 hours after birth (Dershewitz, 1993). The National Child Vaccine Injury Act of 1986 mandates the development and distribution of standard benefit and risk statements for vaccines which should be explained to the parents. This act also requires providers to note in the child's record the date of vaccine administration, manufacturer and lot number, and the name, address, and the title of the person administering the vaccine (Dershewitz, 1993).

In instances of undesired immunizations and screening interventions, parents may be successful when raising religious objections. However, these objections are generally not honored when prophylactic treatment is given to prevent blindness from gonococcal conjunctivitis. Parental objections to neonatal interventions may be overcome by a compelling state interest in the public welfare and prevention of epidemics (Rozovsky, 1990).

Other interventions include but are not limited to intramuscular administration of vitamin K for prophylactic treatment of prolonged coagulation (Pillitteri, 1995); and screening for hypothyroidism, PKU, galactosemia, sickle cell anemia or sickle cell trait, maple syrup urine disease, and homocystinuria (Rozovsky, 1990, 1996). Informed consent must also be obtained for circumcisions and other treatments such as phototherapy for hyperbilirubinemia of the newborn.

ONGOING DISCLOSURE RESPONSIBILITY

The disclosure responsibility pertaining to antenatal screening and testing does not stop with the provision of the information given in the last section. As stated previously, the decision-making process resulting in informed consent, or informed refusal for treatment, is a tiered one. Once the client has undergone testing and screening, she must decide what to do next in light of the results. The provider should continue to disclose material information in order for the expecting woman to have ongoing and sufficient information on which to make a decision about her management options.

Once diagnosis of a congenital anomaly is made, an explanation should be issued as to what impact the anomaly may have on the quality of life, how the child with special needs can be managed, and the life expectancy and morbidity associated with the anomaly. All terms should be explained so that the client can grasp the importance of what is being discussed.

A number of suits have been brought in the courts where parents of a child born with genetic defects, or other severe mental and physical deformities, allege that the provider/physician breached his or her duty to the parents by failing to timely diagnose or inform them of test results. As a result, the parents contend that they were denied the opportunity to decide whether to abort or to continue the pregnancy (Rozovsky, 1990).

When such suits are initiated, the causes of action may be brought for "wrongful pregnancy" or "wrongful birth" by the parents of the affected child, or "wrongful life" by or on behalf of the child. In *Flanagan v. Williams* (1993), the parents and their minor child, claiming an action for wrongful life, sued the physicians for failing to diagnose or inform the parents of the fetus' spina bifida and potential liabilities in time for the parents to terminate the pregnancy. The trial court erred in ruling that Ohio did not allow a cause of action for wrongful birth and found for the defendants. The plaintiffs appealed and the

Court of Appeals reversed the judgment of the lower court in part, stating that the failure of the physicians to diagnose and/or disclose information that is crucial to the exercise of the choice not to procreate was actionable as medical malpractice. However, not all states recognize "wrongful birth" as a cause of action. This case is but one of many that illustrates how an allegation of defective consent can transcend the perinatal period and beyond.

DECISIONS ABOUT PREGNANCY RESOLUTION

Abortion

Deliberations about whether or not to have a pregnancy terminated by abortion are generally heavily laden with religious, moral, legal, ethical, and sometimes financial considerations. The attempt to reach a decision about abortion as the choice of management at this time may also be compounded by such variables as the client's age (teenager or adult), marital status, mental capacity, status of the mother/father relationship, and the circumstances under which the conception occurred. Because of these factors, the decision to abort is often an ambivalent one (Blumberg, Golbus, & Hanson, 1975; Furlong & Black, 1984; Lloyd & Laurence, 1985; Reardon, 1987). Women having abortions for genetic indicators seem to have a more difficult time with ambivalence because their pregnancy is wanted, and pregnancy termination is an end to all their expectations (Blumberg, Golbus, & Hanson, 1975; Furlong & Black, 1984; Lloyd & Laurence, 1985).

Family members also experience psychological reactions to abortion. Men expressed depression and guilt (Blumberg, Golbus, & Hanson, 1975); and some sibling children expressed guilt in thinking that their feelings about the pregnancy or their actions may have caused the pregnancy termination (Furlong & Black, 1984). In light of these factors, it is imperative that information on fetal growth and development as well as the type of procedure to be used for the abortion itself be disclosed to the client with all the risks and benefits. The ambivalence related to the abortion option and the potential impact the decision may have on the client and her family mandate that the provider disclose test results as soon as possible regardless of what they are. In addition to the provider the nurse should be available for support before, during, and after antenatal testing and decisions are made.

Although nurse providers do not perform abortions, they are encouraged to strictly adhere to the protocols and procedures of the facility regarding their role in documenting the informed consent process. Nurses should also be aware that some states require that a qualified individual provide counseling to the pregnant woman prior to the abortion procedure. Under some circumstances, particularly if a minor or client is involved who lacks the mental capacity, the state law may require parental or judicial consent for the intervention (Cohn, 1990). In *Planned Parenthood of Central Missouri v. Danforth* (1976), the United States Supreme Court established minors' rights to consent to abortion. Many state statutes "allow minors to consent to specific types of treatments such as drug and alcohol abuse, venereal disease treatment, pregnancy, contraceptives and abortion" (Feutz-Harter, 1997).

Nonaggressive Management

The decision to consent to nonaggressive management of a less than optimal pregnancy is in effect a right to refuse treatment. Nonaggressive management is a treatment option that limits or withholds obstetrical interventions that would benefit the fetus. Such interventions would be an overt omission of the following: tests for fetal surveillance such as nonstress tests and biophysical profile; tocolytics in the presence of preterm labor; a cesarean section and/or transfer of the mother to a tertiary care unit in the presence of fetal distress.

These actions have been defended ethically in cases where there is a high probability that the diagnosis is correct, a high probability of death as an outcome of the anomaly diagnosed, or a very high probability of severe irreversible deficit of cognitive developmental capacity as a result of the anomaly diagnosed (Gabbe, Niebyl, & Simpson, 1991). The client can only make a true informed decision in this instance after the provider discloses the material risks and benefits, and after the client deals with her own values and feelings regarding this type of nonintervention, which may hasten the death of the fetus.

OTHER ISSUES IMPACTING THE INFORMED CONSENT PROCESS

Although clients generally have a right to refuse treatment, this right does not extend to circumstances where treatment refusal means death. Judicial limits have been placed on the type of acceptable refusal of consent to treatment. Although courts may be more lenient if refusal is based on religious beliefs, many courts have held that states may impose a restriction on religious practices that jeopardize the health, safety, or welfare of the people (Rozovsky, 1990).

There are other areas of medical management of the perinatal client that warrant mentioning as they relate to informed consent. Rozovsky (1990) and Blanpain (1993) articulate several issues that have potential impact on the informed consent process. The list provided here is not exhaustive and will not be covered in detail.

Emergencies

Practitioners may provide emergency treatment without the client's consent when all of the following conditions exist:

- the client is in immediate need of medical intervention,
- the client is unable to consent to medical intervention because of a mental or physical incapacity,
- no surrogate decision maker is available to give consent,
- delay in treatment would increase the risk of death or severed physical impairment,
- the proposed treatment is limited to that necessary to treat the emergency, and
- there is no evidence that the client would object to the treatment.

Emergency treatment without consent warrants documentation of the circumstances, the rationale for treatment, the reason why a surrogate decision maker was not contacted, and other pertinent facts.

Sterilization

Federal regulations require that a special consent form and special consent procedures be followed for sterilization of Medicaid clients. Surrogate decision makers should be reserved for life-threatening or life-saving situations such as cancer. Court orders or specific jurisdictional laws are required for sterilization of incompetent clients.

Physical/Language Challenges

Clients who do not speak English or who are visually or hearing impaired must consent to their own treatment. Reasonable accommodations such as interpreters and visual and hearing devices must be provided.

Incompetent Clients

Most states have laws that allow a surrogate to make decisions on behalf of the incompetent. The surrogate decision maker must be competent and at least 18 years of age. Generally, the following order of surrogate preference should be adhered to: legally appointed guardian or conservator; surrogate or health care agent previously designated by the client, spouse, adult children, parents, adult siblings, or grandparents.

The same disclosure requirement applies when the provider obtains consent from the surrogate. Disagreements among surrogate decision makers may be addressed through ethics committees or the courts. Such disagreements should not be allowed to compromise the client's health.

CONSEQUENCES FOR NONDISCLOSURE

Failure to obtain valid consent may result in litigation if the expectant client or the infant sustains an injury as a result of the provider negligently failing to inform the client of risks that were known at the time consent was obtained.

Rozovsky (1990) states that in order to establish negligent consent, the plaintiff must generally prove that

    (a) a client–provider relationship existed;

    (b) the provider had a duty to disclose certain risk information;

    (c) there was a failure to provide this information, and the failure to do so cannot be excused;

    (d) had the provider furnished the client with the undisclosed information, the client would not have consented to treatment;

    (e) the provider's failure to disclose this information was the proximate cause of the plaintiff's injury and damages claimed.

As in any negligence suit, each element must be proven in order to establish a case against the provider. In *Azzolino v. Dingfelder* (1984), a 36-year-old plaintiff gave birth to a child with Down's syndrome, and brought a wrongful life suit on behalf of the child against a family nurse practitioner (FNP) and the attending obstetrician. Plaintiff maintained that she had specifically inquired about the advisability of having the test done, and that the FNP asked her if she knew that the procedure was dangerous and could produce a miscarriage. Plaintiff also alleged that the FNP interjected her religious beliefs, and that the obstetrician told her the test was not advisable, because only women over the age of 37 were in the at-risk category (Rozovsky, 1990). It was asserted that the FNP failed to further advise the client to discuss amniocentesis with someone else or to inform her of other facilities where she could get the procedure done (Northrop & Kelly, 1987).

The North Carolina Court of Appeals ruled that the defendants had breached their duty to inform the plaintiffs of "material information" regarding genetic abnormalities, and failed to advise them regarding the need for an amniocentesis. The parents claimed that had they been properly advised they would have undergone the test and would have elected a legal abortion had they been informed that the child had Down's syndrome. The Appeals Court reversed the lower court's dismissal of the child's claim for wrongful life (Rozovsky, 1990).

DOCUMENTATION

Not many lawsuits are initiated on the issue of informed consent alone. However, defective consent may be one of the charges that a plaintiff alleges contributed to her current state of health or medical condition. In a malpractice suit one of the best weapons for the party being sued is thorough, accurate documentation (Hahn, 1995). Providers should document orders, treatments, and prescriptive management clearly, competently, and comprehensively. Any matter concerning informed consent should be noted in writing. The written consent is merely a validation that the consent conversation between the provider and the client has occurred (Fiesta, 1994). The writing may be a highly detailed, traditional long-form consent; a less detailed short-form consent; a checklist; or a narrative note.

The short-form consent and the checklist should be accompanied by a complementary narrative note. Each form of documentation should include general information, issues discussed, the date the client gave informed consent, the date on which the document was recorded, and the signatures of the provider and the client (Spindel & Suarez, 1995). Regardless of the form used, in litigation even a signed detailed note may only be highly persuasive of informed consent (Rozovsky, 1990). It is not necessarily concrete evidence that informed consent was obtained.

Northrop and Kelly (1987) state that consent forms used to document a client's informed consent are considered rebuttable evidence that the consent is based on an understanding of the information provided. As a matter of practice the consent form is not usually presented for signature at the same time as the discussion of the intervention. In many instances the person presenting the document for signature may not be the nurse provider or the person who participated in the informed consent discussion.

There have been instances where valid informed consent has been obtained, but the practitioner failed to stay within the scope of the intervention that the client authorized, in the absence of an emergency. In *Millard v. Nagle* (1991), the surgical provider removed the client's remaining ovary during bladder surgery. The court held that generally a provider does not have the authority to extend surgical procedures to areas outside the initial consent unless additional consent is expressly obtained, or an emergency situation exists that requires immediate action to preserve the health or life of the client. This was not deemed an emergency situation, so additional informed consent was required on behalf of the client. There was no documentation of implied or expressed consent for the removal of the ovary.

Documentation of informed consent should also include an evaluation of how well the client understood the procedures or treatments as well as any refusal of treatment. Time frames are always important in verifying when communication between provider and client took place, and when treatment was offered and undertaken. Sometimes when physician providers have engaged the client in the informed consent process, the nurse may be asked to witness the validation document. Fiesta (1994) reminds the nurse to follow the policies of the agency and to actually witness the provider obtaining the client's signature on the form.

In order for a provider to ensure that the appropriate information has been discussed and that the documentation has legal as well as medical sufficiency, the provider should obtain and document the patient's consent according to agency policy and/or prevailing documentation standards. Historically, such responsibility was imputed to the treating physician, but in *Bulman v. Meyers* (1983) it was held that valid informed consent to surgery could be obtained by a nurse assistant who made a full disclosure of the risks rather than the operating surgeon. The critical inquiry was whether the client had been given adequate information, and not the identity of the person giving it (Younger & Conner, 1987). Documentation should include who the parties are, what was discussed, why it was discussed, and when and where the discussion took place, in order to avoid the ambiguities in the aforementioned case.

In addition to the client situations mentioned, specific attention must be given to perinatal clients who fall in the following categories, to ensure that the consent given is not defective: minors, the mentally handicapped and mentally ill, and sedated clients. The provider should also note and document whether the client has a valid advance directive that is readily available.

SUMMARY

Informed consent is a process that is designed to ensure that clients have the opportunity to make an informed decision. There are several steps in the process, and the outcome of the process should be reflected in a signed written document by the client and provider. This writing should be retained in the client's medical record. Clients have a right to refuse treatment, accept a proposed treatment, or request modifications in an ongoing treatment. Clients can also ask to have treatment terminated during the treatment process.

Certain critical information must be disclosed and discussed by the proper person in order for the client or her surrogate to truly participate in the process. The standard of disclosure, what should be disclosed, the responsible party, and documentation of disclosure are all issues that have been litigated. In the event of a lawsuit, documentation of disclosure discussion is the best evidence that the discussion took place. However, even documentary evidence is rebuttable.

The best approach to minimizing litigation is for the practitioner to establish a trusting relationship with the client. The provider must take time with the client and pay attention to her concerns. Clients need to be treated as sensible consumers who have a right to know what management is being proposed and to decide whether or not this is what they want. Finally, providers must remain knowledgeable, current, and competent in their practice.

REFERENCES

ACOG. (1988). Ultrasound in pregnancy. ACOG Technical Bulletin, Number 116. Washington, DC: ACOG.

25

Blanpain, R. (Ed.). (1993). International encyclopedia of laws. Boston: Kluwer Law and Taxation.

Blumberg, B. D., Golbus, M. S., & Hanson, K. H. (1975). The psychological sequelae of abortion for a genetic indication. American Journal of Obstetrics and Gynecology, 122(7), 799–808.

Boyd, P. A. (1994). Serum screening for Down's Syndrome. PBritish Medical Journal (Clinical Research Ed.), 309: 1372.

Calfee, B. E. (1996). Nurses in the courtroom: Cases and commentary for concerned professionals. Huntsburg, OH: ARC.

Chevernak, F. A., & McCullough, L. B. (1992). Ethical issues in obstetric ultrasonography. Clinical Obstetrics and Gynecology, 35(4), 758–762.

Chevernak, F. A., & Gabbe, S. (1991). Obstetric ultrasound: Assessment of fetal growth and anatomy. In S. Gabbe, J. R. Niebyl, & J. L. Simpson. (Eds.). Obstetrics: Normal and problem pregnancies (pp. 269–298).

Clark, S. L., & Devor, G. R. (1989). Prenatal diagnosis for couples who would not consider abortion. Obstetrics and Gynecology, 73(6), 1035–1037.

Cohn, S. D. (1990). Malpractice and liability in clinical obstetrical nursing. Rockville, MD: Aspen.

Consensus Conference. (1984). The use of ultrasound in pregnancy. Journal of American Medical Association, 252(5), 669–672.

Curtis, C. (1989). Crisis pregnancy centers: A study of one center, its clientele, requested services, and services rendered. Unpublished master's thesis. The Catholic University of America, Washington, DC.

Ewigman, B. G., Crane, J. P., Frigiletto, F. D., LeFevre, M. L., Bain, R. P., McNellis, D., & the Radius Study Group. (1993). Effect of prenatal ultrasound screening on perinatal outcome. New England Journal of Medicine, 329(12), 821–827.

Ferguson-Smith, M. A. (1995). Questions of parental anxiety. Prenatal Diagnosis, 15, 1209–1213.

Fentz-Harter, S. A. (1997). Nursing and the law (6th ed.). Rockville, MD: Professional Education.

Fiesta, J. (1994). 20 legal pitfalls for nurses to avoid. Albany, NY: Delmar.

Furlong, R., & Black, R. B. (1984). Pregnancy termination for genetic indications: The impact on families. Social Work Health Care, 10, 17–34.

Gabbe, S., Niebyl, J. R., & Simpson, J. L. (Eds.). (1991). Obstetrics: Normal and problem pregnancies. New York: Churchill Livingston.

Gardner, S. L., & Hagedorn, M. I .E. (1997). Legal aspects of maternal–child nursing practice. Reading, MA: Addison-Wesley.

Goldworth, A., Silverman, W., Stevenson, D. K., Young, E. W. D., & Rivers, R. (1995). Ethics and perinatology. New York: Oxford University Press.

Greenlaw, J. L. (1990). Treatment refusal, noncompliance, and substance abuse in pregnancy: Legal and ethical issues. Birth, 17(3), 152–156.

Hahn, M. S. (1995, July). Practicing "defensive" documentation. ADVANCE for Nurse Practitioners, 41–42, 54.

Hepburn, E. R. (1996). Genetic testing and early diagnosis and intervention: Boon or burden? Journal of Medical Ethics, 22, 105–110.

King, N. M. P. (1994). A guest editorial: Informed consent and the practicing obstetrician-gynecologist. Obstetrical and Gynecological Survey, 49(5), 295–296.

Lichtman, R.I., & Papera, S. (1990). Gynecology: Well woman care. Norwalk, Connecticut: Appleton and Lange.

Lilford, R. J., & Thorton, J. (1993). Ethics and late termination of pregnancy, Lancet, 342(8869), 499.

Lloyd, J., & Lawrence, K. M. (1985). Sequelae and support after termination of pregnancy for fetal malformation. British Medical Journal, 290, 907–909.

Loewy, E. H. (1996). Textbook of healthcare ethics. New York: Plenum Press.

Marceau, T. (1990). Reducing the psychological costs. British Medical Journal, 301, 26–28.

Marceau, T. (1995). Towards informed decisions about prenatal testing: A review. Prenatal Diagnosis, 15, 1215–1226.

Morbidity and Mortality Weekly Report (1995). Chorionic villus sampling and amniocentesis: Recommendations for prenatal counseling. U.S. Department of Health and Human Services (No. RR-9). Atlanta, GA: Public Health Service.

Morbidity and Mortality Weekly Report (1996). Abortion surveillance—United States, 1992. U.S. Department of Health and Human Services (No. 22-3). Atlanta, GA: Public Health Service.

Northrop, C. E., & Kelly, M. E. (1987). Legal issues in nursing. St. Louis, MO: C.V. Mosby.

Nusbaum, J. G., & Chenitz, W. C. (1990). A grounded theory study of the informed consent process for pharmacological research. Western Journal of Nursing Research, 12(2), 215–228.

Olander, J. H. (1986, May–June). Lessons in malpractice. 12 ways to prevent lawsuits. Group Practice Journal, 3–6.

Pillitteri, A. (1995). Maternal and child health nursing (2nd ed.). Philadelphia: J.B. Lippincott.

Pryde, P. G., Drugan, A., Johnson, M. P., Isada, N. B., & Evans, M. I. (1995). Prenatal diagnosis: Choices women make about pursuing testing and acting on abnormal results. Clinical Obstetrics and Gynecology, 36(3), 496–509.

Reardon, D. C. (1987). Aborted women silent no more. Chicago, IL: Loyola Univ. Press.

Rennels, M. B. (1993). Childhood immunizations. R. A. Dershewitz (Ed.), Ambulatory pediatric care. Philadelphia: Lippincott.

Rhodes, A. M., & Miller, R. D. (1984). Nursing and the law (4th ed.). Rockville, MD: Aspen.

Rozovsky, F. A. (1990). (1996, Suppl.). Consent to treatment: A practical guide (2nd ed.). Boston: Little, Brown.

Spindel, P. G., & Suarez, S. H. (1995). Informed consent and home birth. Journal of Nurse Midwifery, 40(6), 541–569.

Stratham, H., & Green, J. (1993). Serum screening for Down's syndrome: Some women's experiences. British Medical Journal, 307, 174–177.

Stubblefield, P. G. (1991). Pregnancy termination. In S. Gabbe, J. R. Niebyl, & J. L Simpson, (Eds.). Obstetrics: Normal and problem pregnancies (pp. 1303–1330).

Sweeney, M. L. (1991, August). Your role in informed consent. RN, 55–60.

Titus, S. L., & Keane, M. A. (1996). Do you understand? An ethical assessment of researchers' description of the consenting process. The Journal of Clinical Ethics, 7(1), 60–68.

White, B. C. (1994). Competence to consent. Washington, DC: Georgetown University Press.

White-Van Mourik, M. C. A., Connor, J. M., & Ferguson-Smith, M. A. (1992). The psychosocial sequelae of a second trimester termination of pregnancy for fetal abnormality. Prenatal Diagnosis, 12, 189–204.

Williams, E. S. (1992). Antenatal screening for Down's syndrome. British Medical Journal, 305, 769–770.

Yeomans, G. (1990). Psychological sequence to abortion. (Letter to the editor) Australian-New Zealand Journal of Psychiatry, March 24 (1), 11.

Younger, P. A., & Conner, C. (Eds.). (1987). Nursing administration and law manual. Rockville, MD: Aspen.

Zamorski, M. S. (1996). Prenatal diagnosis: More than meets the eye. American Family Physician, 52, 2175–2177.

CASE CITATIONS

Azzolino v. Dingfelder, 322 S.E.2d 567 (N.C. App. 1984).

Bulman v. Meyers, 467 A.2d 1353 (Pa. Super. 1983).

Campbell v. Pitt County Memorial Hospital, 352 S.E.2d 902 (N.C. 1987).

Canterbury v. Spence, 464 F.2d 772 (D.C. Cir. 1972).

Flanagan v. Williams, 623 N.E.2d 185 (Ohio App. 4 Dist. 1993).

Planned Parenthood of Central Missouri v. Danforth, 428 U.S. 52 (1976).

Kissenger v. Lofgren, 836F2d678, 1988.

Klink v. G.D. Searle & Co., 26 Wash. App. 951, 614 A.2d 701 (1980).

Millard v. Nagle, 587 A.2d 10 (Pa. Super. 1991).

Schloendorff v. Society of N.Y. Hospital, 105 N.E. 92 (N.Y. 1914).

Shelton v. St. Anthony's Medical Center, 781 S.W.2d 48 (MO. Banc 1989).

Shinn v. James Mercy Hospital, 675 E. Supp. 94 (W.D.N.Y. 1987).

Sinclair by Sinclair v. Block, 594 A.2d 750 (Pa. Super. 1991).

Tisdale v. Pruitt, 394 S.E.2d 857 (S.C. App. 1990).

CHAPTER 16

The HIV-Positive Patient

Barbara Peterson Sinclair

Few diseases or conditions have produced as great a potential for health, moral, ethical, and legal dilemmas as the infection caused by HIV, human immunodeficiency virus. HIV and its progression to end-stage AIDS (acquired immunodeficiency syndrome) burst on the American scene in the early 1980s, at which time it was diagnosed among the male homosexual population. As a consequence, it was labeled a "gay" sex disease and initially its incidence was not of great concern for other populations, especially women and infants (Sinclair, 1990). Researchers found that the infection is caused by a previously unknown retrovirus that depletes the immune system, allowing opportunistic infections and selected cancers to occur. The virus can be found in blood, semen, vaginal secretions, and breast milk, and can be passed vertically from an infected pregnant woman to her fetus. Within a short period of time, the disease quickly spread to intravenous drug users and then to their sexual partners. The populations affected by HIV expanded as the virus was transmitted via needle sharing by drug users, unprotected anal or vaginal intercourse, and crossing the placenta or mixing of maternal/newborn blood at time of birth. As a result, the demographic parameters are changing: Heterosexual transmission continues to increase and the incidence of HIV in women is rising dramatically. This chapter is an overview of the scope and incidence of the disease (especially in relation to women and infants), natural history of the infection in women, selected legal safeguards and issues, and strategies to reduce legal risk.

SCOPE AND INCIDENCE OF HIV/AIDS

According to the Centers for Disease Control and Prevention (CDC), 548,102 cases of AIDS were reported in the United States as of July 1996 (CDC, 1996). Statistics on the number of people infected with HIV but who have not developed AIDS are unavailable as these figures are not collected for those who are asymptomatic, with early illness, or who do not know that they are infected. Surveillance of the HIV/AIDS epidemic has been maintained by analyzing reported AIDS cases from the 50 states, all of which have had mandatory reporting since 1983. However, such reporting has been predicated on a case definition that has changed over time as knowledge about the infection increased. The current classification of the infection (CDCP, 1993) is the third expansion of the case definition and enlarges the base criteria for recognizing HIV-infected persons. By adding CD4 counts under 200 cells/microliter, the definition recognizes the CD4+ T-lymphocyte count as a marker of severe immunosuppression. Also, three new AIDS-defining illnesses are added to the 23 conditions listed previously. The new conditions for those that are HIV-positive are pulmonary tuberculosis, recurrent pneumonia, and invasive cervical cancer. When this definition was expanded in 1993, there was a 151% increase in the number of AIDS cases in women and a 105% increase in cases in men. This is probably due to previous case definitions reflecting clinical characteristics of men and not accurately reflecting clinical manifestations of HIV in women (Abercrombie, 1996). Following this large number of reported cases, a stabilization occurred and after adjusting for definition change, it represents a total case increase of 2–3% per year. (Jaffe, 1996).

Epidemiology of HIV in Women

Evidence of the impact of HIV infection on poor people of color can be seen when one realizes that in 1995, African Americans and Hispanics represented the majority of cases among both men (54%) and women (76%) (Ungvarski, 1997). In the United States, AIDS is the third leading cause of death among women 25 to 44 years of age and the leading cause of death in African American women of the same age. African Americans and Hispanics comprise 21% of the women in the United States, yet they reflect 77% of reported AIDS cases. This represents an AIDS rate for African American and Hispanic women approximately 16 and 7 times greater, respectively, than for White women (CDCP, 1995).

Most cases of AIDS in women can be directly or indirectly related to injection drug use. Women either use themselves or have sex with a partner who uses. Even drugs that are not injected play a role in that the tendency to engage in unsafe sex is increased under the influence of the drugs, which, in turn, increases the possibility of acquiring HIV (Wortley, Chu, & Berkelman, 1997). Injection drug use was the mode of transmission for 41% of women with AIDS in 1994. During the same year, heterosexual transmission approximated 38%, representing a steady increase from 15% in 1983 (CDCP, 1994). Because women with AIDS are twice as likely as men with AIDS to be reported without an established risk factor, it is quite possible,

and in fact likely, that the incidence of heterosexual acquisition is higher due to underreporting. It is expected that the rate of heterosexual transmission will continue to rise.

When considering the time from HIV infection to AIDS diagnosis, it becomes apparent that many women were infected as adolescents. AIDS continues to rise in teens and young adults, ages 13 to 29, accounting for 18% of the nation's cases (CDCP, 1994). These numbers certainly emphasize the need for ongoing and increased vigilance in the promotion of safe sex and educational programs targeted for teenagers. Older women are prone to be overlooked when screening for HIV status. Eight percent of reported cases occur in women over the age of 50 with most infections acquired through unsafe heterosexual contact. Older women do not believe that they need condoms and most do not know how to use them (Wortley, Chu, & Berkelman, 1997).

Although rates vary greatly, current geographic distribution suggests that the infection has reached all parts of the United States. Data regarding prevalence of HIV among women delivering babies were obtained from the 1988 through 1994 Survey of Childbearing Women, a national anonymous serosurvey involving blind testing of the blood samples routinely taken for metabolic screening of newborns. Predicated on maternal antibodies crossing the placenta during pregnancy, a positive finding in the survey indicated an HIV-positive mother. Regional rates suggest a gradual increase in the Northeast with high incidence in urban, metropolitan areas; high rates in urban and rural areas of the South with gradual increase overall; relatively low and stable rates in the Midwest and West. The highest state-specific rates are New York, Florida, Maryland, and New Jersey (CDCP, 1995).

Perinatal Transmission

HIV infection is the fifth leading cause of death in children under the age of 15, and in some high prevalence areas is the number one cause. Perinatal transmission accounts for most HIV infection among children. Without intervention, the majority of pediatric HIV infection is acquired from the mother either in utero, at the time of birth, or in a few instances during postpartum by breastfeeding. Transmission rates have varied from 13 to 40% with an average of 25% in most U.S. cohorts (Bryson, 1996). Several factors are likely to contribute to these variable rates including differences in maternal viral load and immunological response, co-infections, and intrapartum conditions that lengthen exposure of the fetus/newborn to virus in maternal blood or vaginal secretions. However, additional research studies are needed to accurately determine exact mechanisms of the various factors.

Prevention strategies to reduce in utero, intrapartum, and postpartum transmission are being evaluated including antiretroviral therapy, passive immunization, and active immunization. Antiretroviral therapy via zidovudine (ZDV) given to the mother during pregnancy and delivery and to the newborn for 6 weeks after birth reduces transmission to 8.3% from 25.5% in those with placebo, an approximate 70% relative reduction in risk. Although the mechanism of protection is unknown, it is likely to involve a reduction of maternal virus load, especially in women who did not use AIDS drugs previously. ZDV is given to women between 14 and 34 weeks gestation, when their CD4 counts are above 200 cells per microliter, and they have no clinical symptoms that would indicate the need for antiretroviral therapy (Sperling, 1997). Long-term effects on both mother and baby from the use of zidovudine are unknown.

Passive immunization in the form of immune globulin (IG) is being tested on women with advanced immunosuppression. The HIVIG is prepared from donors who are HIV positive, clinically asymptomatic, and with CD4+ cell counts above 400. As a result, the product has high titers of antibodies and high virus-neutralizing activity. Active immunization of the pregnant woman and her newborn is proposed as another option. Ongoing vaccine trials are evaluating several different antigens for safety and immunogenicity (Sperling, 1997).

The timing of transmission (in utero and intrapartum), the extent of early virus replication, the transmitted virus phenotype, and the infant's immune response all seem to be important in determining the onset and course of disease progression in the HIV-infected infant. Studies suggest that early intervention during primary infection in the infant can reduce virus replication. Potent combination therapy may potentially alter long-term outcomes by preserving the immune system during a period of growth and maturation. Obviously, identification of HIV status in the mother would be needed in order to initiate an early prevention regimen for the fetus/newborn.

NATURAL HISTORY OF HIV INFECTION IN WOMEN

Because the initial research on HIV was conducted on men, gender differences were not considered and information about HIV-positive women was extrapolated from these data. Several long-term studies involving women are currently underway but due to the chronic nature of the disease, certain findings will not be available for many years. However, data suggest that disease progression and opportunistic processes in women may be very similar to those in men with the exception of mucosal candidiasis, which appears to be more common in women. Differences do occur in gynecologic manifestations, perinatal implications, and in the need for social services and better family-centered access and systems of care (Clark, 1997; Abercrombie, 1996).

Findings from the few cohort groups that included women and from Centers for Disease Control and Prevention suggest that the most frequent AIDS-defining diagnoses are *Pneumocystis carinii* pneumonia, esophageal candidiasis, and wasting syndrome (Clark, 1996). Other studies concluded that women are more likely than men to develop *candidia esophagitis,* cytomegalo virus, herpes simplex virus, mycobacterial infections, and bacterial pneumonia (especially if they were injection drug users). Men are more likely to have hairy leukoplakia, extrapulmonary tuberculosis, and Kaposi's sarcoma (Melnick et al., 1994; Fleming, Ciesielski, Byers, Castro, & Berkelman, 1993).

Gynecologic Manifestations

In addition to nongynecologic conditions associated with HIV infection, women are at risk for several gynecologic manifestations that are influenced by HIV. These include genital neoplasia, pelvic inflammatory disease, *Candida* vulvovaginitis, and selected sexually transmitted diseases (STDs).

The incidence of squamous intraepithelial lesions (SIL) is reportedly 10 times higher in women who are infected with HIV (Clark, 1996). The majority of cases involve cervical intraepithelial neoplasia (CIN), the severity of which is related to the degree of immunosuppression. Progression to cervical cancer is rapid when compared to non-HIV infected women. Six-month intervals for cervical screening via Pap smear and/or colposcopy are strongly recommended.

Pelvic inflammatory disease (PID) in HIV-positive women has a different clinical presentation when compared to women not HIV infected. Upon admission, they have lower white blood counts and more often require surgical intervention. They are "sicker" as indicated by increased endometritis, higher fevers, more pelvic masses, and greater tenderness. However, response to treatment is not significantly different and there are no significant differences in duration of treatment, length of hospitalization, or endocervical/endometrial cultures (Abercrombie, 1997; Clark, 1996).

Recurrent vaginal candidiasis (defined as four or more discrete episodes per year) is directly related to the degree of immunocompromise. Based on this finding, a hierarchical presentation of mucosal candidiasis is made: Vulvovaginal candidiasis occurs earliest in the disease process and as the CD4+ cell count decreases, it is followed by oral and then esophageal candidiasis. Many believe that a woman with unknown HIV status who presents with recurrent candida vaginitis should be encouraged to test for HIV.

Clark reports on three retrospective studies that demonstrate some increase in selected STDs among HIV-infected women (Clark, 1996). Included are trichomoniasis, chlamydia, syphilis, herpes simplex virus (HSV), human papilloma virus (HPV), and gonorrhea. Syphilis and trichomoniasis occurred more frequently in injection drug users and, as with HSV and HPV, were influenced by reduction of CD4+ cell counts as a measure of immunocompromise. Strains of HPV, different from those causing common genital warts, are also associated with the occurrence of cervical intraepithelial neoplasia and the progression to cervical cancer.

Pregnancy

Controversy exists as to whether or not pregnancy accelerates HIV disease progression. In studies from the United States and Europe, there are no conclusions to suggest that pregnancy is likely to cause a woman to progress more rapidly toward AIDS-defining illnesses or death. This is not the case in studies from developing countries. The effect of the disease on a pregnancy is quite variable depending upon the status of the infection, the general well-being of the mother, and her access to appropriate care. Many symptoms of opportunistic infections overlap with the symptoms of pregnancy; thus, with few exceptions, the same diagnostic tests should be undertaken with the same indications as would be done with nonpregnant women (Watts, 1997). It is highly recommended that in addition to information about both HIV and pregnancy, the risk of perinatal transmission, the need for testing and follow-up, and care of the infant are considered and discussed with the mother.

AN OVERVIEW OF CURRENT TREATMENT

There is no definitive cure for this disease. However, basic research has expanded understanding of the molecular biology and the viral life cycle of HIV. This paved the way for the development of several strategies to interrupt the life cycle of the virus and, as a consequence, to allow for preservation of normal processes within the host cell. Currently, antiretroviral and prophylactic drugs for opportunistic infection are basic standards in the provision of care (Bechtel-Boenning, 1997). Thus far, the mainstay of drug treatment has been nucleoside analogues such as zidovudine (ZDV, AZT, or Retrovir).* Nucleoside analogues prevent the spread of HIV to new cells by inhibiting the activity of reverse transcriptase, an enzyme necessary for viral RNA to be copied into host cell DNA. However, they do not interfere with viral replication in cells already infected (Ungvarski, 1997). When viral particles emerge from an infected cell, they are incomplete and immature and the enzyme, protease, mediates their maturation. When a protease inhibitor is present, a noninfectious virus results. As of December 1996, three protease inhibitors were approved by the FDA: saquinavir (Invirase), indinavir (Crixivan), and ritonavir (Norvir). Combinations of protease inhibitors and nucleoside analogues appear to produce the best results in overall well-being and significant reduction in viral load. A number of other drug categories are currently under study and should be available in the near future.

LEGAL SAFEGUARDS AND ISSUES

The medical, psychological, and social complexities of HIV infection have inspired more legislation, government action, and procedural guidelines than any other known disease. However, law is mutable, and AIDS law in particular is unsettled. Perhaps this is appropriate in order to keep pace with the state of knowledge as it develops. Even so, the law is by nature ambiguous and often arbitrary and as a result, the public and even the judicial system may have difficulty understanding the scope of HIV/AIDS laws (Wood & Marks, 1990). Although it is not possible to cover all of the laws and issues as they relate to HIV/AIDS in all of the jurisdictions, an overview of major legal considerations will be presented.

Disability Benefits

A person with HIV-related disability may be eligible for public assistance through the Social Security Administration (SSA), which supervises the Disability Insurance Benefits program (DIB) and the Supplemental Security Income program (SSI). Disability benefits include monthly payments to a covered employee who is unable to work because of a medically certified illness or condition that has lasted or is expected to last for at least one year or to end in death. SSI is a cash benefit program for low-income persons who are disabled and who meet certain income and resource limits. SSA has established an evaluation process to determine if a person is disabled, including a Listing of Impairments. The newest listing, published in July 1993, more accurately reflects the spectrum of disabling HIV-related impairments including expanded considerations for women (McGovern, 1997). Because assessment of disability includes a review of medical records for information regarding signs, symptoms, and description of physical disabilities, it is important that careful documentation be incorporated by health care providers. Women should be apprised that denials of eligibility can be appealed and that many states or counties provide some assistance for people without other resources or who are not eligible for other programs.

Ryan White Comprehensive AIDS Resources Emergency Act

Passage of the Ryan White CARE Act in 1990 established a number of principles of services for people infected with HIV. (See Display 16-1.) The act has subsequently set the standards for AIDS service programs nationwide and its continued funding has allowed many service centers to remain open and to provide much assistance to persons with HIV/AIDS. Although funding goes directly to the service centers, clients/patients obviously benefit from the programs it supports.

The Americans with Disabilities Act (ADA)

(Note that portions of this section are excerpted from ACLU AIDS Project brochure, 1992.) This

---

* There are five nucleoside analogues approved by the Food and Drug Administration (FDA) for sale in the United States: Didanosine (ddI or Videx), Zalcitabine (ddC or HIvid), Stavudine (d4T or Zerit), and lamivudine (3TC or Epivir).

DISPLAY 16-1

Principles of Services Established by the Ryan White Comprehensive AIDS Resources Emergency Act (CARE)

- Ambulatory services including case management and comprehensive treatment
- Inpatient case management services that reduce unnecessary hospitalization
- Comprehensive continuum of care for individuals and families with HIV disease
- Comprehensive programs that encompass a wide variety of essential health services, plus essential support services, including transportation, attendants, homemaker services, and benefits advocacy.
- Family-centered care for infants, children, women, and families with HIV disease, based on a partnership among parents, professionals, and the community
- Outreach services, especially in reaching people with HIV disease in rural areas
- Home and community-based care assuring the continuity of health insurance coverage
- Public-private partnerships that foster close working relationships among agencies

Source: Adapted from Morrison (1993).

sweeping civil rights law was passed by Congress in 1990 and provides uniform, enforceable, federal protections to persons with disabilities. It protects people from discrimination in private settings such as employment, education, and business services, and prohibits discrimination in governmental programs. Because HIV disease is considered a disability, the ADA protects infected individuals no matter where they are on the continuum from an asymptomatic state to full-blown AIDS. Under this circumstance, the term disability is a legal definition to establish the basis for antidiscrimination protection and does not have the same meaning as that needed for benefit programs. Any business that employs more than 15 people is covered by the ADA. Some states or local jurisdictions have laws that cover employers with smaller numbers.

The ADA specifies that an employer may not discriminate against a qualified person simply because he or she has HIV disease. This includes hiring, promotion, or firing. Of course, the individual must be able to perform all the essential functions of the job on a regular and adequate

basis. The act prohibits an employer from insisting that employees take an HIV test unless it can be proven that the test is necessary to do the job. The ADA also prohibits discrimination against people who associate with those having disabilities. This includes the spouse, friend, lover, family member, or caretaker of a person with HIV. However, to be protected by the ADA it is necessary to prove that discrimination occurred because of the known association.

The employment portion of the ADA is enforced by the Equal Employment Opportunities Commission (EEOC). If an individual believes that rights have been violated, a written complaint should be filed with the EEOC within 180 days of the incident. It would be wise for an individual to consult with an attorney either in private practice or with an AIDS service organization for consultation regarding a complaint; however, a direct contact with EEOC via visit or telephone is possible.

Public accommodations also are prohibited from discriminating against people with disabilities under the ADA. These refer not only to government-funded accommodations, but also to essentially every type of business or service. The list is long and includes doctors, dentists, pharmacists, nurses, and other health care providers; hotels, restaurants, bakeries, movie theaters, convention centers, spas, clothing stores, and any business that provides commercial services; museums, parks, schools, homeless shelters, adoption agencies, and any place that provides social services. These business or service providers may not discriminate in providing goods and services because an individual has HIV or associates with a person having HIV. Businesses and offices of any size are covered. Only religious organizations and private clubs are exempted from public accommodation protection.

Public entities refer to state and local governments, which also are forbidden to exclude people with disabilities from participation in government services, programs, or activities. The public accommodation or public entities provisions of the ADA can be enforced by filing a lawsuit in court or in some instances by filing a complaint with the Department of Justice, which is empowered to undertake an investigation and compliance review. The ADA does not apply to the federal government, but disabled persons are covered under a similar statute, the Rehabilitation Act of 1973. Discrimination in the sale or rental of private housing because of a disability would be covered under the Fair Housing Act as amended by Congress in 1989. In addition to federal mandates, various states have laws that provide protection against discrimination.

Reasonable Accommodation: Standard Precautions

Because of the frequent interaction between persons infected with HIV and those in health care, it should be emphasized that a health care provider may not refuse to treat or care for the infected person. Under the rule established by the United States Supreme Court in *School Board v. Arline* (1987), the risk to others posed by HIV is insufficient to support such a refusal to treat. In that case, the Court held that persons with contagious diseases are handicapped within the meaning of federal disability rights law. Subsequent

cases as well as the passage of the Americans with Disabilities Act have made it clear that persons with HIV or AIDS are disabled and fall within the Court's ruling in *Arline*. As a result, reasonable accommodation must be provided, and in the circumstance of blood-borne diseases, the accommodation means standard precautions. Standard precautions is a strategy of infection control that (1) treats blood and certain other secretions from all patients at all times as potentially infectious; (2) implements appropriate safeguards through the proper use of barriers, disinfection, waste disposal and other workplace practices; and (3) ensures that all health care workers know and follow the safeguards. Standard precautions are required by the U.S. Occupational Safety and Health Agency and are included in the health and safety codes of most states. They apply to the provision of emergency as well as routine care.

Privacy and Confidentiality

Privacy and its associated issue of confidentiality are major ethical and legal considerations for persons with HIV infection. The rule of confidentiality is derived from the ethical principle of autonomy, which affirms the right of self-determination and has become a cornerstone for the relationship between a professional health care provider and a patient. This fiduciary relationship, meaning one of special trust and confidence, has been part of the legal precepts of this country since the late 19th century (Obade, 1991; Benrubi, 1992). Therefore, the provider has a duty to protect patient information given in the context of privacy. This constitutionally based "right to privacy" was recognized by the U.S. Supreme Court in 1965 and has been asserted in a number of states to protect patients from disclosure of medical or psychological information (Obade, 1991). The concept especially applies to those who are HIV infected.

In *Urbaniak v. Newton* (1991), the plaintiff claimed he disclosed his HIV-positive status to a nurse for the sole purpose of protecting her during a procedure that involved blood and asked that his status not be further shared. She informed the physician for whom she worked and he, in turn, included the information in a report to an insurance company. The patient sued. The California appellate court ruled that the nurse's and physician's alleged disclosure violated California's constitutional right to privacy. The court stated:

> In the field of health care, disclosure of information about a patient constitutes 'improper use" when it will subvert a public interest favoring communication of confidential information by violating the patient's reasonable expectations of privacy. We find such a public interest here in a patient's disclosure of HIV positive status for the purpose of alerting a health care worker to the need for safety precautions. The evidence here would support the inference that Urbaniak reasonably anticipated privacy. By enforcing such reasonable expectations of privacy, the courts will simultaneously foster needed disclosures of HIV positive status and protect against their abuses. (*Urbaniak v. Newton*, 1991)

It must be remembered that the potential for harm to the HIV-infected individual through injudicious breaches of confidentiality is very great. Discrimination, isolation, hostility, and stigmatization are all too common when HIV-positive status becomes known to others.

On occasion, however, a breach in the duty to protect information becomes necessary and is ethically and legally sanctioned. Most codes of medical ethics agree that if there is to be such a breach, there must be a well-defined reason for doing so, such as an identified individual or group of individuals who would benefit and, further, that the benefit must override the harm done to the patient whose confidentiality is compromised (Benrubi, 1992). For example, consider the HIV-positive man who has a noninfected sexual partner whom he refuses to notify. Even under this circumstance, the breach of confidence is justified only as a measure of last resort, that is, the health care provider makes extensive efforts to persuade the patient to share information and also determines that failure to pass on the information is likely to result in harm to the partner. On a larger societal scale, public health regulations reflect circumstantial compromise of confidentiality via mandatory reporting of HIV-positive and AIDS patients to public health authorities. This per-

spective is supported on the basis that society has the right and the responsibility to promote general health and safety including accurate epidemiological information (Smith & Martin, 1993).

Not only are individuals admonished to be aware of privacy statutes, but institutional providers are also urged to consider the ethical and legal ramifications of the hospital "grapevine." AIDS cases in particular produce a situation in which discrimination may illegally occur when the "grapevine" passes on confidential information. In the case of *Behringer v. The Medical Center at Princeton* (1991), the court held the hospital liable for the adverse effect of its employees' gossip. The case involved a physician whose hospital privileges were suspended soon after he was diagnosed with *Pneumocystis carinii* pneumonia. The suit involved a breach of confidentiality as well as discrimination against the handicapped. Although the court had several items of which it disapproved, it is particularly important to note its comment that the Medical Center had no written or verbal restriction against any health care worker involved in the delivery of care discussing the plaintiff's diagnosis with others. The court further commented that

> It is not the charting per se [by attending physicians] that generates the issues; it is the easy accessibility to the charts and the lack of any meaningful Medical Center policy or procedure to limit access that causes the breach to occur. . . . It is incumbent on the Medical Center as the custodian of the charts, to take such reasonable measures as are necessary to insure confidentiality. Failure to take such steps is negligence. (*Behringer v. The Medical Center at Princeton*, 1991)

The court rejected the defense's position that physicians and employees were to blame and it was not interested in identifying specific persons who "spread the news." The court commented:

> The information was too easily available, too titillating to disregard. All that was required was a glance at a chart, and the written words became whispers and whispers became roars. And common sense told all that this would happen. (*Behringer v. The Medical Center at Princeton*, 1991)

Obviously, the institution as well as the individual must maintain confidentiality and privacy.

Informed Consent

Informed consent is an important concept in every health care arena. Ethically, every person has the right to know about products, procedures, or treatments that could affect health. Pragmatically, the individual is more likely to conform to directions given when he or she thoroughly understands the actual or potential circumstances in which they will be placed. Legally, the health care provider must provide the patient with sufficient information at a level of understanding that a "reasonable person" would need in order to make a sound and informed decision. Because of the nature of HIV infection given its transmissibility and lack of prevention or cure, informed consent becomes even more important with regards to antibody testing and clinical trials.

Antibody Testing

Although state laws vary, most states have similar testing safeguards in effect. A person must voluntarily consent before being tested for the HIV antibody. (The consent of a parent, guardian or conservator is necessary to test one who is mentally incapacitated or a child.) Following pretest counseling that includes the nature of the procedure, risks, benefits, and alternatives, individuals are asked to sign a written consent in confidential testing settings and are permitted to give oral consent in anonymous testing settings. Posttest counseling is highly recommended for everyone. To assist in providing the best possible information, a mnemonic that can be utilized by HIV pretest and posttest counselors can be found in Display 16-2.

Great debate is ongoing about whether or not testing should remain voluntary or if there are circumstances under which mandatory testing should occur. One of the most frequently heard

DISPLAY 16-2

HIV Test Counseling

A mnemonic that can be utilized in pretest and posttest counseling is:

P: Privacy and confidentiality

R: Risk assessment and risk reduction

- Who: Sexual partners = men, women, or both
  and/or
  Injection drug user

- What: Sites and activities = oral, anal, vaginal, hands, objects
  or
  Sharing of needles with others

- How: Use of condoms and barriers, spermicides and lubricants
  or
  Do not share needles or at least clean them

E: Education and informed consent

P: Privacy and confidentiality

O: Optimism and treatment

S: Support system, suicidality

T: Transmission, partner notification

Source: Adapted from Khalsa (1996).

arguments has to do with the advent of zidovudine as a deterrent to vertical transmission from a pregnant woman to her fetus. The drug's benefit has led some to argue for screening all pregnant women even though long-term consequences of zidovudine treatment during pregnancy are unknown. This argument is vigorously denounced by those who wish to protect the patient's right to privacy. Debate is further complicated by the ethical mandate of the state to protect the medical interests of children, even against parental wishes. Perhaps the best consideration at the present time is that mandatory screening and treatment of pregnant women cannot be ethically justified but it is strongly recommended that all pregnant women be offered HIV testing (Bayer, 1994). Future findings may be speculative at best and the debate will likely continue.

Clinical Trials

Clinical trials are a specific type of clinical research designed to answer a question having therapeutic implications for human subjects. Based on prior test tube and/or animal studies, a protocol is developed that states the problem and its relevance, as well as the design and methods needed to obtain answers to the study question. Inclusion and exclusion criteria are specified and if the protocol involves testing of a drug or biologic agent, the investigator must apply to the Food and Drug Administration (FDA) requesting permission for investigational testing. Needless to say, as basic scientific information is obtained about the biology of HIV and the pathophysiology of the resulting immunodeficiency, the testing of therapeutics to offset the disease process is in great demand. It is through this mechanism that the treatment modalities that are used today have been developed.

Claims have been made by segments of the research community and by women's advocacy groups that the participation of women in clinical trials is exceedingly low. Protocols have been approved that exclude women of childbearing potential or that demand surgical sterilization of childbearing-aged women in order to participate. This exclusion extends to women with life-threatening diseases such as HIV infection. The number of women in HIV clinical research is disproportionately low and, as a result, these studies have not benefited women's health to the same extent as men's health (Mastroianni, Faden, & Federman, 1994; McGovern, 1997). In 1993, adult women numbered 1,952 of the 21,598 participants who were enrolled in AIDS Clinical Trial Group studies (ACTG) even though it was stated that efforts to recruit women had become a priority (McGovern, 1997). Based on information from the ACTG Women's Health Committee, there are insufficient numbers to provide adequate information about the effects of a given drug on women. The committee concludes that more than 15% of participants in large clinical trials must be women in order to detect significant gender differences in toxicity and response to therapy (Eighth International Conference on AIDS, 1992).

Exclusion of pregnant women from clinical trials is particularly dramatic, and has to do with potential liability for injury to offspring. Yet, some experts suggest that teratogenic or mutagenic potential is not a sufficient enough basis for refusing experimental drugs to women who could significantly benefit from them (Mitchell, Mitchell, Tucker, Loftman, & Williams, 1992; McGovern, 1997). An example of this is the recent use of zidovudine during pregnancy, which has been therapeutic for the mother and also has demonstrated over a two-thirds reduction in vertical transmission to the newborn. So far, there have been no identifiable complications, but long-term effects have yet to be proven. The issue is far from being resolved as the law is not yet clear on whether a woman's informed consent to participate in a clinical study is adequate to protect a study sponsor from liability in the event that the offspring is injured.

Advance Directives

Perhaps the greatest concern for HIV-infected women is what will happen to their children when they are no longer able to care for them. Decisions regarding the future should be made when the disease is in an early stage and mothers should be apprised that they have greater control when a plan for custody is arranged legally. The fact that most women with AIDS are minority, poor, and often disenfranchised does not prohibit them from obtaining legal assistance via referrals to appropriate agencies or individuals. Depending upon the state in which the woman lives, there are various legal options available regarding child care, the most common of which is the appointment of a legal guardian. The proposed guardian must be an appropriate caretaker (according to a background check) and, if appointed, can receive public benefits and public assistance for the child, such as Medicaid, food stamps, and shelter allowance. Another option is one of several forms of foster care including voluntary placement with family, friends, or strangers. Financial benefits to the child through foster care may be substantial; however, foster care parents must understand that they are required to attend various training classes and their home may be inspected frequently by state agency representatives (McGovern, 1997). Legal guardians should be apprised of the child's serostatus in order to obtain the best health care possible. Therefore, it is suggested that testing of the child is explained to the mother and informed consent is encouraged.

Almost every state provides for advance directives in the form of a living will. A living will allows a patient to refuse life-prolonging treatment when terminally ill. Also, all states permit a durable power of attorney for health care that allows a patient to assign decision-making authority to another to be implemented when decision-making capacity is lost. Living will statutes typically sanction parental refusal of life-prolonging treatment of minor children who are terminally ill (Chervenak & McCullough, 1996).

In the event that plans for guardianship are not arranged formally, it is possible to designate a guardian in the Last Will and Testament of the parents. The will also allocates real and personal property.

STRATEGIES TO REDUCE RISK

In addition to knowing one's own beliefs about HIV infection and developing an ability to open-ly talk about areas that are socially threatening and ethically puzzling, most legal risk-reducing strategies are predicated on basic information presented earlier in this chapter. Some of the following strategies are meant for individuals, groups, or both. The degree to which the information applies to the individual nurse depends upon the professional role that the nurse assumes.

- Maintain current knowledge about HIV/AIDS, and document when appropriate.
- Ensure privacy and confidentiality at all times and with all people. Institute appropriate safeguards within offices and agencies and maintain guidelines to enhance privacy and confidentiality that are written and periodically reviewed with attending, per diem, and staff personnel. Evoke a duty to disclose (to safeguard others) only when ethical and legal parameters have been met.
- Train staff concerning compliance with antidiscrimination laws and with unique state laws regarding HIV/AIDS. Ensure that current information is available.
- Institute and rigorously enforce universal precautions.
- Assess HIV risk acquisition status of patients, acknowledging the sensitive and confidential nature of questions asked.
- Offer HIV testing as part of routine health promotion. Be especially vigilant to encourage testing for all who fall within a risk category, for all pregnant women, and for women who have recurrent monilial vaginitis. Document the offer.
- Involve the patient in decision making about her or his own care, ensuring that necessary information is shared.
- Utilize standards of care that are determined by standards within the community and by professional organizations. Obviously, standards should meet all legal parameters as well.
- Provide cervical screening (Pap smear or colposcopy) every 6 months for HIV-positive women.
- Discuss the ramifications of perinatal transmission with HIV-positive women and respect their right to make reproductive

decisions. Support whatever decision is made.

- Appreciate demographic information about HIV-infected women, found mostly among poor women of color, in order to enhance positive interactions.
- Refer infected persons to a comprehensive program that includes social services, psychological support, and health care. Know the programs or know the people that know the programs within the community.
- Ensure that patients have appropriate and sufficient information for informed consent for all procedures, treatments, and clinical research protocols.
- Educate regarding the prevention of transmission using specific language and parlance of the intended listener and include concepts at a level understood by the patient. Encourage the public at large to attend educational efforts that highlight prevention.
- Establish institutional contact with an attorney conversant with laws relating to HIV/AIDS so that questions can be posed and suggested policies and procedures can be reviewed prior to implementation.

CONCLUSION

Human immunodeficiency virus infection in the United States continues to grow but at a slower pace than previously. HIV is reaching a more diverse population and is significantly increasing in women. Ethical and legal parameters are being debated as the search continues for methods of prevention and cure. Newer treatment modalities with combinations of drugs are reducing the viral load of individuals and are reducing the advent and severity of opportunistic diseases. The underrepresentation of women in clinical trials has highlighted the need for stronger advocacy, especially at a time when the use of an antiviral drug has reduced vertical transmission by almost 70%. Legal protection has expanded to include wide coverage under antidiscrimination legislation and disability benefits. The constitutional right to privacy and con-

fidentiality has been upheld repeatedly in case law. Issues of informed consent and antibody testing are of special concern to HIV-positive persons and the need for advance directives must be considered. Strategies to reduce legal risks reflect common sense and knowledge about the disease process, legal parameters, and individual preferences.

REFERENCES

Abercrombie, P. D. (1996). Women living with HIV infection. In C. Grady & C. Bechtel-Boenning (Eds.), Nursing clinics of North America (pp. 97–106). Philadelphia: W. B. Saunders.

ACLU AIDS Project. (1992). The Americans with Disabilities Act: What it means for people living with HIV disease [brochure]. New York: Author.

Bayer, R. (1994). Ethical challenges posed by zidovudine treatment to reduce vertical transmission of HIV. New England Journal of Medicine, 331 (Editorial), 1223–1225.

Bechtel-Boenning, C. (1997). State of the art—antiviral treatment of HIV infection. In C. Grady & C. Bechtel-Boenning (Eds.), Nursing clinics of North America (pp. 1–13). Philadelphia: W. B. Saunders.

Benrubi, G. I. (1992). Confidentiality in the age of AIDS. Journal of Reproductive Medicine, 37(12), 969–972.

Bryson, Y. J. (1996). Advances in prevention and treatment of pediatric HIV infection. Proceedings: HIV/AIDS on the front line conference. Costa Mesa, CA.

Centers for Disease Control and Prevention. (1993). Revised classification system for HIVC infection and expanded surveillance case definition for AIDS among adolescents and adults. MMWR, 41(RR-17), 1–19.

Centers for Disease Control and Prevention. (1994). HIV/AIDS Surveillance Report. Atlanta, GA: U.S. Department of Health and Human Services, Public Health Service.

Centers for Disease Control and Prevention. (1995). Facts about women and HIV/AIDS. HIV/AIDS prevention. Atlanta, GA: U.S. Department of Health and Human Services, Public Health Service.

Centers for Disease Control and Prevention. (1996). HIV/AIDS surveillance report. Atlanta, GA: U.S. Department of Health and Human Services, Public Health Service.

Chervenak, F. A., & McCullough, L. B. (1996). Common ethical dilemmas encountered in the management of HIV-infected women and their newborns. Clinical Obstetrics and Gynecology, 39(2), 411–419.

Clark, R. (1997). Clinical manifestations and the natural history of human immunodeficiency virus infection in women. In D. Cotton and D. H. Watts (Eds.). The medical management of AIDS in women (pp. 115–123). New York: Wiley-Liss.

Eighth International Conference on AIDS. (1992, July). Abstract #POC 4507, Amsterdam.

Fleming, P. J., Ciesielski, C. A., Byers, R. H., Castro, K. G., & Berkelman, R. L. (1993). Gender differences in reported AIDS-indicative diagnoses. Journal of Infectious Diseases,168(4), 61–67.

Jaffe, H. W. (1996). Emerging trends in the HIV/AIDS epidemic. Proceedings: HIV/AIDS on the front line conference. Costa Mesa, CA.

Khalsa, A. M. (Ed.). 1996. Common problems in HIV disease (2nd ed.). Los Angeles: Pacific AIDS Education and Training Center, University of Southern California.

Mastroianni, A. C., Faden, R., & Federman, D. (1994). Women and health research: a report from the Institute of Medicine. Kennedy Institute of Ethics Journal, 4(1), 55–63.

McGovern, T. M. (1997). Legal issues affecting women with HIV. In D. Cotton & D. H. Watts (Eds.). The medical management of AIDS in women (pp. 193–204). New York: Wiley-Liss.

Melnick, S. L., Sherer, R., Louis, T. A., Hillman, D., Rodriguez, R. M., Lackman, C., Capps, L., Brown, L. S., Jr., Carlyn, M., Korvick, J. A., & Deyton, L. (1994). Survival and disease progression according to gender of patients with HIV infection. Journal of the American Medical Association, 212(24), 1915–1921.

Mitchell, J. L., Tucker, J., Loftman, P. O., & Williams, S. B. (1992). HIV and women: Current controversies and clinical relevance. Journal of Women's Health, 1(1), 35–39.

Morrison, C. (1993). Delivery systems for the care of persons with HIV infection and AIDS. In M. L. Maas, M. G. Titler, & K. C. Buckwalter (Eds.). The Nursing Clinics of North America: Advances in clinical nursing research (Vol. 28(2), pp. 317–333). Philadelphia: W. B. Saunders.

Obade, C. C. (1991). Whisper down the lane: AIDS, privacy, and the hospital "grapevine." The Journal of Clinical Ethics, 2(2), 133–137.

Sinclair, B. P. (1990). Epidemiology and transmission of infection by human immunodeficiency virus. In B. Sinclair & A. McCormick (Eds.). NAACOG's clinical issues in perinatal and women's health nursing: AIDS in women (Vol. 1, pp. 1–9). Philadelphia: J. B. Lippincott.

Smith, M. L., & Martin, K. P. (1993). Confidentiality in the age of AIDS: A case study in clinical ethics. The Journal of Clinical Ethics, 4(3), 236–241.

Sperling, R. (1997). Perinatal transmission of HIV. In D. Cotton and D. H. Watts (Eds.). The medical management of AIDS in women (pp. 45–54). New York: Wiley-Liss.

Ungvarski, P. J. (1997). Update on HIV infection. American Journal of Nursing, (1), 44–51.

Watts, Heather D. (1997). Care of the HIV positive pregnant woman. In D. Cotton & D. Heather Watts (Eds.). The Medical Management of Aids in Women. New York: Wiley-Liss.

Wood, G. J., & Marks, R. (1990). AIDS law for mental health professionals. San Francisco: The AIDS Health Project, University of California.

Wortley, P. M., Chu, S. Y., & Berkelman, R. L. (1997). Epidemiology of HIV/AIDS in women and the impact of the expanded 1993 CDC surveillance definition of AIDS. In D. Cotton & D. H. Watts (Eds.). The medical management of AIDS in women (pp. 3–14). New York: Wiley-Liss.

CASE CITATIONS

Behringer v. The Medical Center at Princeton, 69321 N.J. Super. Law Division (1991).

School Board v. Arline, 480 U.S. 273 (1987).

Urbaniak v. Newton, 226 Cal. App. 3d 1128 (1991).

Liability Concerns in Perinatal Staffing

Pamela Reidy and Christine Sullivan

In the midst of dramatic changes occurring in the delivery of health care remains the ongoing challenge of staffing maternal–fetal–neonatal units with an adequate number of personnel who are able to perform competently in caring for the childbearing woman, the fetus, and the newborn, under low- and high-risk situations. Staffing issues have historically created some of the greatest ethical dilemmas facing nurse executives (Borawski, 1995). The 1980s introduced mother–baby care and LDRPs, which challenged nurses who were unaccustomed to the concept of caring for the mother–infant dyad. Concern was raised regarding the competency of nurses who were traditionally expert in intrapartum, postpartum, or neonatal care. Cross-training staff to be equally competent in all aspects of maternal–infant care was challenging for many administrators, as well as individual staff who opposed such endeavors. Hospitals incurred liability when poor patient care outcomes were associated with inadequately trained or oriented staff. In fact, most legal cases against nurses are related to the failure to adequately assess, monitor, and communicate findings (Fiesta, 1988). Included in these broad claims are specific acts of negligence such as failure to have appropriate personnel to read monitors, failure to monitor as often as required, failure to interpret the monitor signals, and failure to report results to the

physician (American Law Report, 1995). These failures are often the result of not enough staff or staff without enough training.

As the hospital restructuring and downsizing of the 1990s continues, staffing and resource allocation issues will continue to plague nurse administrators with the increased risk of liability. Borawski (1995) states, "Although patient needs should serve as the underlying justification for staffing, resource allocation, and standard of care decisions, those decisions must be made within the context of a financially healthy institution" (p. 62). Thus the challenge has become to decrease staff numbers in response to lower length of stay and reduced inpatient volume in addition to increased cross-training to provide flexibility in care delivery. With these challenges comes the ongoing need to manage risk and minimize the liability associated with perinatal care. The staffing process requires a planned approach that balances patient needs, resources, professional responsibilities, and the unique considerations of perinatal care.

STAFFING: A PLANNED APPROACH

A well-planned approach to staffing perinatal units is the first step in minimizing liability for any health care organization. Staffing considerations should begin with the overall mission and reflect the standards of the professional community.

With ever increasing external oversight of health care by private and governmental agencies, mechanisms exist that clearly place the responsibility for staffing with the leaders of an organization. The Joint Commission on Accreditation of Health Care Organizations (JCAHO) delineates this theme in the Leadership and Human Resources standards of the *Comprehensive Accreditation Manual for Hospitals* (JCAHO, 1996). These standards place the responsibility and accountability for nurse staffing with the nurse executive. The nurse executive "ensures the continuous and timely availability of nursing services to patients" (JCAHO, 1996, p. 561). The intent implies that a sufficient number of appropriately qualified and competent nursing staff are assigned and present to meet patients' nursing care needs throughout the hospital (JCAHO, 1994, p. 3). This responsibility is usually delegated to nursing care managers who must consider patient care needs and ensure that staff assigned to care for patients have appropriate experience and training to competently care for the patients.

State Nurse Practice Acts also impact staffing needs. Knowledge of specific statutes should be fundamental to policy development in any organization. Although many nurse practice acts are general in nature, some have specific rules and regulations with lists of procedures nurses are allowed to perform (Hansten & Washburn, 1994, p. 52). Nurses as well as organizations should be familiar with such rules. In *Arkansas State Department of Health v. Dr. Thibault and Council* (1984), a nurse was instructed to dose an epidural by a physician who left the hospital. Following complications the court held that the nurse practice act of Arkansas required the physician to be present if the nurse administered the medication (Fiesta, 1988, p. 285).

Specialty guidelines should also be considered in the staffing of inpatient units. The Association of Women's Health Obstetric and Neonatal Nursing (AWHONN) has included its recommendations for staffing in *Guidelines for Perinatal Care* (1992) published by the American Academy of Pediatrics (AAP) and the American College of Obstetricians and Gynecologists (ACOG). These are prudent principles; however, in their text the characterization of staffing is based on assumed conditions, rather than real-life conditions that are unique to each patient, mother–infant dyad, or organizational model. The use of staffing guidelines, patient classification systems, and other staffing methodologies are fundamentally capricious guides. Workload management systems using retrospective data to determine the overall need for staff are just the beginning for staffing any unit. A prospective look at community needs, changes in the market, increased technology, staff turnover, and so on, are other sources of information that must be accounted for in planning for staff. For day-to-day and shift-to-shift staffing, patient classification systems have been used to adjust staff based on current patient needs. Due to the dynamic nature of labor, a universally accepted classification system for labor and delivery is not available; however, patient acuity systems are in place for many other areas in perinatal care (Mandeville & Troiano, 1992, p. 37). All these traditional staffing methods aim to meet the core staffing requirements of a unit and minimize liability for the nurse and organization.

In addition to accrediting agencies holding organizations accountable for staffing, the law also holds hospitals liable to patients for negligence in maintaining adequate staff (Bernzweig, 1996, p. 114). The doctrine of corporate liability requires organizations to ensure that patients receive safe quality care. A safe environment includes enough personnel available to observe, monitor, and care for patients. An Arkansas court held a hospital liable for the brain damage suffered by an infant when nurses in an understaffed nursery failed to notice that he had stopped breathing (Bernzweig, 1996, p. 184). In this case the nursery had 3 nurses on duty and 18 babies, which is within the "staffing ratios" cited in *Guidelines for Perinatal Care* (AAP/ACOG, 1992). Published protocols and guidelines are usually accepted as only a minimal level of care. There are many factors involved in determining staffing requirements for a given situation. Inherent in this is planning for and maintaining adequate numbers of competent staff to meet the needs of the patients served.

PLANNING FOR STAFF COMPETENCE

A key issue in the process of staffing is the competency of staff providing the care to patients. With reengineering, cross-training, and increasing the responsibilities of nurses in perinatal settings, the issue of competency takes on even greater meaning. In addition to providing staff, leaders are also ultimately responsible for ensuring that staff are competent for the positions they hold (JCAHO, 1996, p. 384). Organizations have been held liable under the theory of corporate liability for requiring staff to assume duties which they are not competent to perform. In *Olsen v. Humana* (Fiesta, 1988, p. 256), $7 million was awarded in punitive damages when a nurse responsible for a laboring patient was not adequately trained in fetal monitoring. However, corporate liability does not negate the law's "insistence that a nurse not undertake performing a function she is not qualified or competent to perform" (Bernzweig, 1996, p. 57). It is an inherent responsibility of each staff member to communicate his or her limitation when assigned to care for a patient beyond the scope of that person's competency to perform a specific duty or procedure. For example, a nursery nurse may be asked to cover for the care of a patient in early labor who is being monitored. The nurse must clearly communicate that she is not competent in interpretation of the fetal monitoring strip data or to perform vaginal examinations, though she may be competent in performing vital signs and providing comfort measures, thus being able to provide some assistance in times of short staffing.

COMPETENCY: AN OVERVIEW

Competency attainment is a developmental process that occurs over time (Sullivan, 1994). Competent staff requires that adequate training, competence assessment, and orientation have occurred. The issue of orientation becomes more relevant in relation to cross-training, floating, and use of contract personnel. Staff competency requires familiarity in working in a particular setting. A nurse competent in NICU nursing in one facility is not necessarily competent to work in another NICU that utilizes different equipment and practices under the scope of a particular standard of care or standard of practice developed in different institutions.

Competent staff development is an ongoing process that considers the dynamics of change occurring in health care practice and requires a leadership commitment over time. There is no concrete framework such as length of orientation or number of cases or procedures accomplished that can designate an individual as competent. The achievement of competency to practice and assume care of patients requires a period of time to allow for adequate experience and supervision.

With regard to initial training in perinatal settings, a brief orientation to intrapartum nursing is insufficient, even in the most basic low-risk unit. Competency to practice requires a thorough orientation to the facility, the unit, the standards of practice, familiarity with provider management routines, medication administration, technology used, and safety concerns specific to the unit. Intrapartum nursing requires advanced knowledge and skills beyond the basic nursing program, which can only be acquired with a thorough orientation and a developmental period over time with an experienced clinical expert. Additionally, as with any advancement to critical care nursing, nursing care for the critically ill mother or neonate and use of the highly technological equipment in ICU settings requires education and training beyond basic obstetrics. Orientation and assignment with a preceptor for an extended period of time is needed before a nurse can be regarded as competent. Patricia Benner's (1982) model for staff development, from novice to expert, clearly describes the developmental process for competency achievement. In effect, each nurse must have an individual journey to achieve competency in any specialty area assigned. The following case illustrates a number of points related to staff competency and organizational responsibility. A $98.5 million verdict was awarded in California following a uterine rupture that went unnoticed by nursing staff (Freeman, 1996, p. 41). Although the organization believed they were well staffed with four nurses on duty, the collective obstetric experience of the nurses was fewer than 6 years. The plaintiff argued that hospital cost-cutting measures were responsible for a very young and inexperienced staff. In this case, the staffing issue was not about numbers. The knowledge base, level of experience, and competency of the nurses on duty were considered the responsibility of the organization in providing safe care to patients.

Principles of Staff Competency

- Staff are afforded individualized competency development programs to achieve competence in caring for the patients they will be assigned. The underpinning construct is that competency achievement is individual and cannot be assumed to be attained by a certain period of time or a certain number of experiences.
- Staff are cognizant of their limitations and communicate such limitations to their superior for safe delivery of the patient.
- Staff are properly supervised by a preceptor or mentor in learning new skills or procedures.
- Staff undergo constant education to remain current with standards of practice that are scientifically valid and reliable.

CROSS-TRAINING STAFF

In many hospitals, cross-training staff has been utilized as a cost-effective means of acquiring the flexibility needed to deal with the pressures of cost containment and downsizing. However, cross-training must be carefully considered, with the understanding that the old proverb "a nurse is a nurse" does not fit in today's highly technical arena. Cross-training staff to competently work on different units or to care for a variety of patients requires careful planning and a commitment to properly achieve competent performance of all assigned duties. However,

the liability exists when inadequate orientation, education, and training of staff occurs as a mechanism to further reduce costs. Adverse outcomes have been known to occur when care is rendered by a "float" nurse who is not evaluated for competence prior to the assignment of patient care (Saltus, 1996).

A plan for cross-training must be well thought out with specific objectives for utilization, training, evaluation, and maintenance of skill. For example, is the purpose of cross-training to develop the ability to provide mother–baby care or to utilize nurses from one clinical area to assist in another area during times of short staffing? Defining the objectives will provide the foundation and guidance for the development of a cross-training program. Maintaining the skills needed to provide competent care to a group of patients when called upon requires a different focus than developing clinical expertise for a new population of patients. The former is generally a less in-depth process, but requires increased vigilance to monitor and maintain these skills. Many organizations are utilizing the extensive clinical experience of inpatient perinatal nurses in the home care setting in response to decreasing patient stays and the need for further nursing care beyond discharge (Donlevy & Pietruch, 1996). This use of cross-training builds on patient assessment skills that have developed over time and applies them to a different setting.

One of the liability issues surrounding cross-training relates to the extent of cross-training expected of nurses. Many institutions now have perinatal staff cross-trained to perform surgical nursing functions. These functions may include, but are not limited to, scrubbing for cesarean sections and tubal ligations, circulating, and first assisting. It is prudent to ensure that adequate training and education for surgical nursing duties have been attained. Proper credentialing and documentation of competency achievement for all staff performing specialty nursing duties is essential. It is important to reiterate that competency attainment is not achieved by performing a function or skill a certain number of times; competency is achieved when the performance is *consistently* performed within the standard of practice.

The greatest risk in cross-training today arises when goals are not adequately achieved. The planning methodology to appropriately cross-train staff to other units or specialty care is many times shortchanged due to the high demand to downsize personnel and decrease operating expenses. The goal for one staff member to supervise and properly teach the orienting staff member to thoroughly achieve competency is often not achieved or maintained. This short-sightedness imposes liability risk when untrained personnel are assigned to perform in roles they are not adequately or competently cross-trained for. Many times the error in performing a duty by a nurse or unlicensed personnel lies in deficient knowledge, education, or training, rather than their incompetence. Inadequate cross-training creates problems when staff members have not been given enough training to recognize what they do not know.

Competency assessment tools should be used to appropriately document acquisition of competency through education and training of staff. During the process of cross-training, a competent preceptor should be identified to appropriately educate, orient, and train the RN, LPN, LVN, or unlicensed personnel in the care of parturients and neonates. It is imprudent to assume competence of cross-trained staff without the documentation that skills have been attained and maintained.

CONTINGENCY STAFFING

One of the unique features of perinatal nursing is the unpredictable patient volume that can occur and the unforeseen conditions that can make any low-risk parturient or neonate high-risk. The nature of the unexpected can make even the best-planned approach to staffing substandard for any given day. Perinatal nurses are cognizant of this unpredictable nature of their work. Contingent staffing is the most prudent staffing management plan in a perinatal setting. The liability risk imposed when understaffing results in negligence occurs when standards of practice or standards of care are not met. The cost of malpractice far outweighs the cost of contingency staffing to provide safe and competent care to patients who expect it at all times. A breach of duty occurs when a standard of care is not met with regard to the availability of staff. Organizations cannot afford to routinely staff for the unexpected; however, they should have a planned approach for dealing with staffing crises. Documentation of this plan and ability to rapidly execute it is a significant factor in managing the risk associated with perinatal settings. Organizations have many different ways of dealing with short staffing, such as "floating," contract nurses, overtime (including mandatory), on call personnel, and so on. Large facilities generally have more flexibility due to the size of the organization and number of individuals on duty at any given time. Utilizing trained staff from other areas or reassigning duties within the perinatal unit may not be options in small organizations. Whatever methodology is used, there are a number of key principles that should be considered in any contingency plan.

Criteria that Contingency Staffing Should Include

Contingency staffing should include criteria that indicate understaffing and when to activate contingency plans, such as

- inability of nursing staff to assume care of new admissions
- inability of nursing staff to perform standards of practice/plan of care in a timely manner
- inability of nursing staff to appropriately supervise unlicensed staff
- inability of nursing staff to care for all patients assigned due to development of critical care needs (1:1 care) of a mother or newborn
- a mechanism to obtain competent staff in a timely manner
- careful review of the credentials and performance of out-of-hospital nursing staff if used for contingency staffing
- an efficient process for obtaining contingency staffing without the imposition of greater workload on nurses already in need of assistance
- careful documentation of critical staffing periods (unit communication log) to justify

prioritization of nursing care during interim periods of understaffing

A TEAM APPROACH

Contingency staffing not only deals with a plan to increase numbers of staff, but also relates to team support throughout the shift. The use of fixed staffing ratios does not account for changes that can occur along the continuum of care. For example, a nurse working in an LDRP may be assigned a one-hour postpartum patient and a multipara in early labor. During the course of her shift, the postpartum patient may hemorrhage while the multipara progresses rapidly from 3 cm to 8 cm within the same hour. The nurse cannot adequately care for both patients at the same time as both patients need 1:1 care. Without activation of team support for another provider to assume care for one of the patients, this situation could lead to an adverse patient outcome and liability for the nurse and institution. Another example includes the assignment of only one nurse during the delivery. After birth of the baby, the presence of an additional nurse or competent staff member may be required in the event that the mother needs 1:1 attention while the newborn needs 1:1 attention.

The need for effective teamwork and communication cannot be understated. The essence of success for any team requires effective communication among team members. Perinatal nursing staff are astutely aware of the unstable conditions wherein the low-risk situation can easily become high-risk. Communicating the conditions and adjusting the team based on a contingency approach should take precedence over staffing ratios and reduce the risk of liability, while maintaining a cost-effective approach to staffing.

A team approach to staffing allows for fluid maneuvering of members of the team (licensed and unlicensed) assigned to care for a constituency of patients on a particular unit, area, or department. The following guidelines can be utilized for a team approach:

- All staff should be cognizant of the patients on a particular unit. Staff should hear report on all patients on the unit to be familiar with the conditions and plan of care. Individualized reports impede staff awareness of the conditions of all patients residing on a unit, thus limiting collective familiarity of patients when a staff member may be required to assist with the care of another patient.

- All staff are responsible for the care of all patients on the unit. This translates to the quality principle that all patients are our customers. If a patient call light is on, any staff member should answer and assist as needed. If a staff member is unfamiliar or uncertain as to the appropriateness of an intervention, then the staff member should consult with the primary staff for clarification or instructions. "I'll call your nurse to assist you" is a comment that should be abolished. Ownership or disownership of patients segregates team cohesiveness and is a disservice to patients who need care or assistance during their stay. No patient should be jeopardized because his or her primary provider is unavailable (caring for another).

- Staff should communicate to their immediate superior or charge nurse changes in patient care requirements and the need for assistance to deliver safe patient care.

- Contingency staffing coverage should be outlined at the onset of the shift. This clear delineation of staffing coverage proactively designates crosscoverage of patients within the unit. Patients should never be left without a designated primary nurse provider who is responsible for nursing care. A nurse who has been assigned three mother–infant dyads should not be reassigned to scrub for a c-section without having a designated provider cover her patients during her interim reassignment.

- Team communication throughout the shift is essential for optimal integrated care. Team members should constantly be in communication with each other to ensure that patient care needs are met. Team cohesiveness in caring for the collective group of patients requires constant communication and assessment of care by team leaders to make decisions regarding cross-coverage during times of need. In essence, integrated teamwork requires the astute ability to triage staff to most appropriately care for patients.

STAFF ASSIGNMENTS

When assigning patient care responsibilities, supervisors are held accountable and, therefore, liable for the decisions they make. In addition to decisions relating to staffing numbers and staff competence, the assignments made to individual staff members must be made by individuals with appropriate knowledge of organizational policy, patient requirements, and staff education and training. The Joint Commission (JCAHO, 1994, p. 7) provides criteria to guide the supervisor in assigning staff members:

- What is the complexity of the patient's condition and the required nursing care?
- What are the dynamics of the patient's status, including the frequency with which the need for specific nursing care activities changes?
- What is the complexity of the assessment required by the patient and what knowledge and skills are required of a nursing staff member to effectively complete the assessment?
- What technology is employed in providing nursing care, and what knowledge and skills are required to effectively apply the technology?
- What is the degree of supervision required by each nursing staff member based on his or her previously assessed and current level of competence in relation to the nursing care needs of the patient?
- What is the availability of supervision appropriate to the competence of the nursing staff member being assigned responsibility for providing care to the patient?
- Are there any relevant infection control and safety issues?

Thus, staffing assignments consider the proficiency of the staff to safely assume patient care responsibility and appropriately meet the patient's needs. Once assignment decisions have been made, supervisors must evaluate the outcomes based on the degree of supervision staff members require. Staff members, including registered nurses, may have educational limitations that require supervisory staff to perform or assist with implementation of certain procedures beyond the scope of a particular individual. For example, when a float nurse is assigned to work in an area or assume care for patients that she or he is not adequately oriented to or educated about, direct supervision should be available. RNs supervising other subordinate staff or inexperienced RNs must assess their performance to ensure that competent care is delivered.

Supervisors should be able to defend the assignment decisions they make based on any given situation with full understanding that they are legally responsible to ensure that safe patient care is provided (Bernzweig, 1996, p. 184). Although supervisors and organization leaders are ultimately accountable for staffing assignments, all nursing staff should be assertive in communicating when any assignments are beyond the scope of their practice or educational preparation. Failure to communicate these or any other deficiencies to unit supervisors may impose individual liability for the nursing staff as well as do a great disservice to patients. Unless communication of staffing deficiencies occurs by RNs who are directly accountable to the patients they serve, the hospital leaders cannot implement corrective action to improve staffing conditions. Documentation of such communication is essential for personal liability protection. In situations where nurses are routinely expected to work with inadequate staff, such documentation should be continuously routed to risk management staff. Failure to act by those in leadership positions will lead to increased corporate liability for the organization (Bernzweig, 1996, p. 114).

STAFFING WITH UNLICENSED ASSISTIVE PERSONNEL

The current movement to restructure or redesign patient care delivery challenges organizations to comply with nursing State Practice

Acts and ensure that professional nursing roles and responsibilities are not violated. The use of unlicensed assistive personnel (UAP) has been a mainstay in nursing for decades although use has waxed and waned with varying market and professional fluctuations. Greater utilization of all RN staff or a high ratio of RN staffing resulted in changes in staff mix and increased personnel cost. With the advent of managed care and DRG-based reimbursement, hospitals have responded with changes in staff mix, utilizing more unlicensed assistive personnel. The American Nurses Association (ANA, 1994) defines UAP as "an unlicensed individual who is trained to function in an assistive role to the licensed registered nurse in the provision of patient/client care activities as delegated by and under the supervision of the registered professional nurse." Unlicensed assistive personnel have been utilized extensively as viable members of the health care team in the armed services for many decades. Their unique success is related to leadership involvement in planning and evaluation, comprehensive educational preparation, and clear lines of authority.

UAPs should be trained to practice within a defined scope of practice delineated either in hospital policy and/or nurse practice acts. Within these rules and regulations should be specific guidance defining the relationship between these care providers and the nurses who supervise them.

The concept of team nursing utilizes unlicensed assistive personnel and LPNs for activities within the scope of their education and training, whereas the RN performs more advanced procedures and makes appropriate decisions and assessments for patient care planning. The specific roles of the registered nurse must be clearly understood and differentiated from the roles of other licensed and unlicensed personnel. Those fundamental responsibilities of assessment, planning, and evaluating patient care that define professional nursing must continue to rest with the registered nurse. Clear lines of communication must exist with all members of the nursing care team to ensure that the RN (who is accountable for patient care) is apprised of patient responses to care provided.

All staff should be oriented to the responsibilities of individual roles and communication principles. In addition, nursing education should include the principles of leadership, management, delegation, and supervision. Where entry-level education leaves off, health care organizations must invest in preparing the professional nurse for the changes in care delivery in that organization (McLaughlin, Thomas, & Barter, 1995, p. 45). Delegation of patient care tasks to subordinate members of the nursing care team requires the ability to review performance, provide ongoing education, and develop a trusting relationship that allows the individual to grow. The increased risk associated with delegation can be minimized by following the delegation process correctly and may in fact be less than not having enough personnel available to meet patient needs (Hansten & Washburn, 1994, p. 108). Blousin and Brent (1995, p. 7) outline legal concerns regarding the nurse executive's decision to implement a structure utilizing UAPs:

- training and orientation of the new patient care givers (UAPs)
- patient injury as a result of negligent care allegedly given by the UAP
- adequate staffing
- delegation of patient care
- supervision of the UAP by the registered nurse
- restrictions regarding practices of UAPs by particular state nurse practice acts

Two primary areas of concern relate to the delegation and supervision of the UAPs. Blousin and Brent (1995) emphasize that "the nurse executive must ensure that policies and procedures concerning delegation and supervision by the professional nurse to the UAP are consistent with the state nurse practice act" (p. 8). Additionally, it is imperative that duties assigned to UAPs must clearly be within their scope of practice, and not duties that require a license or certification. The essential components of the nursing process are restricted to licensed nursing personnel, whereas delegation of tasks and low-risk procedures can be assigned to competently trained or oriented UAPs. Supervisors are negligent in their duty if they delegate duties to UAP that they are not competent to perform (Fiesta, 1988, p. 30). Of particular note is the fact that LPNs cannot delegate tasks to unlicensed personnel because they have neither the legal authority nor professional responsibility to supervise subordinates (Bernzweig, 1996, p. 186). Registered nurses should be aware of this limitation and, therefore, not place LPNs in supervisory positions with unlicensed personnel.

Staffing considerations should mandate that adequate supervision of UAPs by the RN is achievable. The staffing ratio of RNs, LPNs or LVNs, and UAPs must appropriately meet patient care needs and the requirement for supervision of subordinate staff. Determination of staffing ratios in perinatal units varies according to the education and training of UAPs and the unique performance of individuals with experience achieved over time. A high rate of staff turnover results in a continual flow of novice or inexperienced UAPs who may require more intensive supervision by licensed nursing personnel. This is in contrast to a more stable institution that may cultivate UAPs to be specialty-trained and expert over time, thus reducing intensive supervision requirements. The point of emphasis relates to competency development and trusting the performance of UAPs. The JCAHO (1996, p. 389) emphasizes that the competence of all staff members must be assessed, maintained, and demonstrated in fulfilling their assigned responsibilities. If they are not competent, direct supervision must be available. The use of a competency assessment tool that clearly delineates the specific skills required for UAP competency attainment is essential.

Negligence in supervision is a growing cause of malpractice claims against nurses although not solely related to UAPs. A supervisor will not be held accountable simply for being the supervisor. The "rule of personal responsibility" holds that every person is legally responsible for his or her own negligent conduct (Bernzweig, 1996, p. 180). Thus in supervising UAPs it is important for nurses to understand the UAP's scope of practice, level of experience, and the skills they are competent to perform when making patient care assignments.

Models of practice that include UAPs are clearly on the rise throughout the country. The profession of nursing must evaluate these models over time to determine the effect on organizational cost, quality of patient care, and risk management.

CONCLUSION

The issues of staffing in relation to perinatal liability are not significantly new issues to the profession of nursing. The effects are more a matter of degree as downsizing and cost cutting are squeezing more and more work out of fewer and fewer nurses. The specifics of adequate numbers, patient needs, trained staff, accurate assignments, and subordinate staff have been with the nursing profession for many years and numerous systems have been devised to deal with them. Changes in the delivery of care in this country and the increase in external oversight will continue to require vigilance in addressing these issues, which all affect perinatal liability. Critical-thinking skills must be developed in all professional nurses to analyze patient care needs and create the long- and short-term solutions to meet those needs. Leadership support, involvement of staff, and a commitment to quality patient care are underlying themes that will encourage innovation and decrease the risk for patients and staff.

References

American Law Report. (1995). (5th, 146, 2b). Rochester: Lawyers Cooperative.

ANA. (1994). Position Paper on Registered Nurse Utilization of Unlicensed Assistive Personnel.

Benner, P. (1982, March). From novice to expert. American Journal of Nursing, 402–412.

Bernzweig, E. (1996). The nurse's liability for malpractice. St. Louis, MO: Mosby.

Blousin, A., & Brent, N. (1995). Unlicensed assistive personnel: Legal considerations. Journal of Nursing Administration, 25(11), 7–8.

Borawski, D. (1995, July/August), Ethical dilemmas for nurse administrators, Journal of Nursing Administration, 25(7/8), 60–62.

Donlevy, J., & Pietruch, B. (1996). The Connection delivery model: Reengineering nursing to provide care across the continuum. Nursing Administration Quarterly, 20(3), 73–78.

Fiesta, (1988). The law and liability—A guide for nurses. NY: Wiley (p. 39).

Freeman, G. (1996, June). OB-GYN malpractice prevention, 3(6), 41–43.

The American Academy of Pediatrics and the American College of Obstetricians and Gynecologists. (1994). Guidelines for perinatal care. AAP/ACOG.

Hansten, R., & Washburn, M. (1994). Clinical delegation skills: A handbook for nurses. Gaithersburg, MD: Aspen.

JCAHO. (1994). Staffing for patient care: Questions and answers for nurse leaders.

JCAHO. (1996). Comprehensive accreditation manual for hospitals.

Mandeville, L., & Troiano, N. (1992). High-risk intrapartum nursing. Philadelphia, PA: J. B. Lippincott.

McLaughlin, F., Thomas, S., & Barter, M. (1995). Changes related to care delivery patterns. JONA, 25(5), 35–46.

Saltus, R. (1996, February 16). Patient's death leads to change at the Brigham. Boston Globe.

Sullivan, C. (1994, July/August). Competency assessment and performance improvement for health care providers. Journal for Health Care Quality, 4.

CASE CITATIONS

Arkansas State Dept. of Health v. Dr. Thibault and Council, P.A. 664 S.W.2d 445 (1984).

Documentation

Trish King-Urbanski and Rebecca Cady

Perinatal nursing is an ever-changing specialty that presents unique clinical problems and issues in the provision of patient care. It is unique from other specialties because any therapy will affect two individuals, each with potentially different outcomes. Although the pregnant woman and her fetus are considered together in the diagnosis of disease process, potential therapies and the desired outcomes must be evaluated separately. The nurse practicing in this area faces extensive demands on professional, technical, and personal resources. With this in mind, perinatal nurses know that the inadequately documented medical record can be their worst liability; conversely the well-documented medical record can be their greatest legal asset. Documentation reflects the character, the competency, and the care delivered by the nurse (Fentz-Harter, 1989). In a courtroom situation the medical record will represent the nurse, rather than the nurse's bedside manner or caring attitude. Due to the delayed time in which cases come through the court system, many nurses are forced to rely entirely on the medical record for information about their care of a patient. The patient likely has vivid memories surrounding the event, but the nurse usually has no independent recollections surrounding the case and must rely solely on the record itself. An additional problem is that it is difficult to predict which medical records will later come under close scrutiny.

In a study regarding malpractice claims, newborn and obstetric claims represented 76.1% of the claims. An analysis of these claims revealed that most involved either deficits with the medical record or system failures. A number of these problems could be prevented by avoiding systems failures and by regarding the medical record as a legal document (Richards & Thomasson, 1992). The court system has issued a warning to nurses that the availability of accurate medical records is not a mere technicality but is a legal requirement (*Valcin v. Public Health Trust of Dade County,* 1984).

An analysis of 294 obstetrical medical malpractice cases confirmed that documentation was a significant problem in medical record-keeping. Failure to document adequately was an important factor in 24% of obstetric cases. In an additional 5% of cases, the records were so poor that this alone mandated settlement (Ward, 1991). According to author Charles Ward, M.D., "in a courtroom the finest care rendered under the best circumstances may be difficult or impossible to defend if it is not documented" (Ward, 1991).

Increased demands for accountability in health care have prompted numerous efforts to measure, monitor, and improve the quality of nursing practice witnessed through documentation. There has been much speculation in the area of quality assurance and risk management about increased malpractice litigation causing demand for accountability of medical practice in documentation (Dworkin, 1989).

The nurse is a key member of the health care team and the nurse's communication skills lay the foundation for the care delivered to the patient. As the complexity of the care nurses provide in perinatal nursing increases so does the complexity of nursing documentation. Aside from actual patient care itself, documentation in the patient record is the single most important part of patient management (Kopf, 1993). Demands for detailed charting are present in everyday practice. Perfecting this skill is just as important as perfecting any other skill used in the clinical setting.

TRENDS IN HEALTH CARE LITIGATION

In the mid-1970s, the risk management environment changed dramatically with what came to be known as "the medical-malpractice crisis" (Danzon, 1990). At that time, a series of reports indicated that increasing numbers of medical malpractice suits with high awards were prompting increases in malpractice insurance premiums and in some cases the cost of the insurance was prohibitive. Total claims by insurers increased 264% from 1980 to 1987 and total medical malpractice insurance premiums paid by physicians grew 235% during that period (Barber, 1991). In 1985, an American College of Obstetricians and Gynecologists (ACOG) survey showed that 77.6% of obstetrician-gynecologists had been sued at least once (ACOG, 1985). As of 1989, obstetric claims represented approximately 10% of all medical malpractice claims nationwide and nearly half of all indemnity payments (Rostow, Osterweis, & Bulger, 1989). This "malpractice crisis" has driven professionals in the obstetric field to take specific steps toward improved quality assurance and risk management measures and documentation (Pearse, 1988; Pegalis, 1991; Ward, 1991). Health care malpractice claims in the United States continue to increase. Every legal action depends on the medical records for evidence that the clinical judgments and actions of the health care team members were timely and appropriate (Eggland & Heinemann, 1994).

RISK MANAGEMENT STRATEGIES

Many physicians and nurses perceive themselves to be at risk for malpractice litigation, either because they are aware of the trends of litigation or because of direct experience. These professionals seek to reduce risks by effecting certain changes in their practices. They have implemented strategies to provide more diagnostic tests and procedures, and to increase record-keeping (Hirsh, 1990).

Poorly kept nursing notes suggest poor communication among the nursing staff about the patient's care and condition. Notes made in an untimely fashion suggest that the patient was poorly monitored and that care of the patient was negligent. The care the patient received will be illustrated by what is and is not in the patient's medical record and specifically what is contained within the nursing notes (*Malonka v. Hermann et al.,* 1980; *Banyas v. Lower Bucks Hospital,* 1981). Failure by nurses to chart on some occasions and to properly chart on other occasions may jeopardize the health and safety of patients under their care. The court can conclude that failure to chart and/or chart accurately can prevent proper care and treatment from being administered to patients by other nurses who treat the same patient (*Alexander v. Department of Health & Human Resources,* 1986).

Despite the fact that the patient is the central focus of the care delivered, the patient's views are often considered external to the process of health care delivery (Prehn, Mayo, & Weisman, 1989). In assessing medical records, often patient satisfaction data are not part of the record. Recent literature suggests that despite minimal technical knowledge or objectivity, patients can make valid assessments of the care they receive (Vouri, 1987). When conducted properly, patient satisfaction surveys are considered an accurate and innovative measure of quality assurance as well as a feedback mechanism for risk management (Prehn, Mayo, & Weisman, 1989; Nelson, Hays, Larson, & Batalden, 1989).

Quality medical care is a logical and definable process. Any valid review of this process requires the transfer of data concerning the process of medical care from the chart to a data collection form. The data reported will aid the health care professional with risk reduction strategies. Linking the quality of care with the patient's outcome is an area just beginning to be studied (Petitti, Hiatt, Chin, & Croughan-Minihane, 1991).

Respectable data on the quality of care delivered and its relationship to medical malpractice is conspicuously absent in the literature (Kapp, 1989). Follow-through is essential in cases where potential litigation may take place. An unusual occurrence report or incident report should be created. The records should be kept together, including any fetal assessment tests such as ultrasound or fetal heart rate tracings. The nurse manager and risk manager should be notified and asked to secure the chart. By securing the chart, the risk manager can ensure that the vital components of the record will remain intact. Documenting "incident report filed" is entirely unnecessary and in fact can create a legal action in which this usually privileged communication is discoverable (*Bernardi v. Community Hospital Association,* 1968). An unusual occurrence report or incident report should contain objective details only, and never admissions of error or placing blame. The creation of the unusual occurrence report does not indicate that malpractice has occurred but merely allows the peer review process within the hospital to occur.

DOCUMENTATION PROBLEMS

Confusion about documentation appears to begin in knowing when to document, what to document, and how to delineate specifics of the care that was rendered. Most nurses begin to learn about documentation in nursing school, where they are instructed to describe what they see, hear, smell, and palpate. Documentation can be defined as written evidence of the interactions between and among health professionals, patients, and their families; the administration of procedures, treatments, and diagnostic tests; the patient's response to them; and education of the patient and family support unit.

Documentation verifies not only the care the patient received but also the status of the patient. Proper documentation clearly depicts the complete picture of the patient as nurses perform an assessment, form a plan of care, implement that plan, and evaluate the care that was delivered. Taking this a step further, nurses also ensure that the quality of care provided is in accordance with professional nursing practice standards. The medical records must therefore be adequate, legible, timely, and complete (Sanbar, Gibofsky, Firestone, & LeBlang, 1995).

Repeated failure to document entries on patient records, falsification of patient records, or making incorrect entries on patient records can lead to the state licensing board suspending or revoking the nurse's license. Documentation has become more vital than ever. Clinical records are subject up to close scrutiny by quality assurance committees, insurance companies, and lawyers as well as professional standards and accrediting committees (*Skillsbook,* 1992). Medical records are essential to resolving issues in nearly every branch of law. It is estimated that medical evidence plays a part in about three quarters of civil cases and in about one quarter of criminal cases brought to trial (Sanbar, Gibofsky, Firestone, & LeBlang, 1995). Although a lot is at stake, documentation errors still occur in many patient records (Betta, 1991).

Inadequacy

Courts have held that the poorly documented record creates a presumption of poor care (Nocon & Coolman, 1987). In the case of *Stack v. Wapner* (1976), the court held that where there were no notations made by the physician of monitoring a woman in labor, the jury could conclude that no monitoring occurred. Other cases have been decided based on the adequacy and the legal importance of good documentation by the nurse (*Malonka v. Herman et al.,* 1980).

When documenting the patient assessment, the nurse must use objective and definitive language. Documentation must be done in ink on the appropriate hospital form. It is best to use concise phrases with proper spelling and grammar. The negative impression that a misspelled, sloppy entry creates allows an opening for a plaintiff's attorney to imply that the nurse is poorly educated, not too bright, or just careless (Iyer, 1991). In *Guigino v. Harvard Community Health Plan* (1980), an expert witness complained that the progress notes were sketchy. Upon reviewing the material, the judge declared the notes totally illegible and barred their use in the court proceedings.

The content of the note should reflect a clear, concise thought process and report symptoms accurately. Ideally the notes should use the patient's words to describe the complaint verbalized or why she is seeking care. The note must describe the complaint objectively utilizing what was seen, heard, smelled, and touched. Medical terms should be used only if they are understood. The nurse must utilize authorized abbreviations only. If an abbreviation can have more than one meaning, for example, AMB for ambulance or ambulate, the abbreviation should not be used.

Late Entries

Information entered into the medical record in a timely fashion creates a picture of the whole series of events that make up the patient's care. By placing activities in the time frame in which they actually occur, important events such as phone calls or changes in the patient's status can be reported and can precipitate the delivery of care to the patient. Because other health care professionals rely upon the clinical record for important information, it is appropriate to make late entries if they are correctly identified and done in a timely manner. They are inappropriate if made after discovery that an adverse patient event has occurred. A plaintiff's lawyer will scrutinize all late entries, looking for evidence that the chart was altered.

A nurse may make late entries when the chart was unavailable at the time the events occurred, the nurse forgot to write notes on a patient's chart, or the nurse needs to add important information that was inadvertently not charted previously. To make such an entry the nurse should (1) begin the entry on the first available line; (2) label the entry LATE ENTRY, timing and dating the entry and indicating it is out of sequence; (3)

indicate the time the entry should have been made; and (4) do not attempt to squeeze just a few words in, especially if squeezing in means utilizing the margins of the chart form. Asking a fellow nurse to leave you a few lines is a dangerous practice. An example of how a late entry should read is: 1200, late entry for 1130 a.m., patient temperature = 101, Dr. Blank notified of T=101, no new orders received.

Inaccuracy

The nurse should begin charting only after checking the name on the patient's chart. The nurse should read the previous nurses' notes on the patient before caring for her, and compare the patient's current status with that of the past.

Falsification of records must never occur. If the nurse should ever falsify a record to cover up a negligent act and the judge or jury were to discover the falsification, doubt would be cast on the entire credibility of the witness and the medical record. The obvious implication of falsifying part of a record is that if the record is erroneous in one area it could be erroneous in other areas as well.

Corrections Versus Alterations

Corrections must be made by crossing through the error with a single line, marking "error," and initialing the entry. Scratching out or obliterating the writing such as with liquid paper so the document cannot be read in full are inappropriate ways of correcting the chart. Improper corrections may suggest that the nurse has tried to hide something with an obscured entry. Document experts can easily determine when records have been altered with white-out by x-raying the pages in question to reveal what is underneath the white-out. Alteration of part of a patient's records calls into question the credibility of the entire record. Revisions made after allegations of negligence arise subject the entire record to suspicions that the revisions were made under consciousness of negligence (*Pisel v. Stamford Hospital*, 1980).

Knowing that the patient has suffered a serious sequela can tempt members of the health care team to append or alter the medical record.

These actions are always improper and will be discovered when a lawsuit is filed. In one case, a 24-year-old woman had a twin gestation with an EDC of 5/29/91. She was scheduled for a repeat cesarian section for 5/20/91. One week prior to her pending surgery she went to her obstetrician's office for a prenatal visit. At that visit she had a blood pressure of 174/80. She had persistent +2 edema in her extremities. She had previously gained 5 pounds in 1 week and had up to 30 milligrams of protein in her urine. On this visit her urine dipstick showed trace protein. Six days later, on the morning of 5/19/91, she developed full tonic-clonic seizures and was diagnosed as suffering from eclampsia. Her twins died in utero.

Suit was brought against the obstetrician, contending he should have diagnosed preeclampsia and taken steps including hospitalization to evaluate the patient's status. Given the elevated blood pressure of 174/80 and the twin gestation, plaintiff's experts testified that this patient's risks were higher for developing eclampsia. The defendant admitted to having changed the note of the patient's blood pressure reading on the last prenatal visit from 174/80 to 124/80 in his medical records by drawing a line at the bottom of the 7 to make it into a 2. The discrepancy in the records was found by comparing a copy of the prenatal chart the doctor had given to the patient with the original. The defendant contended he was merely "correcting" the record.

This plaintiff was not able to recover damages from the death of her fetuses because they were not born alive; however, in other jurisdictions she would have been able to. The plaintiff did recover $885,000.00 for her damages as a result of the eclampsia, which consisted of delusions, psychosis, and permanent partial brain damage (*Washington v. Hollins*, 1993).

Incomplete or Missing Records

Incomplete or lost records pose a significant problem for defense of health care providers in a malpractice proceeding. The unavailability of records creates a strong inference of consciousness of guilt on the defendant's part and/or an inference that there was a purposeful attempt to

conceal what actually occurred. In the case of *Laubach v. Franklin Square Hospital*, the jury found that the hospital had knowingly concealed the fetal heart monitor tracings and awarded the plaintiff $1 million. This concealment of records was in violation of a state law that provided an independent right to recover compensatory and punitive damages against hospitals that hide or refuse to produce records. In the case of *May v. Moore* (1982), an infant died from allegedly negligent treatment during and following its birth. The chart "disappeared" after the hospital administrator had copied it. A suit for malpractice was brought and at the time of trial the hospital administrator produced his copy of the "lost" chart and testified that in other instances, the defendant physician had often "lost" records that showed a poor outcome for his patients. Later the defendant physician "found" the missing records, but they were significantly different from the copy the hospital administrator had made. The jury rendered a verdict for the plaintiff.

FACTORS THAT DEFINE QUALITY DOCUMENTATION

Frequency and Completeness

Gaps and discrepancies in time surrounding the sequence of delivery of care raise red flags. When flow sheets are utilized, they must be filled out correctly and completely, including a time notation for each entry. Boxes that are not filled out create an opportunity for questions about the care delivered. Any box that has no relevance in the patient's care should be marked "not applicable." Frequent irregular checks on the patient should be made to assess her status. Minimal entries made every 2 hours, even when the notation may read "status unchanged," can reflect the level of care received. However, a preferable alternative to "status unchanged" is to reflect on any patient interaction or teaching that has been performed. Nursing notes should be recorded on an ongoing basis during the day and not at the end of the shift. A complete date and time entry should be recorded for each new note. Each entry must be signed. Space must not be left between the signature and the end of the note. Block charting such as "11 P.M. to 7 A.M." should be avoided, as these entries sound vague and imply inattention from the nurse.

The nurse must document clearly and quickly. To ensure the accuracy of the record, the nurse must follow the established rules of documentation. These rules come from federal regulations, state statutes, accreditation boards, policies and procedures of the hospital, and the standards set by professional organizations.

An example of documentation requirements can be obtained from hospital policies, JCAHO accreditation standards, or professional nursing organizations such as the Association of Women's Health Obstetric and Neonatal Nurses (AWHONN). AWHONN standards for frequency and subject of documentation regarding fetal heart rate are illustrated in Display 18-1.

DISPLAY 18-1

Monitoring of the Fetal Heart Rate in Labor

Low-Risk Patients

First Stage of Labor
- q 1 hr in latent phase
- q30 min in active phase

Second Stage of Labor
- q 15 min

High-Risk Patients

First Stage of Labor
- q 30 min in latent phase
- q 15 min in active phase

Second Stage of Labor
- q 5 min

Assess FHR Prior to
- initiation of labor-enhancing procedures (for example, artificial rupture of membranes)
- periods of ambulation
- administration of medications
- administration or initiation of analgesia or anesthesia

Assess Fetal Heart Rate Following
- rupture of membranes
- recognition of abnormal uterine activity patterns, such as increased basal tone or tachysystole
- evaluation of oxytocin (maintenance, increase, or decrease of dosage)
- administration of medications (at time of peak action)
- expulsion of enema
- urinary catheterization
- vaginal examination
- periods of ambulation
- evaluation of analgesia or anesthesia (maintenance, increase, or decrease in dosage)

Source: AWHONN (1993)

Hospital Policies

Each institution has its own policies and procedures about documentation under which the nurse is expected to operate. The hospital's documentation standards can be stricter but not more lenient than those set by agencies regulating the practice of nursing, accreditation, or reimbursement (Yocum, 1993, p. 20).

Nurses should receive the necessary knowledge and skills in their education and orientation to provide safe, quality care. Assistance should be provided with adequate support systems, educational programs, and risk-management resources to decrease the number of poor patient outcomes (Gardner & Hagedorn, 1997). The standard and quality of care is the same despite a variety of practice settings. In one case, a 33-week gravid female presented to the emergency room after being kicked in the abdomen by an unknown assailant. A fetal monitor strip was obtained that showed the child was alive but exhibited a sinusoidal pattern. The emergency room physician failed to identify fetal distress based upon the strip, did not obtain an obstetric consult, and discharged the patient. The child was later delivered stillborn.

A suit was brought against the emergency room physician alleging that had an emergency cesarean been performed, the child would have lived. The defense asserted the patient did not present with signs of fetal distress, an obstetrical consult was not required, and the emergency room staff was not required to interpret the fetal monitor strips. This case resulted in a $160,000 settlement for the wrongful death of the baby and the mother's emotional distress (*Rowell v. Rab,* 1992).

Protocols provide instruction about standardized practice, focusing on problem-solving and decision-making skills. As nurses enter into a new position, they must acquaint themselves with the policies and protocols for that position. In one case a plaintiff was awarded in excess of $7 million after the jury found a hospital totally liable for the failure of its nurses to attach a fetal monitor to a laboring patient when one was available, and when it was standing protocol to do so (*Nelson v. Trinity Medical Center,* 1986).

The nurses in this case testified that they knew of the fetal monitoring policy but had failed to follow it. The defense in this case was made difficult because as there were no fetal monitor strips available, the hospital could not prove that the infant was not in distress during labor.

Hospital policies are one of the most relevant and critical elements in defining the standard of care to be administered to the patient. If the nurse feels that a policy is inappropriate and does not follow it, he or she must be prepared to defend the actions taken. A nurse is required to carry out any nursing or medical policy or procedure he or she is directed to carry out by a duly licensed physician unless the nurse has substantial reason to believe harm will result to the patient from doing so. To meet his or her legal obligation to the patient the nurse must know how to execute the procedure as well as the expected effects of the procedure on the patient. When a lawsuit is brought, the policies in effect at the time of the alleged negligent act are the policies that indicate the standard of care required to have been rendered to the patient (Janulis, 1993). Documentation in the medical record will be examined to see if it reflects care in accordance with the policies in place at the time.

A policy that is too inclusive and stringent may be the "ideal" policy from the development point of view but if it is unattainable for the staff, the policy is inappropriate. Policies should define what the minimal standard is, that is, what is adequate and safe care that can be carried out on a consistent basis. Policies should consistently and clearly define the nurse's duty to the patient. The nurse's notes should reflect that the duty to the patient was carried out and that quality care was maintained according to the applicable protocols.

Legal Standards

Each state's nursing practice act plays a major role in defining the practice of nursing in that state. This law defines, expands, and/or limits the scope of the nurse's legal authority within each state. State nursing practice acts differ in their definitions of nursing practice. Changes have continued to take place since 1979 that reflect increasing emphasis on high standards for nurses; those with superior education and experience often exercise independent judgment about the care of patients, whether in a hospital setting or elsewhere (*Fraijo v. Hartland Hospital,* 1979). Courts have found that the registered nurse is authorized to make an assessment of persons who are ill and to render a nursing diagnosis in her capacity as a professional adjunct to the treating physician (*Cignetti v. Camel,* 1985).

Documentation Systems

The increasing acuity of hospital patients, the complexity of their care, and the expanding responsibilities of the staff nurse place a heavy burden on the documentation and communication skills of the nurse. Patient acuity creates a need for nurses to have timely and accurate data on which to base clinical judgments (Eggland & Heinemann, 1994). Written communication is often the major and occasionally the only medium for data exchange between health care team members (Smith-Temple & Young-Johnson, 1994). Incomplete documentation may come not from lack of observation in the clinical setting but from deficits in the document itself. The format of the record needs to support and prompt the health care professional to document that the standard of care was delivered.

Flow sheets, checklist charting, or charting by exception are different ways to document patient information. The strengths of these documentation tools are that they prompt the nurse as to what information is key to document about his or her assessment of the patient. The weaknesses are that these documents take time to develop, individual nurses interpret the requests for information differently, and the means of noting the time the information is recorded in the medical record are frequently not built into the document. These tools can be a trap for nurses and become their worst nightmare in a courtroom setting when they are not filled out completely or correctly. In addition, interpretation of what constitutes adequate charting varies from nursing department to nursing department and hospital to hospital. "Liability experts are convinced that poor medical records are a lead-

ing reason medically defensible malpractice claims are ultimately filed and ultimately decided in the plaintiff's favor" (Karp, 1992). The key point is that the medical record must accurately reflect the patient's condition and progress no matter what format is used in the clinical setting. These formats must have minimal standards built into the forms themselves as well as in the policies governing their use.

The goals of nursing documentation are that the chart truly reflects that the care delivered to the patient met the standard of care due, that time was spent educating the patient, and that the nurse responded to concerns verbalized by the patient. Source-oriented documentation or narrative documentation is a widely used format in the current clinical system. In this system, the nurse is usually given no guidance as to what each note should contain. In the past nurses were encouraged to chart generally such as "appears to be sleeping," "status report given to physician," or "physician notified." Whenever possible, generalizations should be avoided when referring to physiologic responses such as "vomited copious amounts of bile-colored fluid." Instead the note should read "vomited 350 cc of bile-colored fluid." Vague information regarding the nurse's communication with the health care team should be avoided. The method of communication used such as phone or answering service, the information imparted in the conversation, the nurse's requests, and the physician's responses should be specifically noted. Each nurse will still have to decide what information is descriptive enough to communicate and depict the events occurring during the course of her interaction with the patient and physician.

Each nurse must develop his or her own system to decide on the organization of each note. The nurse should document information that contains the primary patient complaint, assessment of the patient's status and functioning level with daily care activities and patient teaching needs, the patient's agreement to the plan of care, and evaluation of the interventions taken. This documentation most clearly reflects the true status of the patient at a particular moment in time. Years later when asked to recall or review the record the nurse will know what the clinical focus was at that time and what follow-up actions were taken as well as the patient's response to them.

OBSTETRIC DOCUMENTATION ISSUES

Antenatal and Ambulatory Care

Obstetric care involves outpatient antenatal care, management of labor and delivery, and postpartum care. Although malpractice claims and research statistics in obstetrics usually reflect adverse outcomes in the labor and delivery process, antenatal care forms the firm groundwork from which obstetric decisions are made (Chng, Hall, & MacGillivray, 1980; Grabenstein, 1987; Gardner & Hagedorn, 1997). Antenatal care encompasses both the management of problems that arise during the pregnancy and the screening for factors that warrant further action (Guthrie, Songane, Mackenzie, & Lilford, 1989). In the past, perinatal care focused primarily on improvements in fetal testing and advances in newborn care (Kulb & Holtz, 1990). Now the pregnant woman is recognized as part of a much wider social system that involves her family, community, cultural group, and society as a whole. Significant events that occur in her environment affect her health and that of her fetus (Kulb & Holtz, 1990). Demands on the antenatal record are becoming increasingly complex and extensive (Peoples-Sheps et al., 1991).

The increasing number of lawsuits involving obstetrics demonstrates the need for clear documentation to show adequate care was given (Ward, 1991). Despite various reasons for using detailed systematic records in prenatal care, a 1991 survey showed that such records were not in widespread use (Peoples-Sheps et al., 1991). The American College of Obstetricians and Gynecologists (ACOG) conducted a survey of 1,646 members, which represented 39.7% of its membership in 1985, and found that among those ever sued, one of the most frequently reported practice changes was improving the documentation of office visits (ACOG, 1985). Experts state that efforts to create a facility in which medical care is of the highest quality simply cannot be fulfilled if documentation of that care is lacking. "It is critical that there be a record of why something was done. If the record is silent, there is no defense" (Richards & Thomasson, 1992).

In a report covering 591 claims involving allegations of neurologic deficits in newborns caused by negligent medical care during deliveries, investigators found that only 15% of charts reported information on alcohol consumption and that only 27% reported smoking history in the pregnant women. They also observed that whereas prenatal diagnostic tests and procedures were better documented, the results were frequently unavailable. In an effort to apply a simplified risk scoring system, they found that data on at least one risk factor was missing in 45% of the charts. This national survey conducted by Peoples-Sheps et al. (1991) found that a list of risks in the present pregnancy or a checklist for the risk assessment was present in only 30% of the charts analyzed.

Risk screening in pregnancy is an important step in the prevention of bad outcomes. Ongoing, continuous assessment and evaluation of all of the factors that predispose a patient to potential complications should be incorporated in any risk screening program. Because so many factors may influence maternal and infant outcome, standardized risk assessment tools have been designed to formalize this process (Sokol, Rosen, Stokjkov, & Chik, 1977; Holbrook, Laros, & Creasy, 1989; Kulb & Holtz, 1990). The patient's risk factors are evaluated at the first prenatal visit and, depending on the number and/or severity of the conditions found, a score of low, moderate, or high risk is assigned. The patient's risk status is reevaluated at specific time intervals during the pregnancy based on the number of weeks gestation. A patient's risk score may escalate from low to moderate or high risk. However, the score is never reduced from high to moderate risk (Kulb & Holtz, 1990). The nurse may often be the one to identify risk factors that impact outcome and also the one to complete the standardized scoring system. He or she is in an ideal position to coordinate the efforts of the entire health care team in order to provide quality care. From a legal perspective, deficiencies in this risk evaluation leave health care professionals extremely vulnerable in the event of malpractice litigation (Peoples-Sheps et al., 1991).

Studies in which physician's office records were examined suggest that prenatal care may be far from being of even minimally acceptable quality, as audited charts reveal that missing data is common among office practices (Peoples-Sheps et al., 1991; Hansell, 1991). The findings suggest that "the physicians reconsider their pre-natal records in light of the functions that prena-tal record should serve" in the 1990s and beyond (Peoples-Sheps, 1991). In the ambulatory or out-patient office, physicians and health care profes-sionals accept the need to document but they believe that they accomplish more recording than they actually do (Thompson & Osborne, 1976). Frequently, patient complaints are miss-ing from the medical record along with patient concerns and questions. Some offices combat this by asking patients to fill out a form upon entering the office that requests patient com-plaints, concerns, and questions in addition to any signs or symptoms of premature labor, cur-rent self-care needs, or current educational needs. The patient thus becomes an active par-ticipant in formulating her plan of care.

Delay in Performing a Cesarean Section

On June 20, 1988, a laboring mother experienced the onset of severe painful uterine contractions. The obstetrician's office told her to come in imme-diately as the physician was expected to arrive at 1 P.M. The woman waited in the waiting room and was not examined until the doctor arrived at 2:30 P.M. She was then sent to the hospital. Upon admission to the hospital the fetal monitor was applied at 3:04 P.M. and there was evidence of per-sistent late decelerations. Within 20 minutes the nurses began intrauterine fetal resuscitation mea-sures including hydration and position change. At 4:00 P.M. the physician was notified of the pattern of late decelerations with slow recovery to base-line. The physician's response was that he would be up shortly and they were to continue to observe the patient. He did not arrive until 5:00 P.M., whereupon he denied the nurses had previ-ously accurately informed him of the fetal distress. A cesarean section was not performed until 6:23

P.M., as the physician first went to perform an elec-tive D&C on another patient. The nurse docu-mented that the physician's decision to perform this elective surgery delayed setting up for the emergency cesarean section.

At the time of delivery a partial abruption could be seen. At birth, the infant had Apgar scores of 7 and 8 and was hypotonic. The med-ical records had conflicting information about the color of the infant and whether there was a delay in cry. No pH was taken until 3½ hours of life. A $3.5 million settlement was paid to the plaintiff (*Hansen v. Sender,* 1992).

Failure to adequately document when an anesthesiologist was not notified of an emer-gency cesaren delivery resulted in a substantial verdict. In 1991, a gravid female saw her physi-cian in his office and was examined. The doctor advised her that her contractions were 5 minutes apart and she was to go to the hospital. The fol-lowing day the patient's membranes ruptured while she was at home and she was taken to labor and delivery. She was escorted to the restroom where she could change into hospital garb. She was assisted in removing her materni-ty pants and the nurse noticed that 5 inches of the umbilical cord had prolapsed and clumped at the opening of the vagina. The nurse testified that the cord was approximately a 9-inch loop (18 inches of cord) that extended to the knees. An emergency was declared at 5:49 P.M. Entries on the delivery room admission note revealed that the surgeons were called at 5:50 P.M. Cellular phone records verified that the physician returned the call at 5:52 P.M. and arrived at 6:10 P.M. Records showed the anesthesiologist was not paged until 6:02 P.M. The actual arrival time of the anesthesiologist was hotly contested at tri-al. The anesthesiologist testified she arrived before delivery but the physician and nurse tes-tified the anesthesiologist was not present until after delivery. There was evidence that the physi-cian delayed the surgery because of his reluc-tance to operate without an anesthesiologist. The baby was delivered at 6:34 P.M. with Apgar scores of 2, 4, and 5 at 1, 5, and 10 minutes.

Suit was brought against the hospital alleg-ing that the staff delayed in calling the anes-thesiologist and that the facility lacked an adequate protocol to obtain a backup physician. The hospital also allegedly failed in not having a protocol for obtaining a backup surgeon to complete a surgery when it was determined that the surgeon was 20 minutes away. The hospital was also alleged to be at fault as hospital personnel failed to prepare the patient for the operation and did not eliminate cord compression prior to surgery by pushing the presenting parts away from the prolapsed cord. The hospital denied liability and stated it complied with the ACOG standard of making the incision within 30 minutes of the decision to perform a cesarean section. The plaintiff was awarded $1 million (*Song v. Bellflower Doctor's Hospital*, 1993).

Documentation of Fetal Movement

Establishing the presence of fetal well-being is essential for each interaction with the perinatal patient. Documentation of the presence of fetal heart tones, audible accelerations, and fetal movement helps establish that the nurse was thinking about the status of the fetus in his or her interactions with the patient. In one case, a 28-year-old woman was diagnosed as being pregnant but did not return for prenatal care until late in her pregnancy. On 7/3/85 she gave birth to a child that died several days later. In examining the medical record there was a question as to whether antepartum testing should have been performed to determine if intrauterine growth retardation had occurred. The medical records reflected decreased fetal movement 2 weeks prior to delivery. The patient was instructed to conduct home fetal movement counts and contact the clinic if she felt decreased fetal movement. One week later she returned in early labor complaining of no fetal movement and was sent to the hospital for observation. Fetal monitor tracings were not reassuring. Arrangements for an obstetric consultation were made; however, before the physician arrived at the hospital the fetal heart tracing disappeared from the monitor. As soon as the physician arrived, an immediate ultrasound was performed that showed some fetal heart motion. A cesarean section was performed and the baby was resuscitated and remained in the intensive care unit for 5 days before life support was terminated.

Plaintiff brought suit against the clinic, the hospital, and the doctor. The patient denied receiving kick count instructions, and claimed that 1 week prior to the delivery she had complained to the physician of decreased fetal movement. The doctor denied the allegations and the records for the office visit in question contained no references about fetal movement. The defense contended that the care rendered was within the standard of care, and that the infant had suffered irreversible brain damage in utero prior to admission to the hospital. The defense presented strong testimony. The plaintiff's expert was unavailable for trial and the court refused to allow his testimony in deposition to be read to the jury. A verdict was reached in favor of the clinic and the doctor; however, the case is on appeal (*Garcia v. Seattle Indian Health Board*, 1989).

Telephone Triage

Documenting telephone calls to a physician or nurse is essential to maintain continuity of care and to preserve essential information that was provided or conveyed as illustrated in a 1993 case. A case involving problems with telephone triage arose in 1992. A gravida 3 para 1 female delivered following a prolonged second stage of labor. The obstetrician performed a Scanzoni maneuver, which involved the rotation of the baby's head with mid forceps. The delivery was then accomplished with the assistance of low forceps. The mother experienced abdominal pain and difficulty urinating during the postpartum period.

During the next several days she reported by phone to the office that she was experiencing severe pain, hardening of her abdomen, cramps, nausea vomiting, fever, fatigue, and seepage from her vagina. These symptoms were attributed to flu and constipation but the patient was not seen for an examination. Nine days after birth, as her symptoms became worse, she was taken to the hospital. The woman was diagnosed with sepsis, ARDS, and a perforated bladder. She died several days later. Few records of the calls were produced with only one doctor admitting to speaking with the patient. The family was awarded $1.3 million (*Descheness v. Anonymous*, 1992).

Unusual Occurrences in the Operative Delivery

In 1986, a woman died during a cesarean section. Allegations of malpractice surrounded the epidural administration, the subsequent general anesthesia, and the surgery. The surgery was started with a general anesthetic because the obstetrician was in a hurry. Following the delivery of the infant the surgeon noted that the mother's blood seemed to be darkening. He noted this on two occasions to the anesthesiologist with the anesthesiologist insisting the patient was fine. The anesthesiologist did not alter his care. The nurse verified that the obstetrician told the anesthesiologist about the dark blood, that the obstetrician was in a hurry, and that the obstetrician left the room at the time of skin closure, allowing the resident to finish. The patient went into shock, and was comatose for 41 days prior to her death. The husband and baby were awarded $6.55 million (*Cotiletta v. Shin,* 1992).

Informed Consent

In 1980, a 36-year-old woman was in labor and under the care of an obstetrical resident. The patient later brought charges of malpractice as a result of an alleged delay in performing a cesarean section. The plaintiff and her experts felt that due to repeated decelerations, prolonged drops in the fetal heart rate, and meconium staining, a cesarian should have been performed by 2:30 P.M. The physician stated he advised the mother that the cesarean was needed at 3:00 P.M. and the mother withheld her consent until 4:00 P.M. The mother denied withholding her consent. The nurses' notes indicated that the consent of the mother was requested at 3:45 P.M. and the consent was signed shortly after 4 P.M.

The child was born cyanotic with seizures shortly after birth and Apgar scores of 1 at 1 minute and 7 at 5 minutes. The defendant argued that the infant had a maldeveloped brain. The child suffered spastic quadriplegia and profound retardation. The jury awarded $4.5 million to the plaintiff (*Salazar v. New York Hospital,* 1988).

Fetal Monitor Strips

Keeping a verbal accounting of the image of the fetal monitor strip is essential to any obstetrical record. Recording "fetal heart tones 140's" is not a sufficient description of what is occurring in utero with the fetus. A baseline range must be established including the presence of reassuring or nonreassuring signs in the tracing in case the tracing is lost. Although this description may not always prevent recovery from the plaintiff, it is imperative that the document reflect a complete description of the fetal monitor tracings.

In 1981, a 26.5-week gravid female was admitted to the hospital complaining of pain and vaginal bleeding. Her ultrasound indicated a low-lying placenta and breech presentation. Her medical history was of a prior delivery of a 28-week fetus and four previous abortions. The patient continued to bleed on and off for 3 days with heavy bleeding occurring at 5:30 A.M. on the third day. After being seen by a second-year resident, the patient was transferred to labor and delivery. She delivered a footling breech infant with Apgar scores of 1 at 1 minute and 4 at 5 minutes of age. The chief resident and attending physician were not present until just moments before the delivery.

Allegations of malpractice focused on assertions that the delivery of the preterm fetus should have been by cesarean rather than vaginally. The fetal monitor strips were missing at trial but the nurse's notes made reference to late and variable decelerations. Plaintiff contended the late decelerations were secondary to placental insufficiency caused by abruptio placenta and the variable decelerations were present due to cord compromise from the footling breech position. The defendant contended that the child's injuries were caused by prematurity. The plaintiff was awarded $7.5 million (*Ashby v. NYCHHC,* 1993).

The fetal monitor strip is a vital component of any clinical record. There is a controversy surrounding the writing of nursing notes directly on the document. One school of thought is that it verifies the nurse's presence in the patient's room, is readily accessible in emergency situations, and provides evidence that ongoing interpretations and nursing interventions were made in response to the fetal heart tracing pattern. However, there are those who feel that scrawled writing across the paper duplicates information found elsewhere in the medical record. At a minimum, charting on the strip should include proper labeling of the document with the patient's name, patient number, and date of testing. Some facilities require that two RNs read the NST, or that the physician's signature be obtained on the test strip in the 24 hours following the test. A check mark must not be placed above accelerations on a nonstress test, as this eliminates the ability of an expert to impartially view the strip at a later date. If there are any questions regarding an intrapartum fetal monitor tracing, the charge nurse or a senior staff nurse should be consulted to validate the staff nurse's interpretation. Notations should be made as the nurse deems necessary and pertinent without interfering with the FHR tracing or data from the uterine activity monitor.

IMPROVING DOCUMENTATION

Precise attention must be paid to documentation. Documentation must convey objective information in a prompt, concise, and accurate manner. The surest way to prove that the standard of care was delivered is to record and communicate this accurately in the patient record. Clear documentation is the best proof that responsible, well-planned nursing care was given (Smith-Temple & Young-Johnson, 1994).

According to author Barbara Calfee, errors in basic care are usually at the root of negligence lawsuits. These errors can be placed into three categories: assessment errors, planning errors, and intervention errors (Calfee, 1993). Assessment errors in nursing documentation might include failing to adequately gather and document information about the patient or failure to identify the significance of certain information. To avoid errors, an assessment should include the following: the patient's chief complaint, preferably using direct quotes; the primary nursing diagnosis (the most pressing problem or concern for the patient); the patient's history, medication allergies, physical assessment, and emotional status; the patient's assessment of current pain level; and relevant psychosocial data. If the patient divulges information that is part of a risk-taking behavior, the information should be recorded using direct quotes. If the patient is unwilling to tell all the information needed or is evasive in responding to questions, this must be recorded in her chart as well, in objective terms.

Planning errors in nursing documentation are in the form of failure to communicate in a fashion that will ensure continuity of care, failure to deliver discharge instructions in an understandable manner to the patient, and failure to inform the patient of when to call if no improvement is noticed. To avoid planning errors the nurse must clearly communicate to the patient, both verbally and in writing. The nursing notes delineate the necessary steps to be taken for each patient problem, the follow-up delineated by the physician, and the level of understanding achieved by the patient regarding her care. The nurse must assess the patient's level of understanding of the plan of care and discharge instructions. The nurse must assess the patient's level of comfort with the current course of action. The nurse must identify the patient's needs not fulfilled with the current treatment plan. All of these assessments, interventions, and patient responses must be documented. The patient must initial or sign instruction lists that are reviewed. The patient's response to the information received must be recorded.

Intervention errors in nursing documentation might consist of failure to follow up with the physician in a timely manner, fulfill physician orders, or move up the nursing chain of command if the physician's actions or orders are endangering the patient. To avoid intervention errors, the nurse should record physician orders upon receiving them, confirm any orders where the handwriting is illegible, respond to the physiology creating the fetal monitoring tracing, interpret and react to clinical symptoms, carry out appropriate physician orders, use the five rights when administering any medication, utilize good communication when conveying the medical condition of the patient, record both the communication to and the response of the physician to status reports, and when necessary, initiate the nursing chain of command. Continuing to record care or interventions that are ineffective or potentially dangerous is not helpful to the patient or the nurse.

Documentation of the report of patient status given to the physician must also include the response received. When necessary, the nurse must inform the physician he or she is requesting the physician's immediate attendance to the patient or the chain of command will be initiated. All objective dialog must be recorded in the medical record.

Nursing Process and Documentation

The American Nurses Association (ANA) has defined the scope of practice for nurses providing perinatal care (ANA, 1980). Practice is provided within the framework of the nursing process and includes, but is not limited to, the following:

1. Assessment—Assessing the psychosocial and physiological status of the childbearing family by differentiating the level of perinatal risk; by initiating and utilizing multiple sources and assessment tools for data collection, such as history, physical examination, and appropriate laboratory data; and by interpreting data that lead to nursing diagnoses.
2. Plan of care—Establishing an appropriate plan of intervention with the perinatal family based on nursing diagnoses by collaborating with the family and other health care providers; by differentiating immediate and long-term health care goals with the family; and by determining and coordinating the plan of action to meet these identified goals.
3. Intervention—Implementation of interventions with the perinatal family that are based on the plan of care, including initiating technical procedures and therapeutic regimes; teaching, counseling, and facilitating family growth by promoting

optimum health development of the perinatal family.
4. Evaluation—Evaluating the plan of care of the perinatal family by evaluating the interventions, evaluating the effects of the interventions on the family, evaluating the family's progress toward the identified goals, and initiating changes in the plan of care based on new data and resources and on the environment.

The nursing process begins with the assessment of the patient's status including data collection by physical examination, review of history, obtaining responses from the patient and significant others, and review of diagnostic test results. Examination of the medical records, patient risk factors, laboratory data, and medical alert tags are key to formulating and implementing a plan of care. Since 1980, nurses have been empowered to make nursing diagnoses in the care of patients. The use of nursing diagnoses focuses on primary concerns for nursing action. The nursing diagnosis is the identification of patient problems, both actual or potential, as nursing diagnosis is a clinical judgment about the individual or the support system available to the patient. If the nurse fails to utilize nursing diagnoses, it can be construed that there was no primary focus to the care rendered.

In contrast, medical diagnosis is the diagnosis of a pathologic condition. Nurses diagnose and treat the response to the pathologic condition. As an example, with a medical diagnosis of pregnancy-induced hypertension, the nursing diagnosis would include the vasospasm related to hypertension, the impaired venous system with increased permeability, and the high risk for altered blood pressure readings and the hypertension itself. The physician's diagnosis usually stays the same once it is made. The nursing diagnosis changes as the patient's condition deteriorates, improves, or develops complications of a different nature. Eighty-two percent of administrators believe that most of their staff members will utilize nursing diagnosis in documentation (*Skillsbook,* 1992). JCAHO recommends and approves of using nursing diagnoses in documentation, although it does not mandate them.

Documentation must reflect the nurse's assessment, and understanding of the pathophysiology involved in the problem and the potential for the development of problems for both the mother and fetus. As an example, vaginal bleeding at 32 weeks involves not only understanding the abrupt onset of abruptio placenta but also the insidious symptoms of the onset of a marginal detachment or development of a coagulation problem. Documenting the symptoms displayed by the mother and fetus are essential for clear communication on whether the nurse recognized what was going on with the maternal–fetal unit. Nursing diagnoses must indicate a need for nursing care, not a nursing task (Yocum, 1993, p. 26). Nursing diagnosis plays a key role in the identification of real or potential problems. A New Jersey hospital was sued by the family of a maternity patient who died 3 hours after an uncomplicated delivery. An expert witness testified that vital signs were poorly monitored, nurses' notes were poorly kept, and the nursing diagnosis should have led nurses to conclude that hemorrhage was possible (*Malonka v. Herman et al.,* 1980).

Developing and implementing a plan of care is essential for identifying appropriate nursing actions and target times or dates to achieve the care plan. These measurable outcomes must be realistic and attainable. Documentation must reflect this process. Once the plan of care has been established it must be implemented. In considering implementation one must consider the action and the rationale for doing that action. The plan of care has to be reasonable in its expectations for patient improvement. The actions can be nursing- or client-generated and must have clear concise steps toward achieving the plan of care. Good documentation reflects the patient's level of understanding of the plan of care and the patient's agreement to continue on the planned course.

Evaluation occurs as the nurse examines whether the expected outcome or outcomes were achieved. By recording this ongoing process, the care provided to the patient is clearly reflected. By documenting the patient's behavior, the medical record can clearly communicate what the current status of the patient was. Under examination, documentation will reveal if care goals were modified and if expectations were lowered or raised. The prioritized nursing actions must therefore be identified in the medical record. Nursing process is continuous. Nurses document without thinking about their complex decision-making process. Information is reaffirmed continually yet rarely recorded. The priority of care delivered should always be reflected in the medical record. Documentation should reflect the ongoing evaluation process utilized in the clinical situation.

Things to Avoid

The clinical record must not be used to assign blame or to vent anger at a fellow practitioner. Judgmental statements such as "couldn't get Dr. Mathews to see the patient," "the bed was completely saturated with blood," or "apparently the evening shift never checked the mother's fundal tone" must be avoided. Such inflammatory notes increase the potential to create a lawsuit and are unprofessional. Such verbal catharsis is best left unwritten. It is important never to impart such accusations to paper even when requested to do so by the nurse manager under the guise of a peer review process, unless the document is addressed to the risk management department or hospital attorney, as these independently created documents are likely to be subpoenaed in the event of a lawsuit. All objective information should be confined to an incident report and forwarded to the risk manager or defense attorney.

CONCLUSION

"As erroneous as it may seem a great deal of litigation in this field tends to stem from the belief that a child born with any degree of compromised health must have been a victim of physician or nurse malpractice" (Calfee, 1993). Parents are simply reluctant to accept the less than perfect infant or one with any birth defect not disclosed before birth. When patients have unmet expectations they become angry and frustrated and they seek resolution through litigation. Nursing notes and plans of care often will be the only proof in future years that clients were monitored, well cared for, well informed, and in agreement with the plan of care. Well-written notes, plans of care, and flow sheets completed in an accurate and timely manner support the quality all nurses strive for in delivering patient care, and can protect both the nurse and patient.

REFERENCES

American College of Obstetricians and Gynecologists. (1985). Professional liability insurance and its effect: Report of a survey of ACOG's membership. Washington, DC: American College of Obstetricians and Gynecologists.

American Nurses Association. (1980). A statement on the scope of high risk perinatal nursing practice. (American Nurses Association No. MCH-12, p. 2). Washington, DC: ANA.

AWHONN. (1993). Fetal heart monitoring principles and practices. City: AWHONN.

Barber, H. R. K. (1991). The malpractice crisis in obstetrics and gynecology: Is there a solution? Bulletin of the New York Academy of Medicine, 67(2), 162–172.

Betta, P. A. (1991). Documenting to stay out of the courtroom. Imprint, 38(2), 39–40.

Calfee, B. (1993). Nurses in the courtroom. Cleveland, OH: ARC Publishing Company.

Chng, P. K., Hall, M. H., & MacGillivray, I. (1980). An audit of antenatal care: The value of the first antenatal visit. British Medical Journal, 281(11), 1184–1186.

Danzon, P. M. (1990). The "crisis" in medical malpractice: A comparison of trends in the United States, Canada, the United Kingdom and Australia. Law, Medicine & Health Care, 18(1–2), 48–58.

Dworkin, R. B. (1989). Law and the modern obstetrician-gynecologist. American Journal of Obstetrics and Gynecology, 160(6), 1339–1343.

Eggland, E. T., & Heinemann, D. S. (1994). Nursing documentation: Charting, recording and reporting. Philadelphia, PA: J. P. Lippincott.

Fentz-Harter, S. (1989). Legal Insights: Documentation principles and pitfalls. Journal of Nursing Administration, 19(12), 7–9.

Gardner S. L., & Hagedorn, Mary I. E. (1997). Legal aspects of maternal–child nursing practice: Concepts and strategies in risk management. New York: Addison-Wesley.

Grabenstein, J. (1987). Nursing documentation during the perinatal period. Journal of Perinatal Neonatal Nursing, 1(2), 29–38.

Guthrie, K. A., Songane, F. F., Mackenzie, F., & Lilford, R. J. (1989). Audit of medical response to antenatal booking history. British Journal of Obstetrics and Gynecology, 96(5), 552–556.

Hansell, M. J. (1991). Sociodemographic factors and the quality of prenatal care. American Journal of Public Health, 81(8), 1023–1028.

Hirsh, H. L. (1990). Defensive medicine—Friend or foe? Journal of Health and Hospital Law, 23, 145–197.

Holbrook, H. R., Laros, R. K., & Creasy, R. K. (1989). Evaluation of a risk-scoring system for prediction of preterm labor. The American Journal of Perinatology, 6(1), 62–68.

Iyer, P. (1991). New trends in charting. Nursing, 91, 21(1), 48–50.

Janulis, D. M. (1993). Policies and practices guaranteed to make hospital attorneys cry: Part 1. Journal of Nursing Law, 1(1), 15–28.

Kapp, M. (1989). Solving the medical malpractice problem: Difficulties in defining what "works." Law, Medicine & Health Care, 17(2), 156–165.

Karp, D. (1992). Loss minimizer. San Rafael, CA: Author.

Kopf, R. (1993). Are your medical records a legal asset or liability? Legal documentation guidelines. Journal of Nursing Law, 1(1), 5–13.

Kulb, N. W., & Holtz, A. (1990). Perinatal care. In K. Buckley, & N. W. Kulb (Eds.), High risk maternity nursing manual. Baltimore: Williams & Wilkins.

Nelson, E. C., Hays, R. D., Larson, C., & Batalden, P. B. (1989). The patient judgement system: Reliability and validity. Quality Review Bulletin, 15(6), 186–191.

Nocon, J. J., & Coolman, D. A. (1987). Perinatal malpractice risks and prevention. The Journal of Reproductive Medicine, 32(2), 83–90.

Pearse, W. H. (1988). Professional liability: Epidemiology and demography. Clinical Obstetrics and Gynecology, 31, 148–152.

Pegalis, S. E. (1991). The malpractice crisis: An attorney's viewpoint. Bulletin of the New York Academy of Medicine, 67(2), 173–179.

Peoples-Sheps, M. D., Kalsbeek, W. D., Siegel, E., Dewees, C., Rogers, M., & Schwartz, R.

(1991). Prenatal records: A national survey of content. American Journal of Obstetrics and Gynecology, 164(2), 514–521.

Petitti, D. B., Hiatt, R. A., Chin, V., & Croughan-Minihane, M. (1991). An outcome evaluation of the content and quality of prenatal care. Birth, 18(1), 21–25.

Prehn, R. H., Mayo, H., & Weisman, E. (1989). Determining the validity of patient perceptions of quality care. Quality Review Bulletin, 15, 74–76.

Richards, B. C., & Thomasson, G. (1992). Closed liability claims analysis and the medical record. Obstetrics & Gynecology, 80(2), 313–316.

Rostow, V. P., Osterweis, M., & Bulger, R. J. (1989). Medical professional liability and the delivery of obstetrical care [Special report]. The New England Journal of Medicine, 321(15), 1057–1060.

Sanbar, S. S., Gibofsky A., Firestone, M., & LeBlang, T. (Eds.). (1995). Legal Medicine. American College of Legal Medicine. New York: Mosby.

Smith-Temple, J., & Young-Johnson, J. (1994). Nurses' guide to clinical procedures. Philadelphia: J.B. Lippincott.

Sokol, R. J., Rosen, M. G., Stojkov, J., & Chik, L. (1977). Clinical application of high-risk scoring on an obstetric service. American Journal of Obstetrics and Gynecology, 128(6), 652–661.

Thompson, H. C., & Osborne, C. E. (1976). Office records in the evaluation of quality care. Medical Care, 14(4), 294–310.

Vouri, H. (1987). Patient satisfaction—An attribute or indicator of quality of care? Quality Review Bulletin, 13, 106–108.

Ward, C. J. (1991). Analysis of 500 obstetric and gynecologic malpractice claims: Causes and prevention. American Journal of Obstetrics and Gynecology, 165(2), 298–304.

Yocum, R. F. (1993). Documentation skills for quality patient care. Tipp City, OH: Awareness Press.

CASE CITATIONS

Alexander v. Department of Health and Human Resources, 484 So.2d 722 (La., 1986).

Ashby v. NYCHHC, No. 13414/87 Bronx County Superior Court, N.Y. (January 29, 1993).

Banyas v. Lower Bucks Hospital, 437 A.2d 1236 (Pa. Super. 1981).

Bernardi v. Community Hospital Association, 443 P.2d. 708 (1968).

Cignetti v. Camel, 692 S.W.2d 329 (Mo. App. 1985).

Cotiletta v. Shin, No. 32441/87 Kings County Superior Court, Brooklyn, N.Y. (July 1992).

Descheness v. Anonymous, No. 89-2002 Worcester County Superior Court, Mass. (February 13, 1992).

Fraijo v. Hartland Hospital, 99 Cal. App.3d 331 (1979).

Garcia v. Seattle Indian Health Board, No. 86-2-12312-3, King County Superior Court, Seattle, Wash. (March 24, 1989).

Guigino v. Harvard Community Health Plan, 403 N.E.2d 1966 (Mass. 1980).

Hansen v. Sender, No. 89-CV010847 Milwaukee County Circuit Court (Wisc. 1992).

Laubach v. Franklin Square Hospital, No. 85248043 C139548 (Maryland).

Malonka v. Herman et al., 414 A.2d 1350 (N.J. 1980).

May v. Moore, 242 So.2d 596 (Ala. 1982).

Nelson v. Trinity Medical Center, No. 52430 Northwest District Court, Minot, N.D. (July 1986).

Pisel v. Stamford Hospital, 430 A.2d 1 (Conn. 1980).

Rowell v. Rab, No. 91-30621-24 Denton County Judicial District Court, Tex. (May 1992).

Salazar v. New York Hospital, No. 1590/82, N.Y. County Superior Court, N.Y. (September 29, 1988).

Song v. Bellflower Doctor's Hospital, No. VC 006286, Los Angeles County Superior Court, Cal. (September 23, 1993).

Stack v. Wapner, 268 A.2d 292 (Pa. 1976).

Valcin v. Public Health Trust of Dade County, 3rd District Case No. 91-2131 (Fla. 1984).

Washington v. Hollins, No. 92-24665 Harris County Judicial District Court (Tex. 1993).

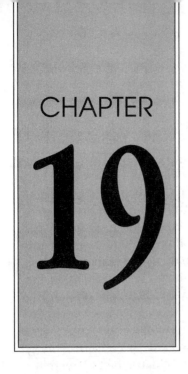

CHAPTER 19

Liability of the Nurse Educator

Jan M. Nick and Lois L. Salmeron

Although the potential for liability has clearly been established for nurses practicing in the clinical area, the issue continues to arise regarding the liability of nurse educators. Nurse educator liability has not been adequately addressed, as evidenced by the paucity of recently published literature on this subject. Due to the changing clinical and academic climate, nurse educator liability remains a cogent and timely issue.

This lack of attention is surprising, particularly when the potential climate for lawsuits is increasing due to four factors: (1) a perceived increase in the number of malpractice suits in the clinical area, (2) an increase in the number of schools of nursing, (3) the ever increasing empowerment and autonomy of the student, and (4) the changing profile of the nursing student. Typically nursing students are older, have graduated with other degrees, have work experience, and have the added responsibility of juggling family, school, and work obligations simultaneously. These four factors have increased the potential liability for the faculty member who instructs in the clinical and academic setting. Because obstetric, gynecological, and neonatal (OGN) nursing is considered a high-risk area for clinical malpractice suits, OGN nurse educators must be especially vigilant.

Nurse educators have been faced with liability issues in the clinical setting for a number of years. As nursing students perform more technical skills due to the complexity of nursing in the 1990s, how can nurse educators protect themselves and their students from lawsuits? How far does a faculty member's liability extend? Is the nurse educator always responsible for a student's actions in the clinical area?

The incidence of lawsuits against nursing personnel is increasing not only in the clinical setting, but also in the academic setting. As student empowerment grows, litigation has also increased in the academic setting. How can OGN nurse educators balance the responsibility they have for removing unsafe or unethical student nurses with the potential for lawsuits from disgruntled students? When student-initiated lawsuits do occur, do the courts favor the faculty, even though the faculty's decision to dismiss the student came from subjective evaluation?

Most faculty find the potential for a lawsuit frightening, whether the lawsuit is generated from clinical malpractice involving negligence or from academic malpractice involving grade disputes. A small portion of academic lawsuits originate from nursing students. Nevertheless, the courts view any student–faculty relationship as falling within guidelines established from previous academic lawsuits (Lessner, 1990). Generally, current and future rulings are based on previous rulings from similar lawsuits. Therefore, it is important for nurse educators to become familiar with appropriate case law and thus anticipate the judgment of the courts.

Articulation of issues such as these acknowledges the dilemma faced by nurse educators in both clinical and academic arenas. This chapter assists in answering questions such as these and hopefully places nurse educator liability in perspective.

RESPONSIBILITY OF THE OGN NURSE EDUCATOR

Several authors indicate that the responsibility of the nurse educator is twofold (Goclowski, 1985; Lessner, 1990; Roch, 1988). The first responsibility includes providing students with a quality education. The second responsibility deals with providing society with competent professionals. Lessner (1990) calls this dual responsibility the standard of care to the patient and standard of conduct to the student. If one or both of these responsibilities is unfulfilled, a breach of duty occurs.

If an injury is proved, the nursing faculty member can be held liable. Roch (1988) refers to a nursing faculty's responsibility as a "multi-faceted accountability" that includes a duty to the student to provide appropriate learning experiences, to the patient to provide safe practitioners, and to administration to perform and uphold the goals, guidelines, and mission of the university.

APPLICATION OF ISSUES TO CLINICAL PRACTICE

Liability in the Clinical Setting

Clinical malpractice is defined as the deviation from a professional standard of care that harms a patient. Malpractice lawsuits are generally initiated by patients or family members against health care workers and the institution. The nurse educator who supervises students in the clinical area is not immune from this clinical liability. Generally, although clinical liability is less for the visiting nurse educator than for the staff nurse assigned to the patient, malpractice can still be alleged and proved against the student nurse *and* the nursing faculty member. Nursing faculty can be held liable for their own actions and/or the actions of their students depending on the facts of the case. Traditionally the principle of *respondeat superior* (translated "let the master respond") holds the employer responsible for negligent acts of employees (Strader, 1985) and is used frequently in malpractice rulings. Because of this principle of ultimate responsibility of the employer, in a faculty–student relationship the faculty member could be held liable for negligent acts of the student.

In *Tarasoff v. The Regents of the University of California* (1976), a psychiatric faculty member was found negligent for harm to a third party due to improper supervision of a psychiatric therapy team (Strader, 1985). Nursing faculty frequently act in a supervisory capacity to their students. Even if the faculty member is not present and knows nothing about the case, the faculty member could still be held liable for a student's negligence. Unfortunately, the onus is on the court to determine whether the student is solely held responsible for the negligent act(s), or whether the faculty is solely held responsible, or both.

Clinical Negligence

Negligence is defined as failure to do, act, or complete a duty in such a manner that harms a person. Strader (1985) identifies four areas of clinical practice in which nurses commonly cause harm to a patient and are found negligent. The most common negligent acts in nursing include (1) errors in administration of medications, (2) failure to communicate clinical information, (3) failure to foresee an event that causes harm, and (4) improper exercise of physical or technical nursing skills. Because nursing students also practice their total learning experience in all four areas, it is reasonable to assume that these are the four areas in which nursing students also make the most mistakes. Nursing faculty must be cognizant of these four areas of potential liability and provide sufficient and appropriate attention to these areas when supervising students.

The first area of nursing negligence involves errors in administration of medications. An error in medication administration can occur when any one (or more) of the five "rights" of medication administration has been violated. Due to the substantial number of medications administered to certain patient populations, intuitively the nurse educator can understand why medication administration errors are so widespread. If harm is done, then the person responsible for the administration of the medicine(s) could be found negligent. Due to the lack of experience in the mixing and administration of medications, nursing students commonly make medication errors.

The second most common nursing error is failure to communicate information important to the care of the patient. If harm to the patient occurs as a result of failure to relay information, liability results. It is easy to understand that due to the many responsibilities of the nurse caring for several patients simultaneously, communication of lab results, information obtained by the patient, or assessment data can be delayed or forgotten. Within the patient–student–faculty triad, the faculty has the responsibility for ensuring that the student accurately relays information to the patient and to other health care providers. Nursing students are often unsure of what is important information, and fail to communicate effectively and thoroughly with appropriate health care providers.

The third most common nursing error is the failure to foresee events that cause harm. Strader (1985) states that this doctrine requires that individuals should reasonably foresee that a certain action or inaction on their part could result in injury to an individual under their care. The nurse, nursing student, or faculty member would be held liable if he or she should have anticipated an occurrence and did not, and that occurrence resulted in harm to the patient. A classic example of negligence involving foreseeability is a failure to restrain a confused patient whose behavior can cause harm to the patient. Another common example involves administration of narcotics to certain patient populations, which caused patient falls due to impaired judgment of musculo-skeletal balance and ability. Strader

(1985) states this type of negligent nursing error should be of particular concern for nursing educators. Due to the intermittent nature of student clinicals, the student and faculty member are at particular risk for these errors of foreseeability due to unfamiliarity of patients who may seem lucid for brief periods of time.

The fourth most common negligent act involves improper techniques of skills. Technical skills range from simple to complex. Perfection of technical skills is gained through repeated practice. Even though instruction and practice may take place in a laboratory setting, the relatively inexperienced nursing student is particularly vulnerable to this potential liability. Technical skills such as injections, IV insertions, urinary catheterizations, sterile dressing changes, and tracheostomy cannula changes are all specific examples of skills that if done improperly could cause harm to the patient, which then results in student nurse and/or faculty negligence. Because of the potential error of improper exercise of technical nursing skills, it is important that the nurse educator emphasize that students should perform only those skills they have had instruction in, and are comfortable and competent to carry out. The nurse educator must encourage students to acknowledge strengths and weaknesses and to seek help whenever in doubt. Of the four potential negligent acts, the first and last errors pose the most threat for the nursing student, and ultimately to the nursing faculty in charge of that student.

Minimizing Clinical Liability

There are many recommendations that nurse educators can follow to minimize or decrease the possibility of malpractice lawsuits during the clinical experience of a student's nursing education. One of the most important, but also one of the easiest interventions, is to *actively supervise* the students in the clinical area. Strader (1985) purports that having a heightened awareness of legal responsibilities will aid the instructor to supervise in an active, thorough manner, thus establishing a positive working relationship with the staff within a clinical facility. Students and nursing staff of a unit can easily determine when a faculty member is actively supervising. Active supervision includes frequent contacts with the student throughout the day, assisting the student with patient care, performing technical skills with the student, supervising charting and documentation, and remaining visible on the unit. These interventions assist the faculty member to supervise in an active manner. Often times, the nursing staff feel the added burden of active supervision and education of the nursing student because the faculty member is not available or rarely visible. Situations such as those just mentioned create a lose–lose situation for the student nurse, the staff nurse, and ultimately the nurse educator as well as a situation of potential harm for the patients. Strader (1985) feels a good working relationship with the staff will do much to minimize the liability risk in the clinical area.

A second recommendation for minimizing the risk is to become familiar with the special medical needs of each patient assigned to a student (Lessner, 1990; Strader, 1985). By becoming familiar with the medical and nursing plans of care, the faculty member will be able to tailor the learning needs and clinical capabilities of each nursing student to a patient. Assignment of a difficult patient to a nursing student who has not been exposed to that clinical situation either in class or in previous clinical days will only frustrate the student and increase the potential for lawsuit to both the student and faculty member. By becoming familiar with the medical diagnoses and idiosyncrasies of each patient assigned to a student, faculty will achieve a good patient–student fit, thus decreasing liability by minimizing the potential of the four common nursing errors.

Another intervention nurse faculty can employ is to interview patients in order to clarify roles of the nursing students (Strader, 1985). During the course of receiving care from health care providers, patients/clients may become confused as to what title and responsibilities go with which health care provider. In the course of a day, a patient/client may see physicians, physical therapists, registered nurses, licensed vocational nurses, nurse aides, nurse techni-cians, student nurses, housekeepers, among others. The patient must know who the student nurse is and have appropriate expectations for the student nurse. Otherwise, due to the student's inexperience at placing boundaries and the additional fervor for learning, the student nurse may attempt skills and duties that he or she is unprepared for. By clarifying roles with the patient, expectations can be appropriately anticipated and met. The patient's needs are cared for, the student nurse meets with success, and the nurse educator is reassured.

Because of the ever changing clinical equipment and expertise required in the acute care setting today, many authors recommend faculty members keep up to date with their own nursing skills and allow students to perform only those procedures that they themselves can competently perform (Roch, 1988; Strader, 1985). Thus, with active supervision and current competency in skills, potential errors in performing the technical aspects of nursing care are greatly minimized.

NURSE EDUCATOR LIABILITY IN THE INSTITUTIONAL SETTING

Nursing faculty can also incur liability in the academic setting. Lawsuits generated by students seeking compensation and reinstatement into academic programs have steadily increased since first appearing in the 1960s. The first case appeared in 1961 when African American students were expelled from school without a hearing for participating in civil rights activities. In the landmark case, *Dixon v. Alabama State Board of Education* (1961), the court ruled that students are guaranteed due process (the right to a hearing) under the 14th Amendment to the U. S. Constitution (Lessner, 1990; Pollok & Poteet, 1983). Since that time, numerous lawsuits claiming academic liability have been filed by students against faculty (*Board of Curators of the University of Missouri v. Horowitz*, 1978; *Eiland v. Wolf*, 1989; *Esteban v. Central Missouri State College*, 1969; *Goss v. Lopez*, 1975; *Nuttleman v. Case Western Reserve University*, 1982; and *Tobias v. University of Texas*, 1992.

Even though most of the academic lawsuits have not been in nursing, the incidence of nursing student lawsuits has blossomed at an alarming rate since the 1980s. In a survey mailed to all NLN accredited nursing schools, Brooke (1988) reported that the majority of schools of nursing (83%) had not been involved in any student-initiated lawsuits. However, what was alarming was of those schools who had incurred litigation from students, *90% of the litigation had been in the five years prior to the survey*. This demonstrates the significant increase in lawsuits by nursing students since the 1980s. The most common student complaint was clinical grades and the timeliness of feedback. Brooke (1988) found that neither the size of the school/program nor the type of degree had any significant impact on the incidence of lawsuits.

Academic Dismissal Liability

An academic dismissal can be effected in one of two ways. Both can carry the risk of liability. A student can be dismissed due to academic failure (poor academic achievement) or as a result of academic misconduct or unsatisfactory clinical performance.

Goclowski (1985) defines academic dismissal as a failure to obtain a specific level of scholarship. Academic grading is generally objective, with well-defined criteria for passing. Because of the objectivity involved with academic grading, it is very difficult for a student to show malice or arbitrary treatment from the instructor/professor. Therefore, the courts do not entitle the student to a hearing (Lessner, 1990), thus making the potential faculty liability for academic dismissal relatively low. Dimond (1992) and Lessner (1990) refer to this area of malpractice as "academic affairs liability." Academic affairs is defined as issues related to the student–university relationship.

Nursing faculty can also incur liability when a student is dismissed due to disciplinary reasons or for poor performance in the clinical area. Goclowski (1985) defines academic misconduct as the violation of institutional codes of conduct. Often, the criteria for academic misconduct is poorly defined; the grading criteria for clinical

performance can be vague. Because both of these can be subjectively evaluated and the criteria can be vague, students are more likely to feel that unfair treatment was received if an unsatisfactory grade was given. Unfair treatment, whether real or imagined, increases the probability of student-initiated lawsuits against faculty. Because academic misconduct and poor clinical evaluations both can incur a high degree of subjectivity, courts will allow a hearing when a suit is brought against an institution due to student dismissal for poor clinical performance. Most of the suits nurse educators face stem from grade disputes over subjectively evaluated clinical grades rather than objectively assigned academic grades.

Brooke (1988) reported from the survey that most often, students filing lawsuits against faculty for clinical failure stated a lack of timely feedback as reason for the suit against the faculty and university. Students who challenge dismissal decisions usually base their suits on the due process clause of the 14th Amendment (Goclowski, 1985). When a lawsuit is filed stating that the due process clause of the 14th Amendment has been violated, the courts must determine if action on the part of the educators and institution was arbitrary and capricious, or in bad faith (Goclowski, 1985). Because disciplinary and clinical dismissals are subjectively based, documentation of due process has to be shown, otherwise the courts tend to look favorably on the student's petition.

Tort Liability and Nursing Educators

A tort is defined as a civil wrong brought about by omission or commission of an act for which courts provide a remedy in the form of damages (Alexander & Solomon, 1972). Tort liability includes allegations of defamation and malpractice. Tort liability would most likely surface in the clinical component of a nursing student's grade. Two factors affect the possibility of liability for tort damages. One factor moderates or dampens the effect of tort liability, and the other factor modulates or increases the possibility.

The dampening effect occurs when nursing faculty hesitate to fail a student or are uncomfortable in evaluating clinical competence, and the faculty err on the side of the student rather than taking the appropriate course of action. The reasons for this hesitancy include (1) subjectivity of the evaluation, (2) limited observations on which assessments are made, (3) allegations of personality clashes that can arise, and finally, (4) fear of litigation (Gocwolski, 1985).

The second effect, which augments the threat of tort liability, deals with the subjective nature of the clinical evaluation. Because of the subjectivity involved, students are more likely to bring suit against an instructor, claiming unfair, arbitrary, and capricious treatment. In addition, because obtaining a failing clinical grade halts progression in the program, students generally seek reinstatement in addition to monetary compensation (Brooke, 1988).

Educator Liability and the 14th Amendment

Students who challenge dismissal decisions usually base their suits on the due process clause of the 14th Amendment (Gocwolski, 1985). Therefore, nursing faculty should understand what the 14th Amendment states and what is expected of the faculty. Then faculty can be confident of their evaluations, and not pass a student simply out of fear of litigation.

The 14th Amendment states that "no state shall deprive any person of life, liberty, or property without due process of the laws" (Thomas, 1987). This amendment provides fair and equal treatment to all persons *at public institutions and some private institutions receiving government aid*. Because public schools and universities are considered extensions of the government, they are subject to the same limitations set forth in the 14th Amendment (Gocwolski, 1985). In cases involving academic liability, the courts look for evidence in the case that either supports or denies due process rights, as stipulated in the 14th Amendment.

Due Process Liability

Due process is defined as the provision of timely feedback and opportunities to correct unsatisfactory behavior before dismissal of a student

can occur. Because of the due process clause of the 14th Amendment, close attention must be given to the nursing school's grading policies and procedures. The student must be given the opportunity to correct behavior prior to dismissal. Providing students with certain constitutional rights in the classroom is not difficult. If faculty can show that they took steps to follow due process, courts favor the faculty's evaluation of the student. Due process liability can be divided into three areas (Gilmore, 1994). These include (1) procedural due process, (2) substantive due process, and (3) equal protection.

Procedural Due Process

Procedural due process issues involve either a disciplinary dismissal or an academic dismissal of a student and arise when liberty or property interests are infringed upon. Procedural due process ensures that with subjective grading, the faculty member is required by federal law to provide the student with oral and written notice, plus an opportunity to respond to the notice prior to dismissal. Due to the nature involved with disciplinary dismissal, the courts have ruled that a fairly structured "procedural due process" is required prior to student dismissal (*Goss v. Lopez*, 1975). In *Board of Curators of the University of Missouri v. Horowitz* (1978), the courts reinforced the need for showing procedural due process, and also recognized the importance for evaluation of clinical and academic competency. In *Connelly v. University of Vermont and State Agricultural College* (1965), a medical student was dismissed from the program and sued the university, claiming capricious motivations on the part of the faculty. The court determined that Connelly did not receive impartial "procedural due process" and ruled in favor of the student.

Substantive Due Process

Substantive due process provides legal protection of an individual from actions that are considered arbitrary and capricious. By using the substantive due process argument, the courts are faced with determining if the faculty's actions were in any way arbitrary and capricious. In a landmark case involving substantive due process, a medical student was dismissed from the program and was denied a hearing at the university. The student then sued the university, claiming capricious motivations on the part of the faculty (*Connelly v. University of Vermont and State Agricultural College,* 1965). The court determined that Connelly did not receive an impartial hearing, and thus ordered the school to provide due process by way of a grievance hearing at the university.

The courts have demonstrated numerous times that they are not anxious to overrule the faculty's actions unless it can be shown that the faculty behaved capriciously (*Board of Curators of the University of Missouri v. Horowitz,* 1978; *Connelly v. University of Vermont and State Agricultural College,* 1965; *Eiland v. Wolf,* 1989; *Lyons v. Salve Regina College,* 1978). If evidence exists (such as documentation of behavior, documentation of counseling sessions) confirming that rational evaluation took place, the substantive due process inquiry ceases because the courts generally do not override the faculty's professional judgment unless there is substantial departure from accepted academic norms (Gilmore, 1994). The judicial system acknowledges the faculty's expertise in setting and maintaining standards for student performance, and defer to that expertise more often than not (Gocwolski, 1985). It can be concluded that even with subjectively graded evaluations, the burden of proof tends to remain with the student to demonstrate arbitrary and/or capricious behavior on the part of the faculty.

In addition to maintaining the *right* to evaluate due process, the courts have also indicated *how* due process must be shown. Because of the 14th Amendment to the U.S. Constitution, before dismissal can occur, demonstrating due process would include conveying well-defined personal and professional goals and objectives at the onset of the student–teacher relationship. The student has a right to know beforehand what behavioral outcomes are expected to be achieved. In addition, documented counseling must be done, and opportunities must be provided for the student to remedy behavioral problems before dismissal can occur. By abiding by these guidelines, faculty can easily demonstrate to the courts that the evaluations leading to dismissal were not capricious and arbitrary.

Equal Protection

Public institutions such as state universities and colleges also are mandated to provide fair and equal protection, treatment, and accommodation regardless of race, creed, color, or abilities. Institutions have dealt with accommodation of student disabilities for several years. During the last quarter of the twentieth century, there has been increased emphasis on the constitutional rights of Americans with disabilities (Parrott, 1994). These constitutional rights, based on the 14th Amendment, include several acts passed by the federal government. These acts require colleges and universities to provide accommodation for educational opportunities for individuals with disabilities. The acts pertinent to equal protection rights include (1) Section 504 of the Rehabilitation Act of 1973, which talks about nondiscrimination on the basis of handicap; (2) Rehabilitation Act Amendments of 1974; and (3) the Americans with Disabilities Act of 1990 (42 U.S.C. 12101).

The Rehabilitation Act of 1973 states that ". . . qualified individuals with disabilities shall not be excluded from participating in, or be denied benefits, or be subjected to discrimination under any federally funded program or activity because of reason of disability." Because of the legal ramifications, typically colleges and universities designate an individual on campus to coordinate requests for accommodations by handicapped students. However, it is considered the responsibility of the individual student to identify the need for the accommodation and to make an official request for such. This request instigates the creation of a plan to provide "reasonable accommodations" for the student. Equal protection issues can be divided into three areas: (1) admission issues, (2) accessibility issues, and (3) reasonable accommodation issues.

Admission issues

Equal protection due process is questioned when an individual is denied admission to a program due to a physical handicap. In suits against institutions, courts tend to rule in favor of students who were denied entrance into an academic program because of their disabilities when admission requirements did not stipulate any special physical abilities. In *Pushkin v. Regents of University of Colorado* (1981), a medical doctor sued the university stating he was rejected admission to a psychiatric residency program because he was confined to a wheelchair. The court ruled that Pushkin was fully qualified for the residency program and thus directed the University of Colorado to admit him into the program (Parrot, 1994).

Accessibility Issues

Starting in the 1970s, and continuing today, public and private institutions have the legal responsibility of providing handicapped accessible ramps, walkways, elevators, and so on, for students. Making the physical layout more accessible for handicapped students is another way institutions must provide fair and equal treatment to students under the guidance of the 14th Amendment.

Reasonable Accommodation Issues

There are several examples in the literature where courts ruled that learning institutions must provide accommodations for individuals with physical disabilities. In *Wynne v. Tufts University School of Medicine* (1992), the university was ordered to provide separate environments for test taking for a handicapped student. In *Crawford v. University of North Carolina* (1977), and *Jones v. Illinois Department of Rehabilitation Services* (1982), the institutions were both ordered to provide interpretive services for the hearing impaired. However, the question remains as to what constitutes "reasonable accommodation." The opinion of the courts seems to affirm that substantive changes in the curriculum requirements are not defined as reasonable accommodations, and that students who have physical disabilities must be qualified to enter the program regardless of type of disability.

Minimizing Nurse Educator Liability

There are many actions that faculty can take to minimize the liability related to student dismissal from a nursing program.

ESTABLISH A HARMONIOUS RELATIONSHIP. Pollok and Poteet (1983) state that first and foremost, a harmonious relationship between faculty and students will reduce faculty liability more than any other single factor. Intuitively, this recommendation is easy to understand. A person is much less likely to sue another if a relationship has not been strained even if the outcome is poor. This phenomenon has been repeated especially in the health care industry. Patients who have a close relationship with their physician or are satisfied with their care are much less likely to sue than those who do not have an established relationship or are dissatisfied with the interaction.

ADDRESS COURSE REQUIREMENTS. Another recommendation to minimize liability in the academic setting is to address both cognitive and noncognitive requirements of the learning experience with the student at the onset of the nursing program and for each semester (Gocwolski, 1985). Because faculty are obligated to evaluate both cognitive and noncognitive aspects of a course, clear and concise criteria from which the evaluation is based provide a platform for evaluations. In this manner, students are aware of course expectations at the onset and are more likely to understand the grading criteria.

CLARIFY EXPECTATIONS FOR ACHIEVEMENT. A third recommendation for decreasing educator liability includes increasing the communication between student and faculty in order to clarify expectations for achievement of personal and professional characteristics (Gocwolski, 1985). Much information has been written about how to role-model nursing students. Mentoring is a positive step toward educating the student in development of the ethical and professional values of nursing. Clarification of expectations is closely related to the second one, which specifies outlining nursing content criteria. However, it differs in that this third recommendation specifies expectations of demonstrating general professional skills that can be germane to a number of health-related professions.

PROMPTLY NOTIFY OF DEFICIENCIES. Because most students filing lawsuits charge that their constitutional rights under the 14th Amendment have been violated because procedural due process was not followed, a fourth recommendation includes promptly notifying the student of deficiencies and providing the student with an opportunity to respond (Gocwolski, 1985). Faculty are obligated to provide the student with information regarding cognitive and noncognitive course expectations and be appraised of their performance frequently.

GRIEVANCE COMMITTEES. A fifth recommendation includes having in place at the college or university both formal and informal committees that deal with disgruntled students (Brooke, 1988). These committees might include university appeals committees, binding union arbitration, and affirmative action hearings. This provides the student with several avenues to pursue before filing a suit against the faculty member or university. In addition, the courts encourage students seeking grievances to begin the grievance procedure at the university level and try to come to an agreement before suits are introduced into the courtroom. Pollok and Poteet (1983) recommend establishing informal student faculty committees. Informal grievance committees may do much to diminish the adversarial tone that develops when working with a formal grievance committee.

ENSURE PROPER DOCUMENTATION. To increase the objectivity of grading and ensure proper documentation of the student's progress, Pollok and Poteet (1983) recommend three actions that faculty can take. The first action includes establishing grading criteria for essays and term papers before students do assignments, then using the criteria when grading student papers. Establishment of grading criteria helps maintain or ensure the faculty's objectivity and fairness toward the student. The second action includes maintaining the student's work in individual files until the student successfully completes the course. By doing this, the faculty has actual copies of the student's work. A third possible action to ensure proper documentation is to write anecdotal notes on each student that address the course requirements, and to share progress in clinical performance with students on a regular basis. Lessner (1990) also recommends maintaining anecdotal notes of the student's clinical progress. These notes should be as factual as possible and recount behaviors, not interpretations of behaviors.

FOLLOW PROCEDURES IN THE SCHOOL CATALOG OR BULLETIN. Because the faculty not only have a responsibility to the student but also to the university, Regan (1983) recommends that faculty follow procedures for evaluation described in the educational catalog or bulletin. Published procedures provide a guide for actions that the university or college expects the faculty member to follow. If faculty follow established school policies regarding student notification of unsatisfactory performance, the responsibility rests with the institution.

DEMONSTRATE INTEGRITY OF CHARACTER. Roch (1988) recommends that faculty comport themselves with integrity. Maintaining honesty and soundness of moral principle will always show fairness and equal treatment to all students. Students can see this and will accept evaluations if done with fairness and integrity (Pollok & Poteet, 1983).

To summarize, faculty members can decrease liability in the educational setting in many ways. In addition, the recommendations provided are interventions often performed by nursing educators. The recommendations may serve only as a conscious reminder. Nursing faculty should realize that few cases have made it into the court system—most grievances have been successfully handled at the institutional level. Of those grievances that do go on to the state or federal court system, courts have continued to uphold the majority of faculty evaluations, and rule in favor of the institution. In the end, Pollok and Poteet (1983) remind nurse educators that

> [I]n some cases careful evaluation, documentation, and sincere effort to respect the

student's rights will not block the student from challenging faculty judgements; the student still may choose to take legal action. In such instances the individual faculty member and the administrator can be reassured that their diligence, foresight, and openness in the evaluation process will undergird their defense before any judicial hearing body.

Even with the most diligent attention to due process, some students may still seek a judgment against the faculty. However, as long as evaluations do not appear arbitrary and capricious, the court will usually uphold the institution's decision.

OTHER LIABILITY ISSUES

Faculty Liability Insurance

The issue of professional insurance for clinical liability is presented in greater detail in Chapter 22.

The issue of professional insurance not only pertains to the clinician but is also germane to the educator. There is support in the literature for the necessity of nurse educators carrying professional liability insurance. Supportive rationales include legal and financial reasons for carrying nurse educator liability insurance.

Often, as a benefit provided by the university or college, blanket coverage is made available for faculty working in the clinical area with students. In fact, because of contractual agreements with clinical agencies used for student clinical experiences, prior to using the agency, students and faculty are required to show proof of malpractice insurance. In a survey mailed to nursing programs in the United States, Brooke (1988) discovered that the majority of faculty and students were required to carry additional professional liability insurance in combination with blanket coverage provided by the educational institution. The literature clearly indicates the need for basic malpractice insurance for faculty and students. However, there is some debate as to whether blanket coverage is sufficient or whether additional insurance should be carried by each individual.

Pollok and Poteet (1983) do not recommend additional liability coverage for nurse educators

as long as the educator is functioning within the parameters of the state Nurse Practice Act and is covered under a blanket policy. Strader (1985), however, recommends that educators carry additional malpractice insurance if they are working in areas with high risk of litigation. OGN nurse educators might consider carrying additional malpractice insurance for legal and financial reasons rather than for minimizing risks of lawsuits. Insurance protects the educator against financial ruin; it does not minimize the liability risk.

Reasons for Carrying Nurse Educator Liability Insurance

Strader (1985) provides three reasons why nurse educators should carry malpractice insurance. They include (1) sovereign immunity—the liability of the employer does not shield the educator from personal liability for negligence; (2) charitable immunity—not-for-profit institutions and their employees are now held liable for their own actions; and (3) *respondeat superior*—historically interpreted to mean that persons in authority were responsible for actions of others under their control.

Of the three reasons listed for carrying additional malpractice insurance, the third reason, *respondeat superior,* has recently begun to have new meaning for the health care industry and especially for nurses. *Respondeat superior* is the doctrine of vicarious liability, which holds the person in charge responsible for others' actions. In the past, this principle has proven problematic to those in authority such as physicians, educators, and nurse managers who are responsible for the actions of others under their supervision. Historically, nurses were not named in lawsuits because of this doctrine, even when the culpability of negligence pointed toward nursing. However, because of increased education and technical skills of many health professions, courts have now begun to rule that *respondeat superior* is not applicable unless the person in authority has a "right to control" the assistant. If the "master" is not in control of the assistant's actions, the culpability rests on the assistant (*Harris v. Miller,* 1994). This change in *respon-*

deat superior is one of the reasons that there is now an increase in the number of nurses being named in lawsuits.

In addition to the legal reasons for carrying some type of malpractice insurance, Pollok and Poteet (1983) mention two financial reasons. The first reason is that in the event of a successful lawsuit against the educator, the insurance company pays the financial judgment. A second reason is that malpractice insurance also provides legal counsel at no additional cost to the nurse who is being sued.

In summary, the need to carry a second policy in addition to an institutional blanket policy may not be necessary if the nurse educator stays within the parameters of the nurse practice act. However, in view of the reasonable costs associated with yearly premiums, it seems reasonable for nursing faculty to obtain some type of additional insurance coverage.

Educational Liability

Several authors have written about the potential liability of institutions when curricula provide incomplete or inappropriate education (Dimond, 1992; Pollok & Poteet, 1983). This liability is a poorly recognized liability potential. However, lawsuits have been filed by students claiming misrepresentation of a program, or for passing a course when either academic or clinical performance was unsatisfactory. Gocwolski (1985) cites two examples of students who sued the institution for misrepresentation. In *Peter W. v. San Francisco Unified School District* (1976), a student filed a suit against a school district for alleged "negligence and intentional misrepresentation." The school kept advancing him the next higher grade and graduated him with only a 5th-grade reading level. However, the court dismissed the case stating that the plaintiff had not suffered injury from this act of negligence. In the second case, *Donahue v. Copiague Union Free School District* (1979), the court did rule in favor of the student, stating that teachers may be held accountable for failure to perform their duties faithfully (Gocwolski, 1985).

When education is viewed as a consumer product, and the consumer is dissatisfied, stu-

dents have filed a lawsuit charging misrepresentation. In *Lidecker v. Kendall College* (1990), nursing students sued the college and its administrators after discovering that the school program was not accredited. The school's defense was the college's catalog, which described a program that would prepare students for licensure as registered nurses and made no reference to accreditation (Tammalleo, 1990). In fact, because it was a new program, accreditation could not be granted until after graduating the first class. The appellate court ruled in favor of the college, stating there was no intent of misrepresentation on the part of the college. Although Kendall College won the suit, this case demonstrates an example of the student awareness of consumer rights and responsibilities of the institution to provide a sound curriculum.

CONCLUSION

Nurse educators are faced with what Roch (1988) coins a "multifaceted" responsibility to ensure quality education to the student, quality care to the client, and quality instruction from the institution. When achievement of this responsibility is questioned, nursing faculty can be charged with breach of contract and thus risk lawsuit. Traditionally, liability in the clinical area has been recognized and faculty have been well informed about the associated risks involved with being in charge of students who are virtually learning while delivering patient care. Now however, due to the recent increase in lawsuits generated from the academic setting, faculty are faced with a dual risk for lawsuit. Nevertheless, many precautions can be taken to minimize the faculty's malpractice risk in the clinical area where direct patient care is given, and also to minimize the liability incurred in the classroom setting. For a multitude of reasons, it is recommended that faculty carry liability insurance in the event that a judgment is ruled against the faculty.

Even though a clinical grade has subjective components and is at times difficult to document, nursing faculty must attempt to provide impartial treatment to all students and to increase their communication and documentation skills for due process to be demonstrated. Nurse educators must be diligent in their attempts to provide the student with clear unambiguous criteria for grading, and must appraise the students of their progress in a systematic manner. However, if faculty exercise good judgment, the courts will continue to recognize the faculty's expertise that is required for evaluation of students and will continue to be reticent to change the outcome of a dismissal. If the dismissal showed due process without regard to malicious or arbitrary treatment, the nurse educator should be confident in the outcome of a trial.

REFERENCES

Alexander, K., & Soloman, E. (1972). College and university law. Charlottesville, VA: Michie.

Brooke, P. S. (1988). Will you be sued? Nurse Educator, 13(4), 5–6.

Creighton, H. (1983). Education of instructors. Nursing Management, 14(5), 48–49.

Dimond, B. (1992). The nurse educator and the legal implications. Nurse Education Today, 12(4), 279–282.

Gilmore, P. (1994). Liability issues for nurse educators. Texas Nursing, 68(1), 10.

Goclowski, J. (1985). Legal implications of academic dismissal and educational malpractice for nursing faculty. Journal of Nursing Education, 24(3), 104–108.

Lessner, M. W. (1990). Avoiding student–faculty litigation. Nurse Educator, 15(6), 29–32.

Parrott, D. (1994). Nursing students with disabilities: An examination of legal issues. Unpublished manuscript, Oklahoma State University, Education Department.

Pollok, C. S., & Poteet, G. W. (1983). Diminishing faculty liability. Nurse Educator, 8(1), 31–34.

Regan, W. A. (1983). Nurse educators: Legal rights and duties. Regan Report on Nursing Law, 24(1), 1.

Roch, S. (1988). Accountability in midwifery education. Midwives Chronicle & Nursing Notes, 101(1205), 182–183.

Strader, M. K. (1985). Malpractice and nurse educators: Defining legal responsibilities. Journal of Nursing Education, 24(9), 363–367.

Tammeleo, A. D. (1990). Nursing students charge fraud: No accreditation. Regan Report on Nursing Law, 31(1), 1.

Tammeleo, A. D. (1994). Surgeon not liable for CRNA: No "borrowed servant." Regan Report on Nursing Law, 34(10), 2.

Thomas, S. B. (1987). Health related legal issues in education. Topeka, Kansas: National Organization on Legal Problems of Education.

CASE CITATIONS

Board of Curators of the University of Missouri v. Horowitz, 435 U.S. 78, 98 S. Ct. 948 (1978).

Connelly v. University of Vermont and State Agricultural College, 244 F. Supp. 156 (District Ct. D. Vt., 1965).

Crawford v. University of North Carolina, 440 F. Supp. 1047 (U.S. District Court, M.D. N.C., Durham division, 1977).

Dixon v. Alabama State Board of Education, 294 F.2d 150 (1961).

Donahue v. Copiague Union Free School District, 418 N.Y. S.2d 375 (1979).

Eiland v. Wolf, 764 S.W.2d 827 (Tex. App. Houston [1st Dist.] 1989).

Esteban v. Central Missouri State College, 415 F.2d 1077 (U.S. Ct. of App. 8th Cir. 1969).

Goss v. Lopez, 419 U.S. 565, 95 S. Ct. 729 (1975).

Harris v. Miller, 335 N.C. 379, 438 S.E.2d 731 (1994).

Jones v. Illinois Department of Rehabilitation Services, 689 F.2d 724 (U.S. Ct of App. 7th Cir. 1982).

Lidecker v. Kendall College, 194 Ill. App. 3d 309, 550 N.E.2d 1121, 141 Ill. Dec. 75 (1990).

Lyons v. Salve Regina College, 435 U.S. 971 (98 S. Ct. 1611, 1978).

Nuttleman v. Case Western Reserve University, 708 F.2d 726 (Ohio Ct. of App. 6th Cir. 1982).

Peter W. v. San Francisco Unified School District, 60 Cal. App. 3d 814, 131 Cal. Rptr. 854 (1976).

Pushkin v. Regents of University of Colorado, 658 F.2d 1372 (1981).

Tarasoff v. The Regents of the University of California, 17 Cal. 3d 425, 551 P.2d 334, 131 Cal. Rptr. 14 (1976).

Tobias v. University of Texas, 824 S.W.2d 201, 73 Ed. Law Rep. 304 (1992).

Wynne v. Tufts University School of Medicine, 976 F.2d 791, United States Court of Appeals, First Circuit (1992).

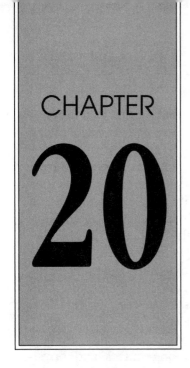

CHAPTER 20

Nurse–Physician Communication

Christine A. Sullivan and Mary A. Bowden

Almost one million dollars was paid in settlement as a result of a breakdown in communication by a doctor and a nurse. In this situation, the patient was instructed by her physician to report to the hospital after she complained of vaginal bleeding. As per hospital procedure, she was placed on a fetal monitor, which showed some variable decelerations. The woman underwent a cesarean delivery but the baby died within 6 hours after birth. An autopsy revealed asphyxia secondary to intrauterine bleeding from a tear in the umbilical cord. The physician claimed that the nurse did not inform him of the variable decelerations. The nurse, on the other hand, was not aware that the patient had told the physician that she experienced vaginal bleeding prior to her hospital admission, as the bleeding had stopped once she was admitted. The inadequate communication between the physician and the nurse, who each failed to adequately assess and communicate their concerns and findings, resulted in the poor defensibility of this case and an $800,000 settlement.

In the American Medical Association's (AMA) 150th anniversary edition of the *Code of Medical Ethics,* 1997, addresses interpersonal relations that specifically involves nurses. Opinion 3.2 Nurses states

> The primary bond between the practices of medicine and nursing is mutual ethical con-

cern for patients. One of the duties in providing reasonable care is fulfilled by a nurse who carries out the order of the attending physician. Where orders appear to the nurse to be in error or contrary to customary medical and nursing practice, the physician has an ethical obligation to hear the nurse's concern and explain those orders to the nurse involved. The ethical physician should neither expect nor insist that nurses follow orders contrary to standards of good medical and nursing practice. In emergencies, when prompt action is necessary and the physician is not immediately available, a nurse may be justified in acting contrary to the physician's standing orders for the safety of the patient. Such occurrences should not be considered to be a breakdown in professional relations. (AMA, 1997)

In the past, the role of the nurse was to carry out the specific orders of the physician. Communication was limited and the nurse was never to question orders (Pillitteri & Ackerman, 1993; Stein, Watts, & Howell, 1990; Porter, 1991). Over the past two decades, changes in nursing education, technology, shared medical–legal responsibility, and collaborative care models have had a positive effect on the image of nursing and the nurse's role as an essential member of the health care team. Some nurses are independent advanced practice nurses, whereas others have had an interdependent relationship with physicians and other health care providers.

Effective communication, which is the ability to understand and to be understood, is the cornerstone of an interdependent nurse–physician/provider relationship. As described in the AMA opinion, this interdependent relationship between the nurse and physician promotes sharing of information and joint decision making with clients, which leads to better health care and clinical outcomes.

COMMUNICATION AND RISK MANAGEMENT

Successful risk management programs focus on reducing or preventing adverse client outcomes, which can and often do lead to legal action. The goal of risk management is to prevent avoidable losses or reduce the severity of those unavoidable losses (Goldman, 1991). Risk management is a collaborative effort by health care providers, nurses, and physicians to plan effective and safe care for their clients. Communication of pertinent clinical information by the nurse and physician with the client about the diagnosis, prognosis, treatment options, and the risks and benefits of each treatment option establishes a relationship of care. Engaging clients in planning and selecting options of care enables them to take responsibility for their choices. Caring by health care providers, especially a genuine feeling transmitted through one's presence and effective communication style, validates a compatible relationship. A genuine and trusting relationship with clients results in fewer medical malpractice claims, even in cases of adverse, unavoidable outcomes.

Effective communication, liability prevention, and risk management are as closely linked as the nurse, physician, and client relationship. Effective communication is an essential risk management measure for nurses and physicians (Killian, 1991).

HISTORICAL VIEWS ON NURSE–PHYSICIAN COMMUNICATION

Stein (1990) described a hierarchial relationship between nurses and physicians with the physi-

cian being superior to the nurse. At that time, he stated that there was clear agreement between nurses and physicians to this type of relationship. Although nurses were often quite knowledgeable, they would make recommendations seemingly initiated by the physician. Stein (1976) called this indirect method of communication "the doctor–nurse game." Stein and colleagues (1990) reviewed changes that have occurred in nurse–physician communications over the past 20 years. They suggest that changes by nurses establish their professional autonomy from physicians. The equal partnership is now found among many health care professionals, not just among nurses and physicians. Stein and colleagues (1990) found that even physicians see the benefits to clients and themselves when the relationship between medicine and nursing is one of mutual respect and interdependence. Additionally, "from ancient times, physicians have recognized that the health and well being of patients depends upon a collaborative effort between physician and patient. Patients share with physicians the responsibility for their own health care" (AMA, 1997, p. xli). Pillitteri and Ackerman (1993) compared journal notes from 1888 to recorded notes in 1990 by two house officers. Although these are very specific observations and cannot be generalized to other physicians, they offer some interesting contrasts and commonalities. In 1888, the physician's journal commented on his role in teaching nurses patient care in contrast to a physician in 1990 who commented in his journal, "we are pretty much responsible for the full care of these patients. It's scary and most of what we learn, we learn from the nursing staff" (Pillitteri & Ackerman, 1993). In both journals, the physicians' recordings demonstrated collaboration and conflicts between themselves and the nurses. In 1888 and 1990, however, both physicians felt that they were the higher authority when the final decision had to be made about patient care.

Porter (1991) feels that the nursing process gives nurses more authority and autonomy in the care of clients. The physician is permitted and expected to diagnose, and this ability gives the physician freedom and authority. The nursing process includes a nursing diagnosis. A study by Porter (1991) found that the formal overt decision-making strategy, which includes the nursing process, was not used by the nurses when communicating with physicians. He found in his study that the most widely practiced strategy to communicate with physicians was informal and overt. Informal overt decision making did not involve the use of the nursing process. Porter (1991) found that formal overt decision-making strategies had little significance compared to the informal strategies. Porter (1990) suggests that involvement by nurses in decision making is less covert than Stein (1967, 1990) implies. Porter's study suggests that if the "doctor–nurse game" existed, nurses and physicians are progressing in their ability to establish more equitable and interdependent relationships to better serve the client. The model of collegiality among various multidisciplinary health care professionals is growing, replacing the traditional hierarchial relationship where the "physician ruled." Direct and factual communication, especially when risk or potential is identified, necessitates expedient communication to circumvent adverse patient outcomes. Stein points out that patients depend on the knowledge of both professions for their safety and are endangered by the unresolved difficulties of the doctor–nurse relationship (Stein, 1990, p. 268).

A MODEL FOR EFFECTIVE COMMUNICATION

To promote effective communication between patients and nurses and thus enhance the data to be passed on the physician, relationships must be established between the patient and the nurse as well as the physician and the nurse.

Arnold and Boggs (1989) describe the concept of "structuring the relationship." "Structuring the relationship" refers to building a professional relationship between the nurse, client, and family (Arnold & Boggs, 1989). The authors describe the therapeutic relationship between the nurse and client as having specific boundaries, purposes, and behaviors in contrast to social relationships.

A successful therapeutic relationship is client-focused, resulting in the personal development of the client and the professional growth of the nurse. This concept is adaptable as a construct for building effective nurse–client–physician communication. This process is characterized by four stages: pre-interaction, engagement, active intervention, and termination (Arnold & Boggs, 1989).

1. Pre-interaction Phase. The nurse, physician and other health care professionals explore goals, assess the environment, and establish priorities in preparation of working with the client. Developing professional goals assists the health care team to select actions that will help the client be successful within the therapeutic relationship. To do this, the interpersonal dimensions of the nurse–physician relationship must be explored to identify environmental variables that foster optimal nurse–physician communication. All participants involved in the therapeutic relationship must view the process as a partnership. Perceiving the relationship as a partnership fosters trust and understanding among the participants and reduces the likelihood of emotional and physical injury to the client.

2. Engagement Phase. This phase establishes the initial contact between the nurse, physician, and client. In preparation for this initial contact, development of a contract between the nurse and physician that defines their role responsibilities and limitations will foster a more interdependent relationship. The assessment done by the nurse and physician identifies the problems and needs of the client. This enables the nurse and physician to assist the client with identifying his or her role responsibilities and limitations within the therapeutic relationship. During this phase, establishment of a trusting and interdependent relationship between the nurse and physician will further promote an optimal client outcome, reducing the risk of an avoidable loss.

3. Active Intervention Phase. This phase is built on mutuality and trust. Strategies and alternative solutions for patient care are negotiated; congruency and incongruence in treatment goals are identified and negotiated; and immediacy of active intervention is prioritized. The nurse and physician collaborate as equal partners with the client to problem solve and develop solutions.

4. Termination Phase. This phase begins when the work of the active intervention phase is completed. This is the phase of closure in the communication process. The nurse–client–physician communication concludes, although it may reenter the engagement phase at subsequent interactions. The primary tasks associated with the termination phase of the relationship include the summarization and evaluation of completed activities and the making of concrete plans for follow-up, when indicated (Arnold & Boggs, 1989, p. 177). If a relationship of mutual respect and trust has developed between the nurse and physician during this communication process, future communication should be successful as well.

This collaborative integrated model demonstrates a relationship of mutual respect between nurse–physician team members and effective communication optimally achieves the goals of client care.

COMMUNICATION STANDARDS

Communication standards delineate requirements for communication among members of the health care team or with administrators in the health care system. Communication standards vary among health care organizations and among individuals in various health care settings (ambulatory settings versus inpatient settings). Communication standards may be components of administrative policies and procedures or practice guidelines. Standards are developed by each health care organization to prospectively assist their employees in performing their duties and responsibilities competently.

Policies and procedures governing nurse–physician communication need to be clearly delineated in organizational standards to carefully guide patient care management. Communication standards written by health care organizations need to clearly delineate the chain of command to ensure that patient care is appropriate and effective to prevent adverse patient outcomes. Failure by the nurse to communicate relevant patient information to the physician, or failure of the physician to respond appropriately to communication regarding a patient's condition, can be viewed as "negligence or breach in duty" (Fiesta, 1993, p. 30).

Documentation of the communication that occurs between the nurse and physician is an essential component of communication standards. Thus it is important to document that communication between the two parties has occurred. In *Gallagher v. Samaritan Hospital* (1992), which settled for $1.02 million against the OB-GYN physician (OB-GYN Malpractice Prevention, 1996, p. 53), documentation by the nurses prevented litigation against the hospital when the obstetrician arrived 2 hours after she was called by the emergency room staff. The patient presented to the hospital bleeding at 34 weeks gestation after she was told by her physician to go to the hospital. The physician claimed that her 2-hour delay in reporting to the hospital occurred because she never received a phone call from the nurses. The nurses' notes in several places in the chart clearly documented each communication with the physician. As a result, the physician was stripped of her defense.

In *Utter v. United Hospital Center, Inc.* (1992), the court found the hospital liable to an injured patient. The nursing manual had a policy that instructed a nurse to call the attending physician if he or she had any doubts about the care provided to any patient or to call the department chairman. In *Utter* the nurse did, in fact, call the attending physician to report that the patient had delirium, but this probably came from OB-GYN malpractice prevention as well the physician did not take action. However, the nurse did not contact the department chairman, per hospital policy. The patient lost his arm, which was amputated at the shoulder. The opinion of the court was that "in the dim hours of night, as well as in the light of day, nurses are frequently charged with the duty to observe the condition of the ill and inform in their care. If that patient, helpless and wholly dependent, shows signs of worsening, the nurse is charged with the obligation of taking some positive action." This case clearly supports the requirement that nurses engage in the chain of command process when patient care is compromised.

Effective communication standards are essential in any health care setting where expectations exist in the provision of patient care, especially when nurse and physician are required to collaborate in the care of the client. Communication standards are often integrated within a policy standard or practice guideline. The following communication standards are provided as samples:

Communication Standard Composed as a Policy Standard:

■ The nurse manager will inform the primary physician (or supervisor) if staffing and patient care assignments fall below the acceptable level of patient monitoring.

For example, an RN on labor and delivery is monitoring two patients who are complete/complete when the standard assignment is for one RN to be assigned only one patient who is in the second stage of labor. The physician or another competent staff member shall be obtained to remain with the patient who is pushing.

Communication Standards Composed Within a Practice Guideline:

■ **Ruptured Membranes:** The nurse shall obtain consent from physician before ambulating any patient after rupture of membranes.

■ **Preterm Labor:** The nurse will notify the attending physician when a preterm patient (<37 weeks) presents with frequent repetitive contractions within 15 minutes of arrival.

Standing orders are written communication standards or verbal orders if approved by the OB-GYN multidisciplinary committee within the hospital. Approved practice standards shall permit activation of nursing interventions based on the nurse's independent assessment and judgment. An example of a standing order follows:

A credentialed L&D nurse may perform the following interventions:

■ Amniotomy to place a fetal scalp electrode if the patient is $\geq$ 4 cm, at least −1 station with a vertex presentation, with decelerations requiring a more accurate tracing.

■ Placement of an intrauterine pressure catheter (IUPC) with ruptured membranes if uterine activity is difficult to assess while on oxytocin or for patients who are undergoing trial of labor for vaginal birth after cesarean.

Communication standards exist to protect the patient, providers, and the institution. Clear communication standards are proactive methods of preventing or reducing liability. Fiesta (1993) says, "The rules, regulations, policies and procedures contained in a hospital employee or nursing manual indicate the standards the hospital requires its employees to meet. Deviation from them suggests that an employee may have failed to meet the standards" (p. 30).

The following case demonstrates a situation in which a standard may not have existed and communication with the obstetrician did not occur to obtain permission to ambulate a patient with known variable fetal heart rate decelerations. In *Miles v. Box Butte County* (1992), the nurse deviated from the applicable standard of care by failing to properly interpret the fetal heart rate pattern, institute fetal resuscitative measures, notify the physician of abnormal fetal heart rate decelerations, and by allowing the patient to walk with a nonreassuring fetal heart rate pattern. The infant was born with mental retardation and cerebral palsy and later died. A jury found that the defendant nurse was negligent and the parents were awarded in the amount of $1,589,280.

FACTORS AFFECTING COMMUNICATION

Arnold & Boggs (1989) believe that faulty communication is hazardous and can result in disordered thinking, feeling and acting. Faulty communication between the nurse and physician may result in poor patient management with less than optimal outcome. Communication pitfalls among providers can result in deficiencies in patient care, thereby affecting optimal outcome. Proactive measures to ensure that communication is clear and relevant to patient care management are essential. Communication standards should be clearly described in policies on patient care processes. Making sure that physicians and nurses are aware of such communication standards is essential for risk management.

Deteriorating changes in the patient's condition must be communicated clearly and promptly and documented as to the time the communication took place.

In *Fairfax Hospital System, Inc. v. McCarty* (1992), a nurse was found negligent in detecting signs of fetal distress and in failing to communicate an abnormal fetal heart rate pattern to the physician. The obstetrician was not notified of abnormal fetal heart rate decelerations during a critical period when irreparable damage to the fetal brain had already occurred. Of significance in this case is the fact that the obstetrician testified that the nurse's failure to inform him of the decelerations once they presented prevented him from appropriately intervening in a timely manner. Thus the obstetrician was exonerated. A jury returned a verdict of for $3.5 million.

Display 20-1 delineates pertinent information the nurse and physician need to communicate

to each other to ensure effective patient management. Display 20-2 lists effective communication techniques.

"Clear, effective oral and written communications among health professionals, patients, and their families are proven deterrents to injury, dissatisfaction and litigation. The value of stressing communication skills must be part of the hospital's risk management program . . . . Courteous, kind, compassionate and sensitive discourse is the gold standard to communication" (Fiesta, 1993, p. 16). These principles apply to nurse–physician communication, as well as to nurse–client–physician communication. The following case demonstrates a catastrophic outcome whereby the nurse failed to properly communicate all relevant facts to the physician, which concealed the diagnosis and delayed emergency intervention.

In a Alabama case, *Baptist Medical Center v. Wilson* (1993), failure of the nurse to communicate all pertinent information to the physician resulted in a delayed diagnosis and cesarean section, resulting in a neonatal death. A patient attempting a vaginal birth after cesarean section had noticed a "sharp pain," followed by vaginal bleeding. The patient told the nurse she felt as though her stomach "had ripped open and the baby had moved up toward the ceiling." The nurse examined the patient, thought she was completely dilated, and noticed that the fetal

DISPLAY 20-1

Nurse–Physician Communication Guidelines

1. Presentation of succinct relevant history and demographic information.
2. Presentation of chief complaint and associated problems identified from the history.
3. Physiologic status (vital signs, contractions, physical examination findings).
4. Presentation of the patient's response to interventions and procedures.
5. Presentation of the ongoing plan of care (goals and expected outcome).
6. Presentation of findings requiring referral to multidisciplinary team members.

heart rate was down to 60–70 beats per minute. The nurse informed the physician about the decelerations and vaginal examination, but failed to report the sharp pain, ripping sensation, and vaginal bleeding. The physician examined the patient but did not find the patient fully dilated. The physician ordered an emergency cesarean section, during which a ruptured uterus was discovered. The neonate suffered brain damage and died 5 months later. The nurse was found negligent and a jury awarded the parents $600,000.

Patient Care and Communication

Coordination and delivery of patient care and services requires optimal communication among members of the multidisciplinary team. The patient's care, whether provided in an ambulatory, inpatient, or home setting, must be planned, coordinated and implemented by the providers involved. Effective communication among the providers of care is essential for optimal delivery of care, evaluation, and ongoing case management. The Joint Commission of Accreditation of Healthcare Organizations (JCAHO, 1997) establishes standards on patient care planning: The care, treatment and rehabilitation planning process is designed to ensure that care is appropriate to the patient's specific needs and the severity level of his or her disease, condition, impairment, or disability. Qualified individuals plan and provide care, treatment, and rehabilitation in a collaborative and interdisciplinary manner, as appropriate to the patient.

Coordination and planning of patient care require effective communication in order to accomplish ongoing evaluation and planning. An Indiana case settled for $725,001, where the failure to properly monitor an obese woman in labor (OB-GYN Malpractice Prevention, 1996, p. 94) resulted in failure to detect fetal distress, resulting in an intrauterine death. A woman in her 42nd week of pregnancy, weighing 314 pounds, appeared in labor. Because of her gross obesity, the nurse was unable to apply the straps to continuously monitor the fetal heart rate. She assessed the fetal heart rate to be approximately 144 bpm during her initial evaluation. During the course of the labor, the heart rate was noted to have poor long- and short-term variability and some occasional variable decelerations. The OB-GYN physician was signing off to his partner and left saying his partner would arrive momentarily. When the

DISPLAY 20-2

Effective Communication Techniques

1. Speak clearly.
2. Speak using a congenial tone.
3. Be courteous and professional.
4. Present facts in a methodical or chronological style.
5. Ask for clarification if communication or orders are unclear.
6. Communicate all relevant facts, abnormal findings, and specific concerns.
7. State your reasons if you disagree with a treatment plan.
8. If the mother or fetus (or both) are at risk, tell the physician to report to the hospital to assess the patient immediately (and document).
9. Inform the physician or provider if you plan to communicate up the chain of command.

oncoming OB physician called 30 minutes later, he spoke with a nurse but was not informed of the status of the fetal heart rate and variable decelerations. Because he was not appraised of the fetal heart rate decelerations and poor variability, he did not arrive for another 50 minutes. Upon his arrival, the FHR dropped to the 40s and a cesarean section was performed. The baby was born without respirations and did not survive. The nurses and physicians in this case were negligent in properly assessing and communicating relevant facts to each other and doing so in a timely manner. Collaborative competent care requires that each member of the health care team continuously assess and initiate appropriate therapy to achieve optimal patient care outcomes. This case clearly demonstrates a breach in fundamental standards of practice (assessment, evaluation, treatment), including inadequate communication.

Verbal and written communication is used between health care providers to share information about the patient. Because the nurse is usually the first health care provider that a patient encounters, the nurse's initial assessment may contain vital information that requires immediate communication to the physician. Health care providers are required to communicate any relevant patient care finding that affects the scope of practice of other members involved in patient care management. For example, if a nurse identifies that a patient is complaining of fever, dysuria, uterine irritability, and flank pain during the initial prenatal patient assessment, and documents these findings in the prenatal record *without* verbally communicating this information to the primary care provider, the nurse might cause harm to the patient. The patient may assume that the nurse communicated this information to her primary care provider and not mention her symptoms again. The physician or certified nurse midwife may fail to read the nurse's note and proceed with a routine prenatal examination without attention to the presenting complaints. This example of faulty communication of relevant findings between health care providers can easily result in an oversight, predisposing the patient to injury and increasing the risk of medical liability. Complete communication of all relevant information between the nurse and physician about the patient is an essential ingredient of risk management and good patient care.

In a case that settled for $750,000, the largest amount recoverable in Indiana at the time, a patient died after the office nurse diagnosed but treated the patient and failed to communicate with the physician (OB-GYN Malpractice Prevention, 1997, p. 76). A 32-year-old patient in her first trimester called her obstetrician office complaining of a possible "strep throat," and relayed symptoms of a sore throat, swollen glands, and a low-grade fever. The office LPN did not consult the physician and gave the woman instructions to gargle with salt water and take over-the-counter medications. After 6 days the patient called back and again talked with the office nurse complaining of no relief in her symptoms. The nurse failed again to consult the physician and told the patient the doctor would evaluate her at her next appointment scheduled for 5 days later. The next day the patient called back stating she was now vomiting. Three hours later the patient called again, and the nurse then consulted the physician who ordered Phenergan suppositories by telephone. After continued vomiting and spotting, the patient came in to be evaluated by the physician who diagnosed the patient with "gastroenteritis," and admitted her to the hospital for intravenous hydration. The patient died within 6 hours after admission, with a diagnosis of group B streptococcus pyogenes.

"This is a classic case of an office LPN doing more than she is trained to do and actually trying to practice medicine," stated Lance D. Cline, JD, the plaintiff's attorney. According to Leslie Iffy, MD, FACOG, who testified as an expert witness for the family, "If the nurse who took the telephone calls relayed the information to the physician before recommending treatment, the physician individually would have been negligent in failing to have the patient come into the office." Failure to communicate pertinent clinical information to the physician in this case was nursing negligence and breach of the State

Nurse Practice Act, resulting in an unfortunate death. Although nurses have a more active role in health care delivery today, they share responsibility in properly assessing and treating clients within the legal scope of their practice, which also requires communicating relevant information to physicians who hold primary responsibility for patient diagnosis, treatment, evaluation of response to treatment, and follow-up.

Patient Care Practice Guidelines

Patient care and communication standards in practice guidelines need to clearly define the scope of practice of all health care providers. The communication standards developed collaboratively by all health care providers and are incorporated into the patient care standards. A section of a sample practice guideline entitled "Care of the Intrapartum Patient," delineating the specific section on communication is set forth in Display 20-3. This guideline clearly delineates patient information the nurse needs to convey to the primary care provider. It is possible that some courts may regard practice standards as the standard of care rather than commonly practiced guidelines. Defendants have been found liable by the courts for violating the standard of care. Fiesta (1993) states that

> While the use of standards could abbreviate the process of establishing fault, standards also must be true and accurate measures of what constitutes reasonable care under the circumstances of the case. . . . [A]s "practice guidelines or guidelines" become more widely accepted in the medical community, they will come to play a greater role in defining the standard of care. State legislatures may enact statutes that explicitly incorporate standards in defining the duty of reasonable care. (p. 16) Although some people fear the guidelines will increase the risks of malpractice by revealing negligence that otherwise would go undetected, they should reduce the incidence of error by enabling physicians to practice in ways that create fewer legal risks . . . . In the cases involving bad outcomes, the use of well developed guidelines focuses attention on the standards of care and defendants' conduct in

relationship to that standard rather than on the claimants' need for compensation. (p. 17)

Patient Care Redesign

The trend in health care today is to streamline operations and avoid redundancy in patient care services. Efforts to redesign patient care services often create upheaval for the organization. Use of industry consultants, unfamiliar with state nurse practice acts, professional organizations' standards of practice, and the health care provider's scope of practice may create operational redesigns that can increase the liability risk for health care providers and health care organizations. Although the focus of change today is on cost containment, health care administrators need to ensure that efforts to save money do not place health care providers and patients at risk of harm and medical liability. Providing quality care and protecting the patient from harm should remain a priority, and the process for delivery of patient care services should be safeguarded.

NURSING PROCESS

In the delivery of patient care services, the nurse is held legally accountable for his or her practice. All elements of the nursing process should be implemented in the delivery of patient care services including assessing, planning, implementing, and evaluating. Ongoing assessment and monitoring of the patient is a fundamental nursing responsibility. If a patient's condition worsens, it is the nurse's duty to report such findings to the primary care provider. Unless defined in the scope of practice in the institutional policy as a "standing order," the nurse is obligated to communicate her findings to a physician for medical management. The assessment is a process that involves the use of nursing judgment. Fiesta (1993) states that "Negligence based on judgement or assessment is always measured prospectively. . . . Based on the available information at the time, did the nurse make a reasonable judgement or assessment of the patient?" (p. 16). This judgment includes informing the physician in a timely manner to ensure the opportunity to take *appropriate* action to properly treat

DISPLAY 20-3

Protocol for Care of the Intrapartum Patient

Purpose   To outline the procedure for admission of the intrapartum patient to the Labor & Delivery Room. Intrapartal care is considered a low-risk health care experience. High-risk conditions are identified early so that appropriate and timely intervention prevents adverse outcome for mother and baby.

Scope   Physicians, Residents
Certified Nurse Midwives
Staff L&D Registered Nurses (within scope of practice)

(Communication Standard)

Conditions to Report to Physician or CNM:

1. BP and Pulse out of patient normal range; T ≥ 100.4.
2. Vaginal bleeding in excess of bloody show.
3. Change in FHR baseline variability—decreased short- & long-term bpm (not related to medication administration).
4. Marked FHR decelerations: severe cord patterns, late decelerations, prolonged bradycardia, suspicious baseline, bradycardia.
5. Meconium-stained fluid.
6. Presenting part other than cephalic.
7. High-risk factors not previously identified.
8. Patient progress or lack of progress in labor.

Documentation

1. Keep accurate, pertinent notes to reflect patient's response to labor, pain assessment, medication administration, and patient response at least hourly.
2. Complete labor flow sheet every hour to note FHR, variability, contraction frequency, medications if administered.
3. Record all medications administered on flow sheet and medication record. Note any effects with pitocin induction or augmentation.
4. Record all anesthesia used.
5. Describe all decelerations noted and interventions applied.
6. Record all communication and consultations with the physician or CNM.
7. Record all telephone and verbal orders.
8. Complete a nursing note or progress note at least every 4 hours during latent phase, every 2 hours during active phase labor, every 1 hour during second stage.

the patient and prevent an adverse outcome. The nursing process is a method of communication that nurses use to ensure successful communication between the nurse–client–physician and includes the following:

ASSESSMENT: Identification of abnormal findings from the history or physical exam or detection of risk factors that might require medical intervention should be communicated to the physician in a timely manner.

PLANNING: The physician should be consulted in a timely manner regarding new patient information that may affect the patient's plan of care.

INTERVENTION: Selection of appropriate interventions to meet the patient's needs is a collaborative process of patient care management. Assessment of the patient's response to interventions must be ongoing. Any adverse patient reaction or unexpected response to interventions should be communicated to the physician. Additionally, if the patient refuses treatment or interventions, the physician should be notified. Any changes in the patient's status (emotional or physiologic) that may alter the course of treatment require communication to the physician. The patient's plan of care should be modified to appropriately meet the patient's needs.

EVALUATION: The nurse has a primary role in continually evaluating the patient. Any adverse patient reaction or unexpected patient response to interventions should be communicated to the physician immediately.

THE CHAIN OF COMMAND

Nurses may encounter physicians who fail to respond to their nursing assessment of a patient's condition. The nurse may feel that medical intervention is indicated, but the physician may not agree to assess the patient. It is critical that the nurse know and use the health care organization's policy that governs situations where the physician's failure to respond could result in harm to the patient. The nurse's

obligation is to the patient, and the nurse must take positive action (Fiesta, 1993). Each institution should have a policy describing the chain of command in order that appropriate care is delivered to prevent adverse outcomes. This should be included in the hospital's quality improvement and risk management program, with emphasis in protecting the health of the clients and the practice of competent health care providers.

The following example demonstrates the failure of the physician to respond to the registered nurse's assessment:

NURSE: "Dr. Smith, Mrs. Lane, the 32 yo G3 P2 at 40 wks gestation was admitted in active labor at 2 A.M. Her prenatal course was uncomplicated by my review of her prenatal record. Vaginal exam reveals that she is 3–4 cm dilated, completely effaced, and the vertex is at 0 station. Her contractions are a minute apart and she is complaining of severe abdominal pain in the lower left quadrant. The FHR baseline is 120s with minimal beat-to-beat variability, with no FHR accelerations for the past 20 minutes. Her BP is 90/50, P 92, R 18, T 98. She has a heavy bloody show."

PHYSICIAN: "If she is in a lot of pain, she may have an epidural or give her some Stadol. Call me when she is 8 cm."

NURSE: "Dr. Smith, I am concerned that she shows signs of possible abruptio placenta. Her contractions are one after another and her pain is severe and localized in the left lower quadrant. I want you to come in to assess her. I think you might need to scan her. Do you want me to draw any coagulation studies while you are on your way in?"

PHYSICIAN: "I think you are overreacting, Nurse Jones. The baby's FHR is fine. Call me when she is 8 cm."

NURSE: "Dr. Smith, I strongly feel that something may be abnormal. I want you to come in to assess her. The FHR is fine now, but if she is abrupting, you know the FHR can drop immediately and the baby and mother can die quickly."

PHYSICIAN: "Nurse Jones, stop this nonsense. Call me when she is 8 cm!"

Dr. Smith hangs up.

In this case, the registered nurse is accountable to act on her nursing assessment of risk or potential risk to the patient and fetus. Although a nurse may recommend medical intervention (such as laboratory studies or other diagnostic studies), he or she is not authorized to order medical studies or medications unless clearly delineated in the policy or procedure of the health care organization. If the hospital policy manual does not authorize nurses to engage in any medical interventions, the communication process or chain of command procedure should clearly delineate what to do when a physician fails to respond to the nurse's assessment of the patient's condition.

Most organizations use a chain of command where the registered nurse consults with the charge nurse and nursing supervisor or director for guidance and action. The case is discussed, and if all concur that the physician's presence is needed to assess the patient and the physician continues to refuse to come in to the hospital, the chief medical officer is notified. Once the decision to contact the chief medical officer is made, after consulting with the appropriate person in the chain of command, the nurse calls the primary physician to inform him or her of their decision to call the chief medical officer. Remaining calm and factual is important. The following is an example of a possible conversation:

NURSE: "Dr. Smith. This is Nurse Jones again. I discussed my concerns about Mrs. Lane with the charge nurse and the supervisor. Both of them agree that she might be having a problem and needs a physician assessment. Would you like to come in or do you want us to call the OB-GYN chairman, or the chief of staff, to come in to assess Mrs. Lane?

PHYSICIAN: "I'll be in."

Effective communication requires maintenance of a calm demeanor with direct communication of facts and concerns. The nurse should not be evasive or vague in communicating desired action or recommendations. If the physician does not respond to the nurse's concerns, the nurse should be firm and assertive in restating the concerns and recommendations. The conversation should be factually and objectively summarized and documented in the medical record.

The standard of care is the legal criterion to determine if a deviation exists sufficient to establish professional negligence. The nursing standard of care includes implementation of the nursing process in the provision of care to all patients. Communication processes among health care professionals and the patient are an internal function in the performance of the standard of care provided to the patient. Failure to properly communicate or to notify the physician of significant findings is a frequent allegation against nurses.

Interdisciplinary collaboration and communication is an integral process in patient care services. Effective and appropriate delivery of patient care requires that health care providers engage in appropriate and timely communication. The patient's progress, response to care, or deterioration should be closely monitored and evaluated by all providers of care. Collaboration between the nurse and physician through effective communication is an integral and key part in providing appropriate and safe patient care services.

Pitfalls in Nurse–Physician Communication

Effective communication is one of the most valuable risk management measures for both physicians and nurses. Pitfalls in nurse–physician communication can lead to liability, often resulting in a judgment providing that the lack of communication demonstrated a deviation from the standard of care. Areas of nurse–physician communication weaknesses include some of the following:

1. *Fear of communicating with the physician or the nurse or fear between physicians or nurses.* Feelings of fear or intimidation between providers can result in avoidance of communication. Unfortunately, lack of communication can result in omission of significant findings, which can delay treatment or emergency interventions. Nurses have been known to say "I don't want to call Dr. So and So, he may yell at me for waking him up!"

2. *Inadequate patient report among nurses and physicians.* Sometimes the communication problems lie in inadequate communication between physicians as they sign off to each other or between nurses as they review information in change of shift reports. Patient reports can be brief and some essential facts may be omitted. Oncoming nurses should thoroughly assess the patient record, her history, and her progress when assuming care. Offgoing nurses should ensure that the nurse's notes clearly and thoroughly reflect the patient's condition and the nurse's final assessment prior to departure. Additionally, it is prudent for the nurse to give a thorough report to the oncoming physician in the event that the offgoing physician left out important facts related to the patient, especially those facts that might affect ongoing management.

3. *Lack of documentation of communication.* In busy times or during inadvertent hallway conversations, pertinent information between providers often is exchanged. Oftentimes in charting or in situations where charting is done via the computer, significant communications may be omitted from the legal document. Unfortunately, if the case progresses to litigation, the pertinent conversations cannot be remembered, much less reproduced as late entries. Nurses should keep track of all communication of adverse findings to providers. At the end of the shift, the time and essence of the conver-sations should be clearly documented. For example, an entry may include the following: "4:00 P.M. Dr. Young notified that the amnioinfusion bolus of 400cc was infused over 30 minutes and repetitive variable decelerations continue. Fetal heart rate remains at 130–140 bpm with adequate beat-to-beat variability and decelerations down to 80 bpm for 40 seconds."

4. *Failure to communicate due to consideration of the physician.* Some nurses do not want to disturb physicians during their busy clinics or while they sleep. Nurses can be too considerate and sometimes hesitate to disturb the physicians or providers, thus withholding pertinent communication about a patient's condition. This kindness or consideration, however, can later haunt the nurse who is found negligent whereas the physician is not because he or she was not notified of a patient's adverse condition. This act of kindness can never be justified when a patient's safety and clinical outcome may be detrimentally affected.

5. *Failure to persist in communication with the physician or provider when there is no response.* Lack of response from the physician does not exempt a nurse from his or her duty to continue to attempt to reach the attending provider. Continual failure to attain a response requires that the nurse initiate the chain of command, especially in emergency situations or progressively deteriorating patient conditions.

6. *Failure to initiate the chain of command when the nurse and physician disagree on the appropriate plan of care.* A nurse who finds that the patient's safety and clinical outcome is at risk should initiate the chain of command communication process *before* there is irreversible damage. The nurse should clearly document each communication attempt, and with whom, in utilizing the chain of command.

CONCLUSION

The importance of nurse–physician communication cannot be overstated. Communication is often taken for granted; however, those who have encountered ineffective and dysfunctional communication know and value effective communication. The lives and clinical outcomes of clients rely on the effectiveness of the health care team to work collectively and competently to continually assess and competently deliver health care. The public entrusts nurses and physicians to provide the best care at all times. There is no excuse for negligence, but most nurses have been in situations where they have simply "forgotten" because they were too busy. Health care systems continue to impose greater and greater demands upon nurses and often result in more responsibilities with fewer resources. Nurses must be ever vigilant in practicing and refining through communication skills.

REFERENCES

American Medical Association. (1997). Code of medical ethics: Current opinions and annotations. Chicago: American Medical Association.

Arnold, E., & Boggs, K. (1989). Interpersonal relationships: Professional communication skills for nurses. Philadelphia: W. B. Saunders.

Comment (1989). Rational health policy and the legal standard of care: A call for judicial deference to medical practice guidelines, 77 Cal. L. Rev. 1483, pp. 1522-28.

Fiesta, J. (1993). Legal aspects—Standards of care: Part I. Nursing Management, 24(7), 30–32.

Fiesta, J. (1993). Legal aspects—Standards of care: Part II. Nursing Management, 24(8), 16–17.

Fiesta, J. (1993). Failure to assess. Nursing Management, 24(9), 16–17.

Fiesta, J. (1994). Communication—The value of an apology. Nursing Management, 25(8), 14–16.

Goldman, T. R. (1991). Risk management concepts and strategies. Journal of Intravenous Nursing, 14(3), 199–204.

JCAHO (1997). Accreditation manual for hospitals. Chicago: Joint Commission of Accreditation of Healthcare Organizations.

Killian, W. H. (1991). Communication is risk management tool for RNs. American Nurse, 24(1), 33–34.

OB-GYN Malpractice Prevention. (1996). Failure to monitor obese mother results in stillbirth. 3(12), 94. Baltimore: Williams & Wilkins.

OB-GYN Malpractice Prevention. (1996). Nurses' notes save hospital from taking rap for OB's late arrival. 3(7), p. 53. Baltimore: Williams & Wilkins.

OB-GYN Malpractice Prevention. (1997). Doctor and nurse don't communicate; parents blame them for baby's death. Special Edition, 5. Baltimore: Williams & Wilkins.

OB-GYN Malpractice Prevention. (1997). Patient Dies After Nurse Gives Diagnosis. 4(10), 76. Baltimore: Williams & Wilkins.

Pillitteri, A., & Ackerman M. (1993). The "doctor-nurse game": A comparison of 100 years—1888–1990. Nursing Outlook, 41(3), 113–116.

Porter, F. (1991). A participant observation study of power relations between nurses and doctors in a general hospital. Journal of Advanced Nursing, 16(6), 728–735.

Stein, L. I., Watts, D. T., & Howell, T. (1990). The doctor–nurse game revisited. Nursing Outlook, 38(6), 264–268.

CASE CITATIONS

Baptist Medical Center v. Wilson 618So2d 135 CAL (1993).

Fairfax Hospital System, Inc. v. McCarty 244Va28, 419SE2d621 (1992).

Gallagher v. Samaritan Hospital, as cited in OB-GYN Malpractice Prevention, 1996, p. 53.

Miles v. Box Butte County, 489 N.W.2d 829 (1992).

Utter v. United Hospital Center, Inc. 236 S.E. 2d 213 (W. Va. Sup. Ct. App., 1977).

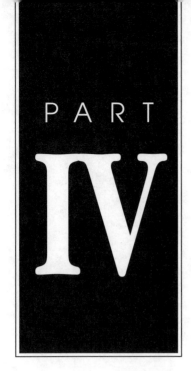

PART IV

Contemporary Perinatal Nursing

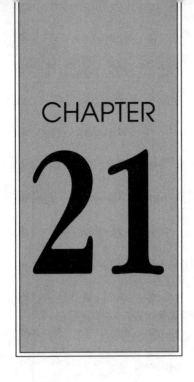

CHAPTER
21

The Nurse as an Expert Witness

Paula DiMeo Grant

This chapter focuses on the purpose and role of the expert nurse witness. Qualifications as well as the importance of case evaluation, expert reports, and testimony are discussed. Case examples are used to illustrate salient points, and suggestions for preparation as an expert are given. For the purposes of this chapter, the terms negligence and malpractice are used interchangeably.

PROFESSIONAL OBLIGATION AND VALUE OF THE EXPERT WITNESS

Does a nurse have a professional obligation to testify as an expert nurse witness? Testifying as an expert nurse witness can add a satisfying dimension to the nurse's practice. The decision, however, rests solely with the professional nurse.

The evolution of the role of the expert nurse witness mirrors the evolution of the profession of nursing in general. Historically, because nursing was not viewed as a profession, nurses were not viewed as professionals. Consequently, nurses were not considered to have the requisite qualifications to serve as expert witnesses. Over the years, however, the profession of nursing has not only gained autonomy but has also demanded more accountability. State laws and court decisions have helped shape the progress that nurses have made on their journey to pro-

fessionalism. Thus, an increase in the use of nurses as expert witnesses has occurred. Nurses who serve as expert witnesses provide an invaluable service to their profession and society as a whole.

Perinatal nursing is among the various specialty groups that enable nurses to acquire the specialized knowledge and skills necessary to maintain competence in their chosen field. Control over nursing practice is paramount to maintaining professionalism. Only nurses can lawfully practice nursing within the parameters of state nurse practice acts. The practice of nursing includes issues of law and ethics; therefore, it is important to examine both areas before making the decision to serve as an expert nurse witness.

In addition to state nurse practice acts, the nurse may look to the ANA's Code for Nurses (hereinafter the Code) as the framework for ethical conduct. The Code addresses the individual nurse's moral obligations and, on a broader scale, the profession's obligation to safeguard society. The Code was adopted by the American Nurse's Association in 1950 and has been revised periodically. It serves to inform both the nurse and society of the profession's expectations and requirements in ethical matters. (See Display 21-1.)

When nursing negligence or malpractice is alleged and a lawsuit is brought by an injured

DISPLAY 21-1

American Nurses Association

Code for Nurses

1. The nurse provides services with respect for human dignity and the uniqueness of the client, unrestricted by consideration of social or economic status, personal attributes, or the nature of health problems.

2. The nurse safeguards the client's right to privacy by judiciously protecting information of a confidential nature.

3. The nurse acts to safeguard the client and the public when health care and safety are affected by the incompetent, unethical, or illegal practice of any person.

4. The nurse assumes responsibility and accountability for individual nursing judgments and actions.

5. The nurse maintains competence in nursing.

6. The nurse exercises informed judgment and uses individual competence and qualifications as criteria in seeking consultation, accepting responsibilities, and delegating nursing activities to others.

7. The nurse participates in activities that contribute to the ongoing development of the profession's body of knowledge.

8. The nurse participates in the profession's efforts to implement and improve standards of nursing.

9. The nurse participates in the profession's efforts to establish and maintain conditions of employment conducive to high quality nursing care.

10. The nurse participates in the profession's effort to protect the public from misinformation and misrepresentation and to maintain the integrity of nursing.

11. The nurse collaborates with members of the health professions and other citizens in promoting community and national efforts to meet the health needs of the public.

Source: American Nurses Association (1985).

party, in many jurisdictions the plaintiff must hire an expert nurse witness to form an opinion and give testimony as to whether or not the standard of care was breached. The expert nurse is uniquely qualified to give such testimony because of his or her knowledge, skill, and expertise. In courts of law, expert nurse witnesses assist the trier of fact (jury) in deciding whether to award damages (monetary compensation) for injuries and losses sustained as a result of alleged nursing negligence or malpractice.

Although courts increasingly look to the nursing profession to define the standards of care for nurses, in addressing issues pertaining to nursing negligence, courts will sometimes allow the profession of medicine to define what the standard of nursing care should be. In these jurisdictions, physicians continue to be allowed to testify as to the standard of care of nursing personnel, largely because of the theory that physicians can be aware of nursing standards because of the physician's quasi-supervisory relationship to the nurse. The wrongful death case of *Haney v. Alexander* (1984) is one case in which this approach was used. The North Carolina Appellate Court upheld a decision by the trial court to allow a physician to testify as to whether or not nurses breached the standard of care by failing to adequately monitor the vital signs of the decedent as his condition worsened.

A review of a series of court rulings on nursing practice traces the nurse's role as an expert witness and begins with a total omission of the nurse's existence, followed by views of the nurse as "borrowed servant," then as one capable of forming an independent judgment, then as a professional, and finally recognition of the nurse as expert (Weiss, 1995, p. 17).

Weiss states: "By the late 1960's the majority of courts had long extended the privilege of expert testimony to the medical and legal professions, but not to nursing. The rationale was based, in part, on the assumption that nurses followed orders and were not expected to make independent decisions" (p. 27). The case of *Richardson v. Doe* (1964) illustrates this principle. The laws of each jurisdiction provide guidance as to the qualifications required of the expert witness.

QUALIFICATIONS OF THE EXPERT WITNESS

The qualifications of expert witnesses are described in Rule 702 of *The Federal Rules of Civil Procedure,* which has been adopted by most state courts. Rule 702, *Testimony by Experts,* states as follows:

> If scientific, technical, or other specialized knowledge will assist the trier of fact to understand the evidence or determine a fact in issue, a witness qualified as an expert by knowledge, skill, experience, training or education, may testify thereto in the form of an opinion or otherwise.

The nurse's knowledge, skill, education and/or training enables him or her to provide testimony in a court of law. The minimum credential is the nursing license. Whether or not the nurse is qualified as an expert witness is a question for the judge to determine. Once qualified as an expert, the credibility of a nurse expert is determined by the jury.

In addition to allowing the expert witness to tell the jury his or her opinion, the law recognizes that an expert during trial may give a dissertation or exposition of scientific or other principles relevant to the case, leaving the jury to apply them to the facts.

The selection of the appropriate expert can be one of the most important factors in the outcome of a case. Because almost all negligence or malpractice cases must be proven by expert testimony, the expert must have a clear understanding of the facts of the case and the applicable standard of care. The expert must be able to communicate effectively to a jury, and in a manner that is understandable.

ROLE OF THE NURSE AS EXPERT WITNESS

Overview of the Nurse's Role

An expert witness is one who by reason of education or specialized experience possesses superior knowledge on a subject about which persons having no particular training are incapable of forming an accurate opinion or deducing correct conclusions (Black's, 1979, p. 519). Expert testimony is necessary when conclusions to be made are dependent upon scientific information that is not based upon common knowledge. Expert nurse witnesses therefore play integral roles in various settings both in and out of the courthouse.

The underlying question in every nursing malpractice action is whether or not the nurse's specific acts or omissions conformed with the standard of care. If the actions did not conform to the standard of care, then the question to be answered is whether the patient suffered injury as a result of the deviation.

As a review, in proving negligence four elements must be present. The elements are (1) a duty owed, (2) a breach of duty, (3) proximate cause, and (4) damages. Therefore, to prove negligence all of the following questions must be answered yes by the jury.

1. Did the nurse owe a duty to the patient?
2. Did the nurse breach that duty by a specific act or omission?

3. Was that breach of duty the proximate cause of the injury?
4. Was there actual loss or damage?

Three Phases of the Nurse Expert Role

The role of the expert nurse witness consists of three phases: (1) the *initial phase,* (2) the *pretrial phase,* and (3) the *trial phase.* (See Display 21-2.)

The Initial Phase

The *initial phase* of the nurse expert's role commences when the attorney has contacted the expert seeking advice as to whether or not nursing malpractice has occurred. It is important at this point to ascertain whether or not any con-

flicts of interest exist, such as having already been contacted by another party to the litigation, or some relationship with the hospital or nurse involved. This initial phase should include an interview with the attorney and a preliminary review of the pertinent medical records and witness statements if available.

In addition, there may be a contract signed by the expert nurse and attorney outlining the terms of the agreement with clarification of responsibilities, time frame for completion of tasks, and compensation for services rendered. The expert will determine an hourly fee structure based upon his or her educational background and experience. The nature of the case and the number of parties will dictate the

DISPLAY 21-2

Expert Nurse Witness Review Sheet

THREE PHASES

Initial Phase

1. Meet with counsel to discuss and review case. Ascertain whether any conflicts of interest exist.
2. Agreement should be in writing signed by both parties. Agreement should contain
   a. Terms clearly defined
   b. Hourly compensation specified
   c. Number of hours anticipated

Pretrial Phase

1. Thorough preparation is the key;
2. Review all pertinent medical records and other relevant materials;
3. Know who, what, when, where, and why;
4. Know allegations and defenses;
5. Prepare for deposition with counsel;
6. If deposed, review deposition testimony prior to trial.

Trial Phase

1. Review all pretrial records and documents you prepared for counsel;
2. Read your deposition (if one was taken);
3. Be familiar with opposing parties' testimony and also *prepare with counsel* for
4. Direct examination (by counsel);
5. Cross-examination (by opposing counsel);
6. Re-direct examination (by counsel).

Verdict at End of Trial

Please note: There may be settlement negotiations between the pretrial phase and trial phase. In some instances, mediation or arbitration is mandated.

amount of time and effort needed for preparation of the case. Thorough case evaluation is crucial at this juncture because the nurse expert must determine whether or not the standard of care was breached, that is, whether or not the nurse acted as a reasonably prudent nurse would have acted in similar circumstances.

For example, in a typical obstetrical case the plaintiff's claims may include the following:

1. a failure to diagnose [assess] risk factors or conditions;
2. a failure to carry out physician's orders;
3. a failure to observe or monitor properly;
4. a failure to give the appropriate medication;
5. a failure to refer or report untoward symptoms; and
6. a failure in the delay of delivery or failure to consult the appropriate specialists. (Apfel, 1996)

This list is by no means exhaustive; however, it does provide examples of possible elements of nursing malpractice actions. A malpractice action may include complaints regarding one or more acts or omissions by the nurse. The expert nurse should be familiar with the allegations and the defendant's answers, otherwise known as defenses, to those allegations to assist in preparation of the case.

The Pretrial Phase

During the pretrial phase of the case, the nurse expert is required to draw upon all his or her expertise and knowledge to adequately assess and evaluate the case. Thorough preparation is mandatory.

It is imperative that the medical records be carefully reviewed and a time line of events established when necessary. In addition to the medical records, other sources such as the Nurse Practice Act, agency policies and procedures, nursing textbooks and journals, and legal precedent are helpful in forming opinions. (See Display 21-3.)

Depending upon the jurisdiction, the nurse expert may be required to write a report substantiating his or her opinions that negligence occurred. Unless the states have opted out of the mandatory expert witness disclosure, they must also produce a written report repared and signed by the witness. The report must contain a "complete statement of all opinions to be expressed" by the expert, and "the basis and reasons therefor" (Hirt, 1996, p. 46). However, in many other states this written report is not required.

The case of *Kruck v. St. John's Episcopal Hospital* (1996) illustrates the importance of an expert signing the report. In Kruck, the appellate division reversed the judgment of the trial court and granted the hospital's motion for summary judgment dismissing the lawsuit against the hospital.

The New York Supreme Court held that parents of an infant diagnosed with a fractured leg after delivery failed to prove that malpractice by the hospital was the cause of the injury. The court looked to expert testimony, in part, to render its decision. The hospital's expert indicated that the injury could have occurred in utero

DISPLAY 21-3

Sources Used in Preparing Expert Nurse Opinion

1. Agency policy and procedure manuals
2. State Nurse Practice Act and regulations
3. American Nurses' Association Code for Nurses
4. American Nurses' Association Standards of Practice
5. Joint Commission on Accreditation of Hospitals Standards
6. Other accreditation standards
7. Agency licensing regulations
8. Specialty nursing group standards
9. Nursing textbooks and journals
10. Continuing education and education program curriculum

Source: Northrop & Kelly (1987).

even in the absence of negligence. The only evidence submitted by the parents was an expert affirmation, which was *unsigned* and had the expert's name *deleted*. Because the report was not signed by an expert and the expert was not identified, the hospital was precluded from testing the validity of the cause of action and from ensuring that the purported expert existed; therefore, the court dismissed the claim against the hospital.

The pretrial phase is also known as the discovery phase. Discovery enables the parties to learn more about the facts and issues of the case. It allows the parties to discover all there is to know about the case to prevent "surprise" at the trial. One means of accomplishing this task is by deposing witnesses. It is likely that the expert witness will be deposed by opposing counsel. The expert witness should be aware that any testimony given during a deposition may be used for impeachment should the expert's testimony at trial conflict with the earlier deposition testimony.

Deposition is the testimony of a person taken under oath. Its purpose is to make a record of certain information and opinions to be used in settlement negotiations or at trial. The deposition requires diligent preparation with counsel. At the deposition, the expert witness has an opportunity to meet opposing counsel and vice versa. It also gives all parties a preview of what to expect at trial. The deposition is recorded and a written transcript is provided. The expert is allowed to review the transcript for accuracy before signing under penalty of perjury. Depositions may also be videotaped. It is important to remember that the deposition establishes a record to be used during negotiations or trial. See Display 21-4 for tips on giving a deposition.

During the pretrial phase, the case may be dismissed as it was in the *Kruck* case. This is sometimes accomplished by filing pretrial motions with the court. Expert reports, affidavits, and deposition testimony can be used to support any written arguments made by counsel during this phase. The expert's appearance in court is usually not necessary at this stage.

Trial Phase

After the initial and pretrial phases have been completed and if the case has not been settled or dismissed, the third or trial phase begins. Prior to this stage, the attorney has spent many hours of preparation and has developed a theory and theme of the case. The theory and theme of the case are closely related concepts and many times are used interchangeably. Basically, the theory of the case is its legal or factual justifications and the theme is its "story line" (Purver, Young, Davis, & Kerper, 1990, p. 16).

In order to prevail, the plaintiff has the burden of proving each of the required elements of malpractice by a preponderance of the evidence (more than 50%). The expert witness's courtroom testimony is crucial in meeting this burden of proof. In deciding the case, the jury will evaluate and determine each expert's credibility.

It is therefore essential that the nurse expert establish credibility with the jury. Jurors begin assessing the credibility of attorneys from the first moment they see them in the courtroom. The same is true for expert witnesses. The jury's assessment of the nurse expert's credibility will be influenced by the images presented during testimony. The following factors contribute to the nurse expert's credibility:

DISPLAY 21-4

Tips on Giving a Deposition

- Understand the process
- Be prepared
- Be sure to understand the question
- Answer *only* what is asked
- Be truthful
- Do not guess
- Do not volunteer information
- Be polite
- Speak clearly

1. competence or expertise,
2. knowledge of the facts, and
3. trustworthiness (Purver, Young, Davis, & Kerper, 1990).

The image the nurse expert projects is important. The general rule regarding physical appearance is to dress conservatively and neatly.

The jury will believe the nurse expert is trustworthy if they perceive the nurse expert as being a reliable source of information, honest, and polite. As a general rule, the fundamentals of good communication should be used in the courtroom. The expert should also be cognizant of the body language exhibited as well as the tone of voice used in responding to questions.

Although trial testimony is more formal than deposition testimony, the same general rules apply when answering questions. In addition to those rules, the nurse expert must be aware of objections made during his or her testimony. Should an objection be made by either side, the nurse expert must not answer until the judge rules on the objection. If the judge overrules the objection, the nurse expert may proceed with the answer. If the judge sustains the objection, the question is not answered and the attorney must proceed with another question.

If it is possible, the nurse expert should visit the courthouse prior to trial because courtrooms can be somewhat intimidating. It is important for the nurse expert to be comfortable and familiar with the surroundings. A schematic drawing of the inside of a courtroom provides an idea of where the players are situated (see Figure 21-1).

DIRECT EXAMINATION. The direct examination at trial is usually conducted by the attorney who has hired the nurse expert. The following are sample questions on direct examination to illustrate (1) establishing the witness's qualifications as an expert, and (2) the methodology employed for presenting the expert's opinion.

Establishing the Witness's Qualifications as an Expert

Would you please state your name and address for the court?

What is your profession?

What is your educational background?

Where have you been employed?

Where are you currently employed?

What is your current position?

What is your nursing experience?

What is your nursing expertise or specialty?

Are you certified as a specialist in that area?

What, if any, professional associations do you belong to?

Have you held any leadership positions in these groups?

What, if any, awards or certificates have you received?

Presenting the Expert's Opinion.

Method 1: You've had the opportunity to review the medical records that are in evidence before the court and have heard the testimony of the plaintiff. What is your opinion as to the defendant's actions in this case? (Further questions would elicit the standard of care and explain the basis of the opinion.)

Method 2: The expert witness is given a hypothetical situation which is similar to the actual case and then asked to give an opinion (Northrop & Kelly, 1987, p. 532).

During direct examination the expert should provide the jury with enough information to fully understand what occurred and why it is or is not malpractice. To achieve this goal, open-ended questions may be used.

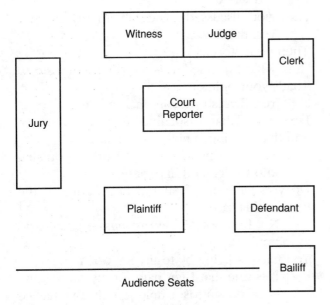

Figure 20-1. Court room diagram

To enhance the testimony and assist the jury to visualize what happened, exhibits are sometimes introduced. According to Mauet (1986, pp. 233–234) there are three basic methods of giving the witness an exhibit:

1. The attorney walks to the witness stand and hands the exhibit to the expert to establish a foundation.
2. The witness may be asked to read or mark parts of the exhibit.
3. The witness may be asked to leave the stand to illustrate testimony using an enlargement of a document such as the patient's chart.

Permission is needed from the court for the witness to step down from the stand.

Example:

COUNSEL: Your Honor, may the witness leave the stand and continue his testimony by the exhibit?

COURT: He may. (Mauet, 1986, p. 235)

Upon the court granting permission to the witness to step down, the witness should then step down and stand at one side of the exhibit. The key is not to block the jury's view of the exhibit.

Many expert witnesses use a pointer to illustrate key points in their testimony and mark the exhibit whenever possible. This approach can be very compelling and hold the jury's attention. The educational component of the nursing process is operative at this stage for it is the expert nurse's role to educate the judge and jury.

CROSS-EXAMINATION. After counsel completes the direct examination, in all but a few circumstances, opposing counsel will conduct the cross-examination.

There are two basic purposes of cross-examination:

a. Whenever possible, to elicit favorable testimony to enhance your own client's position;
b. To discredit the witness or the witness's testimony.

Opposing counsel will want to elicit favorable testimony to support his/her client's the-ory of the case. The second method that may be employed is to destroy the witness's credibility so that the jury will disregard their testimony. Traditionally speaking, the areas used to discredit witnesses are motive, interest, bias, and prejudice. The expert's credibility can also be impeached by pointing out a prior inconsistent statement. This can be accomplished if the expert gave a different opinion in earlier testimony, such as the deposition. It is therefore wise to carefully review all affidavits and deposition testimony in the current case prior to trial to minimize the risk of impeachment. Opposing counsel may also have obtained transcripts of depositions or trial testimony given by the expert in other cases so the expert also needs to keep in mind the testimony he or she has given in previous cases with similar facts, as counsel will point out any inconsistencies.

Cross-examination of a witness by opposing counsel may include only subjects that were testified about on direct examination. Sample questions and responses to cross-examination are as follows:

Who told you to say that?

   No one. I was told to tell the truth.

Are you being paid to testify?

   Yes, I am being compensated for my time and work.

Have you discussed this case with anyone?

   Yes, the lawyer.

Then your story is . . . ?

   What I testified to is the truth, not a story.

That's your opinion?

   Yes, that is my opinion.

Do you find that reasonable people can disagree and that nursing is not an exact science?

   Yes, my opinion is based on my nursing knowledge and experience.

Do you have any firsthand knowledge of the facts in this case?

   No, I do not. (Expert witnesses usually do not.)

You make a living by testifying, don't you?

   It is true that I get paid for my time, however, nursing is a unique field of practice with its own standards of practice, which require expert testimony.

Off the record, would you tell me why . . . ?

No.

(There are no off-the-record questions. Refer the opposing attorney to the attorney who called you to testify.) (Northrop & Kelly, 1987, p. 532)

Following cross-examination, redirect examination by "friendly" counsel is sometimes necessary for clarification or rehabilitation purposes. The decision to conduct redirect examination of the expert is usually determined by counsel during cross-examination. At the end of redirect, the expert witness will hear counsel say "Your Honor, I have no further questions." That is the expert's cue that his or her testimony has ended.

CONCLUSION

What qualities make a good witness? Eight trial lawyers identified eight characteristics of a good witness, as follows:

1. Willing to spend time to prepare.
2. Answers the question asked.
3. Is comfortable with not knowing all the answers.
4. Grasps the big picture.
5. Persuades the jury.
6. Possesses the right demeanor.
7. Believability.
8. Sincerity. (McElhaney, 1993, p. 66)

As rapid changes in health care continue, the need for expert nurse witnesses will become even greater both in and out of the courthouse. Expert nurse witnesses are charged with imparting knowledge regarding nursing practice to the judge and jury. This knowledge, which impacts on decisions, has a lasting effect on our system of jurisprudence. The physician testifying as to the nursing standard is still common, although this trend is changing as nursing takes a more center-stage role in managed care.

The future of the role of expert nurse witnesses rests within the nursing profession. It is up to nurses to maintain control over nursing practice. Expert nurse witnesses provide a mechanism to control not only the practice of nursing, but also the public's perceptions of nursing as an integral part of today's health care system.

REFERENCES

American Nurses Association. (1985). Code for nurses with interpretive statements. Kansas City, MO: Author.

Apfel, D. (1992). Obstetrical negligence: Hypertension in pregnancy. Trial (28), 32.

Black's Law Dictionary. (1979). (5th ed.). St. Paul, MN: West.

Brown, L. A. (1996). Trial tips: How to prepare a witness for deposition. Inside TAANA, Journal of Nursing Law, (3).

Carroll, M. M. (1996). Nursing malpractice and corporate negligence: How is the standard of care determined? Journal of Nursing Law, 3(3), 53–59.

Federal Civil Judicial Procedure and Rules. (1996). (pp. 372–373). St. Paul, MN: West.

5 Health Law Week 731, citing Kruck v. St. John's Episcopal Hosp. 644 N.Y. S.2d 325 (App. Div. 1996).

Hirt, T. C. (1996). Expert reports. Litigation. The Journal of the Section of Litigation, American Bar Association, 22(4), 46–50.

Josberger, M., & Reis, D. (1985). Nurse experts. Trial 21, 68–71.

Mauet, T. A. (1986). Fundamentals of trial techniques. Boston: Little, Brown.

McElhaney, J. W. (1993). A good witness. Litigation. The Journal of The Section of Litigation, American Bar Association, 19, (4), 65–66.

Northrop, C., & Grant, P. D. (1986). Connecticut Nurses Association. The expert nurse witness seminar: Glossary. (pp. 6–8). (unpublished material used as handout).

Northrop, C., & Kelly, M. (1987). Expert nurse witnesses. In Cynthia E. Northrop & Mary E. Kelly (Eds.), Legal issues in nursing. (pp. 525–532). St. Louis, MO: Mosby).

Prosser, W. (1980). Negligence: Standard of conduct. The law of torts (5th ed., pp. 160–168). St. Paul, MN: West.

Purver, J. M., Young, D. R., Davis, J. J., & Kerper, J. (1990). The trial lawyer's book: Preparing and winning cases. Rochester, NY: Lawyers Cooperative.

Tammelleo, D. A. (1994). Can a nurse testify as to "nursing negligence"? The Regan Report on Nursing Law, 37(5), 1.

Tammelleo, D. A. (1996). Can a nurse "expert" testify against a physician? The Regan Report on Nursing Law, 37(7), 2. (See Carolan v. Hill, 553 N.W.2d 882, Iowa 1996).

Weiss, J. P. (1995). Nursing practice: A legal and historical perspective. Journal of Nursing Law, (2), 17–36.

CASE CITATIONS

Haney v. Alexander, 323 S.E.2d 430 (N.C. App. 1984).

Kruck v. St. John's Episcopal Hospital, 644 N.Y. S.2d 325 (App. Div. 1996).

Richardson v. Doe, 199 N.E.2d 878 (Ohio 1964)

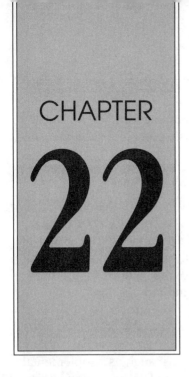

22

Professional Liability Insurance

Paula Lashenske Burgess
and Beverly Butler Karasick

Whether nurses should purchase their own insurance coverage or solely depend on their employer's insurance coverage is a question that should be analyzed carefully by every nurse. The nurse who is not adequately insured voluntarily personally accepts the risk of any settlements or judgments. Without adequate protection, the nurse is responsible for any damage award not covered. If the nurse is unable to pay the amount awarded, then the court may rule that liens be placed on personal property and/or future income be garnished. In addition, defending against a claim or lawsuit is very expensive with attorney fees now well over $100 per hour. As some advertisements suggest, only one malpractice suit is all it takes to sentence you to a life of debt if you are unprepared.

Unfortunately, insurance contrasts are generally complicated or boring at best and most people do not have the time or the interest to study the terms of the contract to any degree. However, key points basic to survival when navigating the insurance policy can be easily dissected for discussion. Although this chapter is not an exhaustive exploration of the concept of liability insurance, it is intended to prepare the nurse to make more informed decisions about insurance coverage or to identify areas where additional research is needed.

PURPOSES OF LIABILITY INSURANCE COVERAGE

The fundamental structure of insurance is the sharing of payment for losses within a group made possible by combining resources of the group, or in insurance terms, "pooling." Pooling is the sharing of losses incurred by the few over the entire group, so that average loss is substituted for actual loss (Rejda, 1989). The insurance agreement process dates back to 4000 B.C. in China, when rice farmers pooled their produce to reduce risk during transportation. Today, nurses pay premiums that are combined with others so that when a loss occurs, expenses are paid from the pool rather than by the individual. When a covered loss occurs, the nurse is protected against a claim that would be financially catastrophic.

In 1989 the American Association of Nurse Attorneys published a booklet entitled *Demonstrating Financial Responsibility for Nursing Practice,* which set forth the following statements:

> All professional nurses engaged in the practice of nursing should be insured against liabilities to third parties arising out of their professional practice.
>
> The means by which a nursing professional elects to insure professional practice should

be based on an informed decision. (American Association of Nurse Attorneys, 1989)

This means that each nurse should make the decision about how much personal coverage to carry in the same manner as other professionals. Unfortunately, many nurses do not learn about the importance of coverage until they are involved in potential or actual litigation.

ANATOMY OF A LIABILITY INSURANCE POLICY

There are many issues to consider when studying of a liability insurance policy. This chapter focuses on the major parts that are common to insurance in general and how these relate to professional liability insurance. Each section includes clinical and case examples, as well as recommendations.

It should be understood that each insurance company contract has a different policy format but the essential elements should be present in all policies (sometimes referred to as certificates of insurance). However, the nurse should be cautious when comparing the different forms available, because even minor differences in wording or phrases, which will be described in this chapter, can result in major coverage varia-

tions (John Liner Organization, 1994). Display 22-1 illustrates the basic parts of a liability insurance policy.

Declarations

The declarations section of a professional liability insurance policy is the part that personalizes and individualizes the contract. On a personal policy, the nurse's full name will appear in print. If a nurse is insured by her employer, the nurse may not be named individually but would be insured within the nursing group.

The declarations section also identifies other types of coverage besides professional liability coverage if it is included, such as supplemental liability coverage and medical payments coverage. Supplemental liability coverage and medical payments coverage are important for coverage of occurrences that are nonbusiness related or those occurrences not involved with professional issues. This additional coverage may provide for those instances when you help an accident victim and the victim or family makes allegations about your assistance requiring legal and financial support. This coverage is described as coverage that fills in any gaps between standard professional liability coverage and homeowner, renters, or premises insurance. Specifically, the declarations most likely would include those in Display 22-2.

Although the declarations appear to be self-explanatory, lawsuits are sometimes brought to determine who the "insured" is when a group or more than one individual may be an insured. In *Legler v. Meriwether* (1965), a nurse anesthetist found that anesthesiologist group practice policies do not automatically include nurses as additional insureds unless there is a specific endorsement included. In this case, the nurse learned too late that a nurse who is employed by a group of physicians needs to actually review the insurance documents to determine coverage rather than rely on verbal statements for confirmation. Another example of whether coverage should be afforded a defendant is illustrated by *The University of North Carolina v. Shoemate* (1994), where it was found that the hospital's liability insurance trust fund covered

DISPLAY 22-1

Generic Insurance Policy

Declarations
Coverage Agreement
Supplementary Payments
Limits of Liability
Defense and Settlement
Policy Territory
Exclusions/Restrictions
Conditions

an impostor resident (physician) who had never been to medical school. The court found that because the defendant acted as an agent of the University of North Carolina (UNC), then the trust fund is responsible for medical malpractice coverage even though the contract between UNC and the defendant was void because of the false information in the defendant's application.

Coverage (Insuring) Agreement

The coverage (insuring) agreement summarizes what the insurer intends to cover and what it agrees to do. Although stated in broad terms, the coverage agreement includes key phrases that have major implications for the nurse. The nurse should keep in mind when reviewing the coverage agreement that it does not cover the full scope of the policy because the limits of liability, exclusions, and conditions found in the entire document will modify or further detail the policy.

DISPLAY 22-2

Declarations

- The name and address of the underwriting insurance company
- The insured's (nurse's) name and address
- The producer's (agent's) name and address
- Occupation/nursing specialty to be covered
- Policy period
- Policy number
- Category of coverage provided and the limits for each category:
  - Professional Liability Coverage
  - Supplemental Liability Coverage (nonbusiness exposure)
  - Medical Payments Coverage (nonbusiness exposure)

Key Phrase Indicates Types of Coverage

One of the most important distinctions in the insuring agreement is whether the coverage provided is *occurrence-based* or *claims-made*. In an occurrence policy, the nurse will have coverage for any incident that happened during the policy period even if the claim is filed after the policy period ends. For example, if a child is diagnosed with cerebral palsy when he turns 5 years old and the OB nurse is named as a defendant for having failed to identify fetal distress while the child's mother was in labor, the nurse will be covered by the occurrence policy. The nurse should review the insuring agreement to see if it states "caused by an incident that occurs during the policy period," which would indicate that the policy is occurrence-based. The occurrence-based policy is the preferred coverage even if the premiums are more expensive. The nurse should be aware that some insurance companies no longer offer occurrence-based coverage.

In contrast, the claims-made policy only covers the nurse for any incident that developed into a claim during the period of time covered by the policy. If the policy is claims-made, it is recommended that the nurse seek expert advice on what type of endorsement (tail or rider) to add to the policy for complete coverage. The nurse should understand that claims-made coverage with the appropriate tail or rider can be comparable to occurrence coverage but does pose more of a challenge when purchasing. The nurse should be most persistent in detailing this type of coverage and how it compares to an occurrence policy.

Key Phrase Indicates Supervisory Coverage

The insuring agreement may also include coverage for actions by those people the nurse supervises, whether they are nursing students, nursing aides, licensed practical nurses, or other registered nurses. This may be stated as "any injury or damage caused by a medical incident by you or anyone for whose professional acts or omissions you are legally responsible."

Key Phrase Indicates Extent of Coverage

Another area for consideration is how the coverage for nursing activities is worded. Typically, the individual nurse's professional liability coverage policy usually encompasses all activities that are performed as a nursing professional. The policy should indicate that the nurse will be covered for "professional acts or omissions for which you are legally responsible." This would include nursing advice to a neighbor or volunteer work. However, the institutional or employer coverage may be limited to include only those acts "within the scope of your employment" and would only cover those acts done on behalf of the institution or employer. This means that the institution or employer coverage will not cover all activities that are performed by nursing professionals but only those activities that it assigns. For example, if you are qualified for advanced practice nursing but your institution does not recognize advanced activities and you perform these activities, in a subsequent lawsuit the institution might refuse to defend your actions. Thus it is important to know what the nurse's job description includes, and what acts may be considered within the scope of employment.

Supplementary Payments

The supplementary payments are for expenses the insurance company will assume that are incurred by the nurse personally. Supplementary payments are in addition to defense costs and are separate from the limits applicable to awards or settlements. Supplementary payments (not supplemental liability) can pay for partial or complete loss of the nurse's income up to a maximum amount for attendance at trial proceedings, expenses incurred by the nurse in discovery investigations, or attorney fees and other costs up to a maximum amount for defense before a state licensing board or governmental regulatory body. Because supplementary payments are additional optional benefits, this part of the insurance policy varies among the types of coverages. The institutional/employer coverage may not offer supplementary payments or may have stipulations that if the nurse is no longer employed at the institution, then the loss of income would not be reimbursed. Although supplementary payments may not be as critical to a nurse working for an institution because of vacation or discretionary paid time off, the self-employed nurse may suffer serious hardship by a loss of wages.

The nurse should be sure of the procedure to follow if there is a possibility that supplementary payments will be needed. The requirements may include a pre-authorization by the insurer or defense attorney to attend a trial or other proceedings for coverage to be activated. The employer may agree to be responsible for the nurse's salary but the nurse might have to complete some type of request form. How supplementary benefits are initiated and what they include needs to be understood by the nurse when she purchases the policy or becomes employed by an institution.

Limits of Liability

The limits of liability describe how much the insurance company will pay for each occurrence up to a maximum amount (aggregate). It is usually written as a maximum dollar award per incident with a maximum amount (aggregate) per policy period or $1 million/$3 million. The nurse should be aware, however, that many insurance companies group all claims for a single incident under "one occurrence." Generally, if the policy specifically states "all claims arising from the same or related incident shall be considered a single claim for the purpose of this insurance and shall be subject to the same limit of liability" then it is deemed to be one occurrence. If the coverage is $1 million per occurrence/$3 million per aggregate with this statement in the policy, then the limits of coverage for a single incident where several claims are asserted would be $1 million only and not $3 million.

It is up to the nurse to decide whether the limits provide the amount of coverage sought. The amount of coverage for the nurse practicing in obstetrics is very important because obstetrics is a high-risk specialty in which multi-million dollar verdicts do occur. The nurse should determine the amount of coverage provided by her employer. When an obstetrical nurse is determining what an adequate amount of insurance should be, consider current verdicts for the most debilitating obstetrical injury cases. There should be concern if the coverage today is less than $1 million per incident for an obstetrical nurse even if there is a cap, which in some states limits liability per defendant. The caps may rise because of inflation and other factors, and possibly could exceed the limits many years later. The insurance company will pay no more than the maximum coverage stated in the policy and the nurse must personally pay any damages not covered by the policy. Because of high exposure risks in obstetrical nursing, premiums are higher than those of other areas of practice. The self-employed obstetrical nurse will experience even higher premiums. The liability exposure is heightened by the lengthy statute of limitations, which in most states extends to the age of majority plus one or two years depending on the individual state.

Defense and Settlement

In connection with the limits of liability is the issue of defense and settlement authority. Under an institutional policy, the nurse will not be able to authorize or refuse settlement. However, with an individual policy, the nurse may have the right to make this decision depending on the policy language. Statements that may be found in individual policies limiting the right to decide on settlement may be written as "The company will settle any claim as we feel appropriate." Statements that my be found in individual policies promoting this right may include "The company will not commit the insured to any settlement without written consent." There are no clear-cut guidelines on when to settle a case and when to defend it. If the nurse is not in agreement with the insurer, whether it is an institutional or individual policy, the nurse may need to retain a personal attorney for advice. Although hiring an attorney may be thought of as extremely expensive, it really depends on what advice is needed. Before hiring an attorney, though, the nurse should let the insurer know of any dissatisfaction, which may facilitate a reasonable resolution.

The nurse should also determine whether or not the policy limitations are reduced by defense expenses. Defense expenses can add up very quickly and the right to select counsel for the nurse's defense is usually not an option with the institutional policy or individual policy, which is usually stated as "an attorney of our choice" or "the company, at its option, shall select and assign defense counsel." If the policy limitations are reduced by defense expenses, the nurse should know that the nurse would have to make up the difference if the jury verdict and defense expenses were higher than the policy limitations. For example, a $1 million policy could be reduced $200,000 for defense expenses leaving coverage of only $800,000 for settlement or a jury verdict. Therefore, the nurse should look for phrases such as "claim expenses incurred shall be paid in addition to the applicable limits of liability," so the nurse will not have to worry about defense expenses cutting into the limits of coverage.

Whether or not the defense expenses are in addition to the limits of liability, the nurse should be an active participant in any claim or lawsuit and is responsible for helping educate the attorney about the specifics of the case and spending the time necessary to gather the information needed for adequate defense of the case. However, this does not mean that for either an institutional policy or an individual policy the nurse is prevented from questioning the quality of the legal services provided and requesting another attorney for an appropriate reason. If the nurse is not satisfied with the appointed attorney and the insurance company does not reevaluate the situation, the nurse can retain or confer with independent counsel but again at personal expense. The nurse may also find that separate defense may not be provided with institutional coverage when others from the same institution are defendants. The nurse should also be aware that if a conflict of interest exists between the nurse and the insurance company and its attorney, there are situations in which the nurse may be permitted to select the defense attorney of choice to be paid by the insurance company. In the case of *Ladner v. American Home Assurance Company* (1994), a psychologist was granted the right to choose her own defense attorney. The psychologist's insurance policy included coverage for sexual claims

($25,000 limit) and professional liability claims ($1 million limit). Because it was obvious to the psychologist that it would be to the insurance company's benefit to argue that the allegations in the claim were sexually based (because of the lower monetary limit of $25,000), the psychologist argued that independent counsel should be afforded her to protect her legal and financial interests (defending the claim on the professional liability level with a limit of $1 million) rather than accepting an attorney assigned by the insurance company who would be protecting the insurance company's best interest first.

Policy Territory and Worldwide Protection

Professional liability policies may or may not provide for overseas coverage. If the nurse works outside the continental United States, then worldwide coverage needs to be seriously considered. However, even if the insurance includes injury or medical incidents that occur anywhere in the world, the claim or suit may only be covered if it is brought within the United States, its territories or possessions, or Canada. If the policy states the "claim and suit must be made against the nurse in the coverage territory," the definition section for "coverage territory" becomes critical. (There is a "definition section" in all policies that explains the insurance terms as the insurance company interprets them.)

Exclusions and Restrictions

The exclusion/restriction section identifies what the insurer does not intend to cover. Exclusions often generate negative publicity for the insurance company because when the insured does not read the policy until it is activated, the coverage may be significantly different than expected and may be specifically excluded with one small phrase. Needless to say, particular attention should be given to exclusions by the nurse so that there are no misunderstandings or surprises. Without a doubt, exclusions are laborious to review but the fine print in this section should never be overlooked. Basically, exclusions are necessary to

1. Eliminate coverage for exposures that are considered uninsurable.
2. Eliminate coverage for intentional acts of the insured (moral hazard) or extreme carelessness (moral hazard).
3. Reduce the likelihood of duplicate coverage.
4. Eliminate coverage not needed.
5. Eliminate coverage requiring special treatment or coverage that the insurance company is unqualified to offer.
6. Keep insurance premiums affordable. (Head, 1993)

Some activities that nursing professional liability policies usually do not cover are set forth in Display 22-3. These exclusions as analyzed by professional nursing organizations, were found in policies provided by the Chicago Insurance Company.

Conditions

Conditions describe the actions that the nurse (insured) must perform for coverage protection. The nurse must understand and abide by the policy conditions in order to avoid coverage cancellation. If the nurse does not act as set forth in the policy, the insurer may be released from its obligation to honor some or all of the otherwise enforceable promises in the contract. For example, the failure to provide timely notice of a claim to the insurance company may void the insurer's obligation under the policy. In *Hasbrouck v. St. Paul Fire & Marine Ins.* (1993), a physician was denied coverage under a claims-made policy because he did not notify the insurance company of a lawsuit, which alleged negligent performance of a colonoscopy, while the policy was still active. Instead, the physician hired his own private attorney and did not notify the insurance company until after the policy had expired. It was found that coverage was appropriately denied and the physician was personally responsible for the attorney expenses and settlement amount because he did not meet the condition of timely notice.

Common conditions included in a professional liability policy that will be further elaborated on are

1. Notice of an adverse occurrence
2. If a claim occurs
3. Cancellation process
4. Endorsements
5. Transfer of policy
6. Multiple policies
7. Subrogation
8. Insured and insurer limitations

Notice of an Adverse Occurrence

The nurse should notify the insurance company in writing whenever an adverse occurrence, accident, or incident occurs involving patients or others the nurse has cared for even before a claim is made. Immediate notification of an incident is not only required for coverage for some policies, but prompt investigation of the facts is also necessary to obtain the best information possible to determine the nurse's liability exposure. If a claim is subsequently filed, the nurse's position will already be formulated and an answer to the complaint will not be as difficult.

If a Claim Occurs

Depending on the policy, the specific duties of a nurse in the event of a claim or lawsuit may be straightforward or enmeshed within the other policy conditions. Some examples of general policy conditions regarding the duties of an insured in the event of a claim or possibility of a claim may include:

- Notifying your insurance company and your insurance agent in writing as soon as possible.
- Specifying the names and addresses of the injured person(s) and any witnesses.
- Providing information on the time, place, and nature of the event.
- Forwarding all documents that you receive in connection with the claim or lawsuit immediately.

DISPLAY 22-3

Exclusions

- Worker's compensation, unemployment compensation, disability benefits
- When acting as an uncovered professional, that is, those related professions stated in the policy as exclusions
- The act of loading or unloading patients for transfer
- Actual, alleged, or threatened exposure to asbestos
- Injury resulting from the hazardous properties of nuclear material
- Claims arising out of actual or alleged involvement in any antitrust law violation
- Any liability as a proprietor, superintendent, director, administrative, or executive officer
- Any claim alleging any act of sexual intimacy, sexual molestation, or sexual assault
- Personal injury arising out of the publication or utterance of a libel or slander or a publication or utterance in violation of an individual's right of privacy
- Any claim, action, judgment, settlement, loss defense, cost, or expense in any way arising out of actual, alleged, or threatened pollution, contamination, or any environmental impairment
- Any dishonest, fraudulent, criminal, or malicious acts or omissions
- Any unlawful action

- Fully cooperating in the making of settlement, the conduct of suits, or other proceedings, enforcing any right of contribution or indemnity against another who may be liable to you because of injury or damage. Attending hearings and trials, assisting in securing and giving evidence, and obtaining the attendance of witnesses.

- Refusing, except at your own cost, to voluntarily make any payment, to assume any obligation, or to incur any expense other than reasonable medical expenses incurred at the time of an event. (Nurses Service Organization, 1992, p. 1)

If You Wish to Cancel

The policy can be canceled either by the nurse or insurance company within the guidelines set forth in the policy conditions. Cancellation by the company should be sent to the nurse in writing and may be based on nonpayment of the premium, policy obtained through material misrepresentation, violation of any of the terms and conditions of the policy, the risk originally accepted significantly increased, or loss by the insurance company of reinsurance that provided coverage for all or a substantial part of the risk involved.

The insured nurse can cancel the policy at any time. In order to cancel the policy, the nurse must either return the policy to the insurance company or agent and/or mail a written notice to the company stating when the cancellation is to be effective.

The "cancellation provision" in the conditions provides further details for the process of cancellation. The number of business days to expect notification and cancellation are set forth. The insured may be entitled to refunds, which will also be explained in this section.

Endorsements

An endorsement is a document attached to the policy that can modify the original policy in some way. One reason for an endorsement is to protect the nurse against claims after coverage has expired, which is necessary with a claims-made policy. The insurance policy may state that "the terms of the policy will not be waived or changed except by written endorsement" issued as a part of the policy. The terms "reporting endorsement coverage," "tail coverage," "riders," or "prior acts coverage" are types of endorsements. However, endorsements can complicate coverage and require a court decision if more than one insurance company is involved. In the case of *Doctor's Co. v. Insurance Corporation of America* (1993), a physician had two claims-made policies. The first policy purchased by the physician was with Insurance Corp. of America and the second (or later) policy was purchased from Doctor's Company. The second policy that was purchased, from Doctor's Company, included a retroactive date or prior acts coverage. Before the first coverage expired, the physician notified Insurance Corp. of America that a lawsuit had been filed although the physician had not been named as a defendant at that time. After Insurance Corp. of America's policy expired and the Doctor's Company policy became active, the physician was added to the lawsuit as a defendant. Although both insurance companies argued that the other was responsible, the court ruled that the physician's knowledge of the lawsuit did not constitute a claim but the "notice of a demand" did. The result was that the Doctor's Company policy, with a retroactive date, was in effect when the actual demand was received and, therefore, was ordered to provide the physician's coverage.

If You Want to Transfer Coverage

In order to transfer or assign the insurance policy to anyone else, written consent must be obtained from the insurance company. In the event of the insured's death, the policy usually will continue for the benefit of the insured's legal representative. This means that if the nurse dies and a claim is brought against the nurse's estate, the individual insurance policy will continue to be valid for as long as the policy stipulates.

If You Have Multiple Policies

If the nurse is covered by an institutional or employer policy and decides to purchase individual professional liability insurance, the nurse should be aware that individual insurance conditions may transform the individual coverage to that of excess insurance. If the insurance is considered excess, then the individual coverage policy *may not* defend the claim or lawsuit. However, if the nurse's institution or employer is "self-insured," then the nurse with individual coverage might discover that the employer's self-insurance is considered excess especially if the money in reserve is lower than the nurse's coverage. Being self-insured means that the institution sets aside a certain amount of earned money to cover losses rather than buying an insurance policy and paying premiums.

If You Want to Subrogate

Subrogation is technically substituting the insurer in the place of the insured (nurse) for the purpose of collecting from a third party. The insurer becomes entitled to the insured's legal rights against a third party if the insurance company pays the entire claim and others were negligent but not insured. If several nurses were found liable for the same incident but only the insured's nurse's insurance paid, then the insured nurse's company may collect money from the other nurses through legal action. However, the nurse should understand that the insurer cannot subrogate against the insured nurse; otherwise, the purpose of owning insurance would be worthless. Whether the institution or employer will try to pursue reimbursement from the nurse for settlements or judgments paid is always a question, but one that may convince a nurse to obtain individual coverage.

Understanding Limitations of Insured and Insurer

The insurance company must cover the nurse under the terms of the policy. Because a properly executed insurance policy is a legally enforceable contract, there is legal recourse for the nurse if the insurance company fails to fulfill the terms of the policy. However, the nurse must fully comply with all the provisions of the policy to be successful in a legal action against the insurance company.

GUIDELINES FOR SELECTION OF A POLICY

After being introduced to the different parts of a professional liability policy, the nurse is ready to actively move toward selection. If the nurse already has coverage, the guidelines for selection may prove useful for evaluating the coverage already in place or for future selection. When selecting professional liability insurance, it is recommended that the nurse investigate what policies are available. Nurses may not even be aware that their institution provides an amount of liability coverage for them as the premiums are not deducted from paychecks. Other avenues to obtain coverage information are through independent insurance agents and nursing professional societies, such as The Association for Women's Health, Obstetrics and Neonatal Nursing (AWHONN), The American Association of Nurse Attorneys, Inc. (TAANA), or American Nurses Association (ANA). The nurse should try to obtain samples of actual policy documents in order to conduct a detailed examination of all parts of the policy.

Selection of a policy is an individual decision and guided by a nurse's scope of practice. Scope of practice determines exposure risk and coverage. The nurse's responsibilities and privileges are directed by each state's Nurse Practice Act. Even though policy and procedures are established within an institutional setting, they should not conflict with the standards set forth by the state in which you practice. Liability coverage should mirror the level of nursing practice you are permitted to perform. All responsibilities listed in the nurse's performance standards should be consistent with the nurse's preparation. Analysis of exposure risk and coverage begins with a comprehensive review of the job description.

Outlined in Display 22-4 are the basic guidelines that provide a framework to assist in determining which policy is appropriate for the individual nurse. Whatever type of coverage the nurse purchases, it is advised that the policy document itself be stored as long as possible and not be discarded without legal guidance.

DISPLAY 22-4

Guidelines

- Discuss institutional coverage provided by the employer with the risk manager; obtain a copy for your records if possible.
- Access the commercial market through professional organizations, insurance agents, and colleagues.
- Compare premiums; mass plans may offer savings but offer less choice in coverage.
- Identify your exposures; compare the job description with the scope of practice limits in your state.
- Insure for the biggest exposures and broadest coverage; use this chapter as a reference.
- Check the insurance carriers' financial standing by reviewing the ratings put out by A. M. Best, Moody's, or Standard & Poor's. Your agent may be able to give you a list of these ratings or check your library.
- Determine if there are any premium reductions for educational attendance.
- Investigate whether the insurance company provides additional services such as consultations, newsletters, educational programs, or any insurance reports.

THE APPLICATION PROCESS

Purchasing an insurance policy requires it to be correctly processed with the basic elements of any legal contract: offer and acceptance, consideration, competent parties, and legal purpose. To initiate the process for an individual policy, the nurse must first fill out and sign the application. Payment of a premium may be required. The act of completing the application and remittance of a premium constitutes an offer. The underwriter for the insurance company decides to accept or reject an application for insurance coverage based on specific criteria. If the nurse is found insurable according to the underwriting standards, the insurance will be effective on the date the application and premium were received and accepted. If at any time the application information changes for the nurse, such as changing employment status from "employed only" to "self-employed, solo practice," the agent of the policy must be notified immediately because this may void the policy and the nurse

may not be covered. The consideration given by the nurse is payment of the premium and agreement to abide by the requirements specified in the policy, whereas the consideration given by the insurer is to pay for injury, damage, or loss incurred by the nurse, as well as defend the nurse in a lawsuit. Although the values are not equal, this is a recognized and legally accepted difference of an insurance contract. For example, a hospital-based obstetrical nurse may pay a premium of $385.00 whereas the insurance company promises to provide $1 million liability insurance coverage for an occurrence. Finally, for the contract to be valid, the nurse must be an adult and of sound mind to be viewed as competent or the contract can be challenged.

SUMMARY

In this chapter we explored the purposes for liability coverage, its component parts, and recommendations on what to consider when purchasing malpractice liability coverage. Purchase of an individual insurance policy is not mandatory for a staff nurse because the employer usually provides coverage. However, all nurses whether they are staff nurses, inactive retired nurses, certified, advanced practice, practicing outside of an institution, or volunteering within the United States and/or abroad need to consider the advantages and disadvantages of individual personal coverage. For nurse entrepreneurs, even more extensive study is needed. If the nurse ever has any questions with the policy meaning, the nurse should not hesitate to contact the insurance company, insurance agent, or a personal attorney. Without complete knowledge, the best interest of the nurse cannot be accomplished. The nurse should not be intimidated by the insurance industry or its terminology. The nurse's choice today on what type of insurance to purchase or maintain can make a great difference for his or her future.

REFERENCES

American Association of Nurse Attorneys, Inc. (1989). Demonstrating financial responsibility for nursing practice (p. 1).

American Nurses Association. (1995). Chicago insurance company. Chicago, IL, POP2028 (1/95) (elec).

Head, George. (1993). Essentials of risk financing, Volume I (2nd ed., p. 184). Malvern, PA: Insurance Institute of America.

The John Liner Organization. (1994). The risk manager's guide to the new insurance market (p. 51). Boston: Standard Publishing.

Nurses Service Organization. (1992, March). CNA insurance company. Chicago, IL, G-58032-B(ED 03/92), (pp. 1, 5).

Rejda, George. (1989). Principles of insurance (p. 20). Glenview, IL: Scott, Foresman.

CASE CITATIONS

Doctor's Co. v. Insurance Corporation of America, 864 P.2d 1018 (Wyo. 1993).

Hasbrouck v. St. Paul Fire & Marine Ins., 511 N.W.2d 364 (Iowa 1993).

Ladner v. American Home Assurance Company, 607 N.Y. S.2d 276 (A.D. 1 Dept 19).

Legler v. Meriwether, 391 S.W.2d 599 (1965).

The University of North Carolina v. Shoemate, 437 S.E.2d 892 (N.C. App. Ct. App. 1994).

CHAPTER
23

Advanced Practice Nursing

Teresa Dossey James

Debates on health care reform have been going on in the United States since 1917. In the late 1980s, however, increasing costs of health care started to impact the middle class for the first time. It was no longer an attitude of "something we should do for someone else." In the early 1990s, it seemed the federal government would be the source of changing health care delivery through federal legislation. Although many of the promised reforms did not occur, health care delivery did undergo significant changes as a result of market forces. Managed care became the method to provide comprehensive health care while keeping costs contained.

One of the major goals of managed care is to keep patients out of hospitals or shorten the stay as much as possible in order to be more cost effective. This has led to a decreased need for nurses in hospitals. Many of these nurses are moving to alternative settings for health care and expanding their practices. Advanced practice nurses are in great demand for health promotion activities, case management of chronically ill and complicated acute care patients, and providing primary care as an integral member of the health care team. These expanded roles carry with them unique liability issues.

DEFINING ADVANCED PRACTICE NURSING

Advanced practice nurses are registered nurses with additional formal education and clinical preparation, resulting in either a certificate or master's degree. Many states have recently passed legislation to phase out the acceptance of certificates for advanced practice nurses and instead require additional formal education to achieve advanced practice status. The recognized advanced practice specialties are certified registered nurse anesthetist, certified nurse midwife, nurse practitioner, and clinical nurse specialist.

Although recently there has been a strong move towards increasing the use of advanced practiced nurses, prohibitions against nurses practicing in advanced roles have a long history in this country. Prohibitions against nurses practicing in advanced roles have a long history in this country. The earliest recorded case was *Commonwealth v. Porn* in 1907, when the Massachusetts state court upheld the conviction of a nurse midwife for practicing medicine without a license.

Certified Registered Nurse Anesthetist (CRNA)

Nurse anesthesia was the first expanded role for nurses. In the 1900s, nurse anesthetists attained legal recognition through certification and education. They won the first challenge to their practice in 1936 when the California Supreme Court ruled in the case of *Chalmers-Francis v. Nelson* that providing anesthesia was not within the definition of diagnosing or prescribing, which were actions prohibited to nurses by the medical practice act.

Certified Nurse Midwife (CNM)

A short time later, nurse midwifery was legally recognized as a profession. These advanced practice nurses have also encountered frequent opposition to their practice. A Massachusetts case *Leigh v. Board of Registration in Nursing,* (1985) decided that the basis for conviction in the previously cited *Commonwealth v. Porn* (1907) was not the actual practice of midwifery, but rather the use of obstetric instruments and prescription formulas. The profession continues to try to clearly define the practice of midwifery.

Nurse Practitioner (NP)

A shortage of primary care physicians in the 1960s led to the development of an expanded nursing role. In 1965, the first nurse practitioner program was started to teach nurses advanced patient care skills. Nurse practitioners now regularly perform functions that were once exclusively within the scope of medical practice, including the diagnosis and management of common acute health problems, as well as chronic diseases.

In *Bellegie, M.D. v. Texas Board of Nurse Examiners* (1985), the Texas Medical Association and Texas Hospital Association challenged the right of the Board of Nurse Examiners to set rules regulating advanced nursing practice. The court ruled the board had the authority to create a class of advanced nurse practitioner based on educational preparation, and to regulate the activities of nurses holding themselves out as having advanced training. This ruling was upheld by the Texas Court of Appeals in 1996.

Clinical Nurse Specialist (CNS)

The most recent category of advanced practice nurse is the clinical nurse specialist. This role evolved in the 1960s as nurses with clinical expertise who did not want to move into the tradition-

al fields of administration or education looked for other areas of clinical nursing so they could continue to work directly with patients and families. The clinical nurse specialist was defined by the American Nurses Association (ANA) in 1974 as a practitioner holding a master's degree with a concentration in a specific area of clinical nursing. This expanded role also includes proficiency in teaching, research, and consultation. Most clinical nurse specialists are certified through the ANA or a professional specialty organization. Unlike other advanced practice nurses, the clinical nurse specialist is more likely to be a hospital employee rather than an independent practitioner.

STATE NURSE PRACTICE ACTS AND ADVANCED PRACTICE NURSING

There have been nurse practice acts in every state since 1952. These acts are designed to protect the public by defining the practice of nursing, establishing the legal scope of nursing, and setting standards for the nursing profession. Each act includes the minimal qualifications a nurse must have to acquire and retain a nursing license. They also list any violations that could lead to disciplinary action against a nurse.

Nurse practice acts generally fall within three classifications: traditional, transitional, and administrative. The first nurse practice acts were all traditional, based on the model proposed by the American Nurses Association (ANA) in 1955. They prohibited nurses from performing tasks that were considered to be medical practice. For advanced practice nursing, most significant were the exclusion of independent diagnosis and treatment of medical conditions from the scope of nursing practice. The few states still using this approach usually do not address advanced practice roles. However, some do include expanded roles for nurses in their medical practice acts.

Next evolved the transitional approach. These states often permit evaluation and diagnosis, but do not allow independent treatment by nurses. They authorize advanced nursing with physician supervision and/or standing orders. As of 1996, there were 15 states in this category. Occasionally, committees of physicians, nurses, and other health professionals issue joint statements recommending that nurses be allowed to diagnosis and treat under certain circumstances. These statements have no legal standing until the state legislature amends its nurse practice act to broaden the definition of nursing.

Most states now use the administrative approach. This allows both physicians and nurses to diagnose and treat patients. The state board of nursing is usually given authority to devise the rules for advanced nursing practice, eliminating the need for legislative action.

Considerable time is required to investigate, draft, and enact laws, so most nurse practice acts are broadly worded to prevent the need for frequent revisions as technology changes. When necessary, amendments can be used to change a nurse practice act. Amendments may give nurses legal permission to perform certain procedures or functions that have become accepted practice in the community. Redefinition is a legislative action where the actual definition of nursing is rewritten. For example, if the definition of "diagnosis" is changed to include "nursing diagnosis," the meaning of the entire nurse practice act may be altered. It is vital that a definition of the term "nursing diagnosis" is included. Many nurse practice acts contain such confusing language that it is difficult to determine the difference between nursing and medical diagnosis.

It is the responsibility of every nurse to be familiar with the legal scope of nursing practice in his or her state. Except in life-threatening emergencies, those limits cannot be exceeded without risk of disciplinary action. Nurses must be aware of not only the current nurse practice act, but also any newly adopted rules and amendments. Although nurse practice acts are used for guidance during legal actions, the court always has the ultimate decision in interpreting the rules and regulations.

Licensure

In 1985, the National Council of State Boards of Nursing (NCSBN) recommended that each state develop regulations for advanced clinical nursing practice. They proposed mandatory licensure of the "Advanced Practice Registered Nurse." These proposals influenced the policy of state boards of nursing but led to wide diversity in regulations among states.

In March 1992, NCSBN released a draft of model legislation and a position statement calling for a second license for nurses in advanced practice. The model was designed to provide guidance to state boards on the regulation of nurses in advanced practice. The goal of the NCSBN was the national standardization of requirements, philosophies, and policies for advanced practice nursing.

The model specified three levels of practice within the profession of nursing that would be regulated and controlled: licensed practical nurse, registered nurse, and licensed "other" nurse, which would include the four categories of advanced practice nurses. The advanced practice of nursing is defined as "practice based on the knowledge and skills acquired in a basic nursing education, through licensure as a registered nurse, and in graduate education and experience, including advanced nursing theory, physical and psycho-social assessment, and treatment of illness." The definition also specified that advanced practice nurses make independent decisions in solving complex patient care problems, and performing acts of diagnosis and prescription of therapeutic measures. Requirements for advanced practice licensure included a graduate level academic degree with a major in nursing and professional certification.

One goal of the proposal was to provide clear authority for advanced practice and thus offer protection from inadvertently performing beyond the legal scope of nursing practice. The NCSBN believes that standard policies will facilitate direct reimbursement from third-party payors, provide title protection, and promote the highest level of public protection.

Certification

The NCSBN is concerned about the variety and lack of consistency in professional certification. There can be significant differences in title, educational requirements, and scope of practice among advanced practice nurses. This inconsistency makes it difficult for boards to develop criteria broad enough to accommodate the variations yet specific enough to be effective. Certification exams have traditionally been designed for professional recognition and may not be useful in legal regulation. In August 1996, a subcommittee of NCSBN recommended the development of standardized core competency exams for advanced practice nursing, with state boards as the certifying bodies, rather than specialty organization. The suggestion that boards of nursing would determine who is an advanced practice nurse has implications for educational curricula, standards of practice, and scope of practice.

Hospital Privileges

Merging the roles of nurse practitioner and clinical nurse specialist has expanded the definition of advanced practice nursing beyond the traditional ambulatory primary care provider role. Many advanced practice nurses also provide care for patients in tertiary care settings that require hospital privileges.

Most states now require hospitals to award clinical privileges to qualified advanced practice nurses based on education and demonstrated competence. Health care institutions cannot defend a credentialing system that excludes licensed providers who are not physicians, thus interfering with those providers' ability to compete in the marketplace. A hospital that refuses privileges has a legal responsibility to notify the individual of the reason. The hospital may be sued for restraint of trade if it is determined the denial was based on the medical staff's attempt to limit competition. *Bhan v. National Medical Enterprises Hospitals, Inc.* (1985) and *Nurse Midwifery Associates v. Hibbett* (1988) upheld the right to practice for nurse anesthetists and nurse midwives, respectively.

The hospital credentials committee is responsible for evaluating each applicant applying for hospital privileges and reviewing matters concerning the clinical or ethical conduct of health providers. Advanced practice nurses are usually required to provide such basic items as current licensure, proof of liability insurance, and personal and/or professional references. Also needed may be national certification by a profes-

sional organization, documentation of credentials to practice as an advanced practice nurse, and a sponsoring physician from the hospital staff. The credentials committee may request submission of advanced practice nursing protocols for their review if none are currently in use. Peer review and due process protection should be available to all staff on the same basis.

Nurses who request privileges to perform more complicated procedures should be able to provide documentation of training and demonstration of competence. The request for privileges should clarify which advanced skills are performed according to nursing judgment, after physician consultation, according to established practice guidelines, or with more than one qualified provider present. Probationary or initial observation periods should be consistent with those required for physicians.

SCOPE OF PRACTICE

Scope of practice refers to the legal limits within which a health professional is permitted to perform. State legislatures often use the national standards of a profession or specialty to help them define the scope of practice. Legal boundaries of the scope of nursing practice frequently do not clearly delineate between the practice of nursing and that of other health professions, nor between the expanded role of the advanced practice nurse and nurses in general. The ANA states that the scope of advanced practice nursing is distinguished by autonomy of practice and self-initiated treatment regimens.

Physicians were the first health care practitioners to gain legislative recognition of their practice. In the 1800s, a well-organized effort ensured that only physicians were granted the exclusive right to practice, establishing themselves as the legal and official medical profession. Their scope of practice was defined by statute as curing, diagnosing, treating, and prescribing. This all-encompassing definition also made it illegal for anyone not licensed as a physician to perform these acts.

In the early 1900s, the first nursing laws mandated registration or certification by the state. Tasks not specifically included in the medical scope of practice were selected for legal recognition of the nursing role. Nurses' independent functions were the supervision of patients, observation of symptoms and reactions, and accurate recording of facts. The remainder of the nursing scope of practice was subordinate to the physician. In 1955, the ANA developed a definition of nursing that did not require physician supervision of all nursing functions, but did prohibit diagnosis and treatment. This definition was amended in 1970 to include the right of nurses to take on expanded roles with proper preparation and to eliminate the prohibition on nursing diagnosis. In 1971, Idaho became the first state to include diagnosis and treatment within the scope of advanced practice nurses. They required every institution that employed nurse practitioners to develop guidelines for their expanded role.

There are two legal areas where nursing scope of practice issues commonly occur: when there is negligence within the scope of practice or when there is a possibility that practice boundaries have been exceeded.

The first situation is illustrated by a case in California. *Cooper v. National Motor Bearing Co.* (1955) involved an occupational health nurse who failed to recognize that a patient's signs and symptoms were consistent with cancer and did not refer the patient to his physician for treatment. The court ruled the nurse had sufficient education to be able to diagnose whether to treat or refer the patient. Although diagnosis was legally outside the scope of nursing practice at that time, the court decided it was called for to a limited extent. In a later case, *Stahlin v. Hilton Hotels Corp.* (1973), a federal court in Illinois found that the nurse should have determined that the patient's complaints indicated a subdural hematoma, not alcohol intoxication. Here again, the court found limited diagnosis to be within the nursing scope of practice. Courts expect nurses at all educational levels to possess some degree of competency in medical diagnosis and evaluation of treatment. These courts also held that nurses with greater degrees of formal education should possess greater expertise.

The second scope of practice situation is an accusation that the advanced practice nurse breached the boundaries of nursing practice. A Florida court in *Hernicz v. Florida Dept. of Professional Regulation* (1980), ruled that a nurse practitioner should have his license suspended for examining and treating patients without a physician's supervision. In a case in Missouri, *Sermchief v. Gonzalez* (1983), physicians from the state medical board accused two nurse practitioners of practicing medicine illegally. The physicians who signed standing orders for the nurses were also sued. The state court dismissed the case, stating that diagnosis and treatment by nurses, according to standing orders and protocols, were within the nursing scope of practice. It ruled that professional nurses have a right to practice within the limits of their education and experience, which placed considerable emphasis on the nurses' graduate education. Recognizing the trend of independence in nursing practice, the court declared that the functions of diagnosis and prescription were no longer the exclusive territory of physicians.

Occasionally state nurse practice acts and hospital policy are not in agreement on the scope of nursing practice. Although hospital policy often is more detailed, an employer cannot legally expand the scope of practice to include tasks prohibited by the nurse practice act. In *O'Neill v. Montefiore Hospital* (1960), the court ruled that when there is a discrepancy, the nurse must choose the practice act over hospital policy. This was later reinforced in the case of *Lunsford v. Board of Nurse Examiners* (1983).

STANDARDS OF CARE

Standards of care are the minimum skills a nurse must possess in order to provide an acceptable level of care. They are not the ideal, as is often thought, but rather are the minimum common skills and education considered adequate by the profession. Although standards of care are not law, they have important legal significance. An accusation of malpractice is based on the premise that the standard of care was not met. The nurse's actions are judged against reasonable standards of care. The classic test is "What would a reasonably prudent nurse, with similar education and experience, do under similar circumstances?"

Advanced practice nurses are often judged by the standards for physicians, rather than for other nurses. As early as 1925, the court used the medical standard to judge the actions of a nurse midwife. In *Olson v. Bolstad* (1925), a suit against the midwife's consulting physician was disallowed. The court found that the physician relied on the midwife to perform her duties properly and thus incurred no liability. In *Mohr v. Jenkins* (1980), a nurse anesthetist was accused of incorrectly injecting a medication, which resulted in phlebitis. The suit was dismissed because the court found that the nurse performed the procedure correctly and conformed to accepted medical practice. A similar case in Michigan, *Whitney v. Day* (1980), held that nurse anesthetists are professionals with expertise similar to medical practice. Therefore, they can be held to the same practice standards as physicians.

Other courts have used advanced practice nursing as the standard. In *Fein v. Permanente Medical Group* (1985), a nurse practitioner misdiagnosed myocardial infarction as muscle spasm and gave the patient Valium. The trial court determined that because the nurse practitioner made a diagnosis, the applicable standard of care was the medical standard. The California Supreme Court disagreed and ruled that a nurse practitioner should be held to the standard of a reasonably prudent nurse practitioner. In *Harrison v. Michael Reese Hospital* (1988), a clinical nurse specialist failed to notify the physician of an infant's jaundice for the first 5 days of life. The court found malpractice because the standard of care for the nursing specialty was not met. The New York State Court of Appeals held advanced practice nurses to a higher standard of care in *Toth v. Community Hospital at Glen Cove* (1968). This case involved premature twins whose blindness was caused by an excessive level of oxygen administered by the clinical nurse specialist. The court found that practitioners must use any advanced skill and knowledge they possess. Just meeting the acceptable practice of a prudent nurse is insufficient.

STANDARDIZED PROCEDURES/ PROTOCOLS/GUIDELINES

State regulation of advanced practice nurses usually includes a requirement for written guidelines to direct the practice. These may include standardized procedures and protocols, scope of practice statements, and standing orders. Courts use these guidelines to help determine the nursing standard of care and scope of practice. If the guideline is vague or too broad, the court may interpret it very restrictively. Too detailed a protocol may be impossible to meet. Guidelines must reflect the actual practice and be specific for the patient population. All protocols should be reviewed on an annual basis to ensure that they reflect the current practice provided, as well as community standards. Any deviation from community practice not supported by appropriate medical and scientific principles may expose the advanced practice nurse to liability. It is the responsibility of the nurse to ensure compliance with state statutes on written guidelines, and not the responsibility of the facility or collaborating physician in the practice.

Whenever there is a charge of negligence, malpractice, or other liability action, attorneys may request copies of any pertinent guidelines in existence at the time of the incident. It is important to keep all protocols including any revisions. These guidelines will be compared to the documentation of care for the patient to see if they were followed.

In those states requiring that advanced practice nurses work under a collaborative agreement or in practice with a physician, it is extremely important that the physician be clearly identified and co-sign the protocol. The guideline should also describe the situations requiring physician referral or consultation.

Although standardized protocols and standing orders have become common practice, their legality is still often challenged. In 1988, the attorney general of Georgia issued an opinion that public health nurses had no statutory authority to prescribe medications such as birth control pills under the guidelines of a written protocol (1988

Op. Att'y Gen. 9). Although the attorney general acknowledged that prescribing by protocol was a common nursing practice in public health clinics in the state, he interpreted the nurse practice act to authorize only the administration of medications that had been ordered by physicians. It is advisable to review protocols from a legal standpoint to ensure they fall within the permissible scope of nursing practice.

LIABILITY

Nurses in expanded roles face dual legal liabilities. They are licensed as registered nurses, so their scope of practice still includes those skills expected of all nurses. As such, they are accountable to the rules and regulations of the state board of nursing. Added to that are the expanded knowledge and skills required to direct patient care and those increased responsibilities. There is no published information on the number of advanced practice nurses named as defendants in malpractice actions. However, the number of nurses in general named as defendants in medical malpractice cases rose 500% from 1983 to 1989, and the number of nurses named as sole defendants has also increased significantly.

The National Practitioner Data Bank was established as a result of the Health Care Quality Improvement Act of 1986 and became effective September 1, 1990. It requires that physicians and dentists, but not nurses, report results of peer-review activities that suggest substandard care. However, all medical malpractice payments made on behalf of any licensed health care professional and any adverse actions against their license to practice must be reported to the Data Bank.

Advanced practice nurses often provide the same patient care as physicians. This does not mean they are guilty of unauthorized medical practice, but they cannot always be sure how their actions will be interpreted by the courts. As expanded roles become better understood, this legal risk should decrease. In order to protect themselves, nurses must be familiar with the statutory definitions of expanded roles. One way

this can be done is to request an opinion from the state attorney general to clarify what procedures are allowed or prohibited. Another is to review recent judicial decisions that include definitions of roles. Professional organizations may issue joint statements on scope of practice. It may also be helpful to review the state medical practice act and pharmacy act. These acts sometime contain language that expands the nurse's role, especially in those states that do not specify advanced practice in their nurse practice acts.

Informed consent is one of the traditional areas of physician responsibility now shared by advanced practice nurses. Essential elements to relate to the patient include the diagnosis, recommended care or treatment, risks involved, benefits of treatment and prospect for success, prognosis if care or treatment is not provided, and alternative care or treatment, if any. Defense lawyers recommend a brief progress note describing the informed consent discussion. Such a note would have been helpful for two nurse anesthetists were found liable for failure to fully inform the patient of all the risks of the anesthesia procedure in *Steele v. Ft. Sanders Anesthesia Group*, 1995.

Advanced practice nursing offers flexibility and responsiveness to clients as an alternative to the medical model, which is one reason for the low number of lawsuits. Unfortunately, this flexibility sometimes attracts patients with unrealistic or unsafe expectations. It is important to maintain minimum standards of safety. If the patient and nurse cannot agree on a mutually acceptable level of care, the patient should be encouraged to seek care elsewhere, with adequate time to find substitute care in order to prevent a charge of abandonment.

Primary Liability

Every professional is responsible for his or her own actions. This is known as direct or primary liability, based upon one's own conduct. The amount of liability of the advanced practice nurse is determined by the degree of independence in the nurse's practice. The Joint Commission on Accreditation of Healthcare Organizations (JCAHO) defines an independent practitioner as an individual who is permitted by law and hospital policy to provide patient care services without direction or supervision, within the scope of license and individually granted clinical privileges. The authority of the advanced practice nurse does not come from the authority of a physician's license. When functioning as an independent practitioner, the nurse has total responsibility in the event of a lawsuit.

Vicarious Liability

Vicarious liability is a legal liability based upon a relationship rather than upon individual conduct. Many insurers have claimed that a physician who works with an advanced practice nurse is at risk of being held liable for any negligence by the nurse. Hospitals have also used vicarious liability to hold consulting physicians liable for the advanced practice nurse. When a hospital requires an employment relationship between an advanced practice nurse and the consulting physician as a condition of granting privileges, this may violate federal antitrust law. It forces two independent contractors to function as a single entity, preventing any possibility of competition between them. Sometimes an insurer or hospital will require strict personal supervision, thus creating a basis for vicarious liability. Without such a rule, the consultant/referral relationship would be the same as when two physicians care for the same patient. In *Kavanaugh v. Nussbaum* (1988), the court did not find the first doctor liable for the second, on the basis that he had no right or authority to control the actions of the physician on call. When two professionals treat a patient, neither is vicariously liable for the other's negligence. Unless there is a right to control, however, one may be found liable if he or she observed malpractice and negligently allowed it to continue. This is direct liability, not vicarious.

Independent Practice

Consultation is a mechanism for an advanced practice nurse, who maintains primary management responsibility for the patient's care, to seek the advice of a physician or another health care team member. Collaboration occurs when an advanced practice nurse and physician jointly manage the care of a patient who has become medically complicated. When the physician must assume a dominant role, the nurse may continue to participate in physical care, counseling, guidance, teaching, and support. Referral is the process by which the advanced practice nurse directs the patient to a physician or another health care professional for management of a particular problem or aspect of the care.

Hospital or Physician Employee

Courts used to assume that the physician had total control of a patient's care, like a ship's captain. Thus the physician was liable for anything that went wrong, no matter who was negligent. This was known as the doctrine of "captain of the ship." Another doctrine, the "borrowed servant," held that when the physician admitted patients to the hospital, the hospital employees were borrowed to help provide care, again making the physician liable rather than the hospital. Although still existing in a few jurisdictions, both of these legal doctrines are nearly obsolete. When the nurse is an employee of an institution or physician, the doctrine of *respondeat superior* applies. The employer is usually held liable when the employee's negligent act or omission occurred within the scope of employment.

Sometimes it is unclear when an advanced practice nurse and a physician provide services to the same patient whether one is the employee of the other, or whether they are independent contractors working in collaboration. The court will consider to what extent one controls the actions of the other; which party supplies the instruments, tools, and place of work; the length of the relationship; the method of payment; and whether they regard themselves as employer and employee. Another consideration is the apparent agent principle, which holds that whether the patient perceives the nurse is an employee is more important than whether it is true. Advanced practice nurses should always clarify for patients their independent role, and the relationship between the nurse and the consulting physician. In *Hernicz v. State of Florida, Dept. of Professional Regulation* (1980), a nurse was held liable for failure to inform a patient of the expanded nursing role and that the expanded nurse practitioner was not a physician.

Impact of Managed Care

Third-party payers have had a significant impact on liability for all health care professionals. One area seen more frequently is denial of hospitalization or early discharge of patients when payers refuse reimbursement. In a landmark case, *Wickline v. State of California* (1986), the physician requested an 8-day extension of hospitalization, but Medicare approved only 4 days. Although the physician did not agree with the decision, he did not utilize the process in place to appeal the decision by Medicare. The patient was discharged at the end of the 4-day extension and later developed serious complications after discharge. The California Appellate court found that Medicare was not liable because the ultimate decision to discharge was the physician's. The court held that it was the provider's duty to protest adverse payment decisions. Another case, *Wilson v. Blue Cross of Southern California* (1990), involved a physician request for inpatient psychiatric care. The payor ruled that hospitalization was not required, and the patient later committed suicide. The court held that payors are liable for injury to patients regardless of whether the provider protests.

Corcoran v. United Heathcare Inc. (1992) involved a case of a high-risk pregnancy. The physician recommended complete bedrest, but the payor decided hospitalization was not necessary. Complications developed and the fetus died. The payor was found liable for making negligent medical decisions that the patient followed due to financial constraints. With these conflicting court decisions, the best risk management for the advanced practice nurse is to protest all adverse payment decisions. Using the appropriate procedural process, experienced providers have learned that payors will often pay if providers persistently protest.

EXPANDED SCOPE OF PRACTICE

Advanced practice nursing includes many roles beyond that of direct patient care provider. These may include education for patients and their families, as well as other health care providers, consultation, and clinical research.

Patient Educator

Advanced practice nurses are often responsible for providing patient education. As early as 1898, the court found that health care providers had a duty to give the patient or family all necessary and proper instructions as to the care of the patient and the precautions to be observed (*Pike v. Honsinger,* 1898). Patient instruction must be thorough, and the nurse should ensure that the individual understands and can perform the procedures. Including a family member in the teaching and documenting the entire process is extremely helpful. In *Kyslinger v. United States* (1975), it was alleged that a patient and spouse did not receive adequate instruction in operation of a home dialysis unit. The court rejected the claim when it was proven that the patient received ten months of instruction. Reevaluation of self-care skills is also important, especially for chronic patients. Regardless of specific patient outcomes, patients and families are less likely to sue if they have been actively involved in the treatment regimen.

In Idaho, the Board of Nursing suspended a nurse's license because she discussed alternative therapy with a cancer patient. The Idaho Supreme Court revoked the suspension and ordered reinstatement of the license because the nurse practice act had no provision that patient education was outside the scope of practice (*Tuma v. Board of Nursing* 1979).

Professional Educator

JCAHO requires that all members of the nursing staff are competent to fulfill their assigned responsibilities. Often the advanced practice nurse is given the task of verifying nursing staff competency prior to independent practice. If the advanced practice nurse becomes aware that a staff nurse is not complying with a standard of care and does not try to correct the situation, the expert nurse may be held individually liable. In providing staff education, the advanced practice nurse must be aware of professional standards and document staff participation in training.

Consultant

The advanced practice nurse is frequently used as a consultant in the development of institutional policies and procedures, which must ensure compliance with federal, state, and local law, as well as JCAHO and professional organization standards. Each policy should reflect actual practice and be revised periodically to reflect clinical advancements. A well-written policy that reflects acceptable standards of care, combined with documentation of adherence to the policy, is a vital tool in the successful defense of a malpractice case.

Many advanced practice nurses are serving in consultant roles, making them increasingly accountable for their knowledge and problem-solving skills. Nurses are covered for consultation services under their professional liability policies only when these duties are within the scope of their employment or assigned to them by their employer. Nurses providing independent consultation services for a fee should check with their insurance carrier to be certain that they are covered for their extended role. Liability insurance designed specifically for the consultation process does exist. This coverage, however, usually is available only through the national counseling organizations that serve various types of consultants.

The best defense for independent consultants is to maintain an open relationship with clients, including feedback to determine if expectations are being met. A written contract should include the expectations of both parties and the agreed-upon outcomes. Careful adherence to a predeveloped set of guidelines may provide some legal protection.

Clinical Research

The advanced practice nurse plays a significant role in enhancing nursing practice through clinical research. This responsibility has been clearly identified by the nursing profession for nurse specialists. However, the nurse must be aware that when they treat a patient in whom they also have a research interest there is a high potential for conflict of interest.

Any nurse who engages in clinical research is required to obtain informed consent, which includes a description of the treatment being proposed, any potential risks, and alternative methods of treatment and their risks. The patient must also be advised that participation is voluntary, confidential, will have no effect on any other medical or nursing services they receive, and they may withdraw from the study at any time.

PRESCRIPTIVE AUTHORITY

Less than 60 years ago, not only did consumers have access to all the drugs now classified as nonnarcotic prescriptive drugs, but many nurses also worked independently from physicians and made drug therapy recommendations within their normal scope of practice. All that was changed by the 1938 Federal Food, Drug and Cosmetic Act. Physicians were chosen as the providers to prescribe medications.

In many states, prescriptive authority for advanced practice nurses remains controversial. Laws for prescriptive authority may be found in nursing, medical, and pharmacy practice acts or controlled substance acts. The Boards of Pharmacy and Medicine are often involved, either as advisors or on a joint committee, in the development of the rules and regulations for prescriptive authority for nurses. Although there may be written legal authority to prescribe, state attorney generals have issued opposing statements, or pharmacists have refused to honor nurse prescriptions because of conflicting pharmacy regulations. Occasionally, vague nurse and medical practice acts have facilitated the expansion of nursing practice by allowing physicians to delegate their activities to nurses without violating the acts of either profession.

A variety of techniques have been used to enable advanced practice nurses to "prescribe" for their patients in those states that do not grant prescriptive privileges. These include using prescription pads pre-signed by a physician, calling the prescription into a pharmacy, co-signing the prescription with the physician's and nurse name, utilizing standing order protocols, or distributing stocked medication. Some of these methods are explicitly prohibited by law in some states; all are potentially in conflict with pharmacy or nursing regulations and of ambiguous legality.

There are two types of prescriptive authority: substitutive and complementary. Substitutive jurisdictions are states in which advanced practice nurses have the authority to prescribe without the supervision of a physician and therefore function as "substitutes" for physicians. As of 1996, 15 states allow this independent authority. States where advanced practice nurses may prescribe drugs, but only in conjunction with a supervising physician, are called complementary jurisdictions. There is much controversy over the definition of the word "supervise" and the use of standard protocols.

Regulations may require the development of a formulary or written practice guidelines to identify the medications and circumstances under which they can be prescribed. A recent trend is the requirement for additional educational courses in pharmacology for advanced practice nurses. Some states require application for prescriptive authority separate from that necessary for practice. The first limited prescriptive authority was granted to advanced practice nurses in North Carolina in 1975. As of 1996, only two states, Illinois and Oklahoma, still specifically prohibited nurse prescriptions. For state-by-state information about prescriptive authority, see Table 23-1.

The major law regulating the prescription and administration of drugs is the Federal Controlled Substance Act. Practitioners who dispense controlled substances are required to register with the Drug Enforcement Agency (DEA) of the United States Department of Justice. The DEA determines who is authorized to prescribe, dispense, administer, or conduct research with controlled substances under the laws of the state in which they practice. They also have the authority to take disciplinary actions of revocation, denial, and suspension.

The lack of standard definitions in federal and state statutes has been a major obstacle to advanced practice nurses' efforts to prescribe. The DEA requires independent authority as a prerequisite to the issuance of a DEA registration. If the advanced practice nurse is employed by a physician with DEA registration, the nurse is not entitled to a personal DEA registration. If the nurse prescribed a drug that resulted in harm to the patient and was sued, the physician could also be sued, so many physicians are unwilling to accept this risk.

REIMBURSEMENT

Many reimbursement laws at both the federal and state levels have been unfair to advanced practice nurses. The Comprehensive Omnibus Budget Reconciliation Act (COBRA) of 1985 severely limited reimbursement to advanced practice nurses. Nurse midwives were covered only for services throughout the maternity cycle, not for family planning or gynecological care. These maternity services were reimbursed at 65% of the physician fee schedule amount. Nurse practitioner services covered under Medicare were limited to specified basic situations, and each required that the nurse work in collaboration with a physician. Their reimbursement was also capped at a percentage of the physician fee schedule. The COBRA 1989 specified Medicaid coverage only for family and pediatric nurse practitioners. This restrictive language was a problem because of the variety of advanced practice nurse titles and designations. The law also granted direct reimbursement only for services by nurse practitioners in rural areas. States have broad discretion in determining both fee levels and payment methodology to advanced practice nurses under Medicaid. Recently, states that mandate direct third-party reimbursement have ruled that any service covered for other providers will be covered for advanced practice nurses operating within their state-defined scope of practice. However, this ruling has been preempted by new federal legislation allowing block grant funding to states for Medicaid patients.

TABLE 23-1. American Nurses Association© 1997 Prescriptive Authority Chart

State	Type of Practitioner	Drug Schedules Under Which Practitioner Has Authority to Prescribe	Is Practice Agreement Collaboration, or Protocol Required to Prescribe?	Remarks
Alabama	NP, CNM	Noncontrolled drugs only	Yes	Must be in collaborative relationship, working under a protocol.
Alaska*	NP[1], CRNA	II–V	No	Must have an approved consultation plan.
Arizona*	NP	II–V[2]	No	Must have "collaborative," i.e., consultative or referral, relationship with a physician. No specific protocol required. Schedules IV–V: 34-day supply.
Arkansas	NP, CNS+	II–V◊	Yes	Law allows certified NPs to prescribe drugs when in collaborative practice agreement, to include protocols.
California	NP	Noncontrolled drugs only	Yes	Protocol is required to prescribe. (Although NPs cannot apply for DEA Registration numbers in California, they can be issued "furnishing numbers" by the state.)

[1]NP includes NP and CNMs

NP = Nurse Practitioner, CNS = Clinical Nurse Specialist, CNM = Nurse Midwife, CRNA = Certified Registered Nurse Anesthetist.

Both controlled and noncontrolled drugs require a prescription. Controlled drugs are organized according to schedule (II–V), with the lowest schedule number having the highest potential for abuse. Noncontrolled drugs include antibiotics, analgesics, and anti-inflammatory medications, among others.

*States where nurses can apply for their own DEA numbers

+As long as CNS is licensed as an ARNP

◊DEA numbers on hold

[2]Previously Arizona limited schedule II–III to 48-hr supply in 1996 to amend law for consistency in schedule IV–V authority.

TABLE 23-1. *(cont.)*				
Colorado*	NP, CNS, CNM, CRNA	II–V	No	Prescriptive authority collaborative agreement must exist; however, law specifically states that nothing shall be construed to limit the liability of the APN to make an independent judgment, or to require supervision by a physician.
Connecticut*	NP, CNM, CNS, NA	II–V	Yes	Limitations on scope of prescriptive authority of CRNA based upon certification. Limitations on Schedules II & III for NP and CNS.
Delaware	APN, CNS, NP	II–V under drug schedules and can apply for their own DEA numbers	Yes	Must be under collaborative arrangement and in compliance with joint practice committee rules.
District of Columbia*	NP, CNM, CRNA, CNS	II–V	Yes	Must be in collaborative relationship with appropriate health care provider.
Florida (M)	NP, CNS	Noncontrolled drugs only	Yes	Under statutory-authorized protocol and practice agreement. CNS can prescribe only if licensed as ARNP.
Georgia	NP	None	Yes	No independent prescriptive authority, but APN can be delegated authority to order controlled substances and dangerous drugs under formulary.
Hawaii	APN	Noncontrolled drugs only	Yes	Per formulary.
Idaho	NP	Noncontrolled drugs only	Yes	Joint regulation of prescriptive authority; w/protocol, inclusive formulary.

(continued)

TABLE 23-1. *(cont.)*

State	Type of Practitioner	Drug Schedules Under Which Practitioner Has Authority to Prescribe	Is Practice Agreement Collaboration, or Protocol Required to Prescribe?	Remarks
Illinois				Legislative efforts are underway for 1998.
Indiana[3]	NP, CNS	II–V	Yes	In collaboration with licensed MDs as evidenced by practice agreement or privileges.
Iowa*	NP, CRNA, NMW, CNS	II–V	No	Physician's assistant or registered nurse may supply when pharmacist services are not reasonably available or when it is in the best interests of the patient, on the direct order of the supervising physician, a quantity of properly packaged and labeled prescription drugs, controlled substances, or contraceptive devices necessary to complete a course of therapy.
Kansas	NP, CNS+	Noncontrolled drugs only	Yes	NPs and CNSs may prescribe under jointly adopted protocols between the nurse and "the responsible physician," excluding controlled drugs.
Kentucky	ARNP (NP, CNM, CNS, CRNA) Legal designation is ARNP	Noncontrolled drugs only Nonscheduled legend drugs	Yes Does not affect CRNA practice.	ARNPs have non-scheduled legend drugs (noncontrolled) prescriptive authority. Use designated Board of Nursing ARNP number to track ARNP prescriptive authority.

[3]Burns Ind. Code Ann. §25-23-1-30 (1995) specifically states that prescriptive authority not required for administration of anesthesia.

TABLE 23-1. *(cont.)*				
Louisiana[4]	CNM, NP, CNS	Non-controlled drugs only except as specifically authorized by the Joint Administration Committee	Yes	Joint promulgation of rules by Board of Nursing and Board of Medical Examiners. BON has total enforcement authority.
Maine*	NP, CNM	III–V	Yes	New NP works with a collaborating physician for the first two years.[5]
Maryland*	NP[6]	II–V	Yes	Written agreement between MD and NP.
Massachusetts*	NP, CNS[7]	II–VI	Yes	Orders to manufacturer/wholesalers limited to schedule VI only.
Michigan	NP	Noncontrolled drugs only	Yes	Physicians may delegate the prescribing of drugs to RNs, excluding controlled substances.[9]
Minnesota*	NP, CNS	II–V	Yes	NPs must have agreement with physician in order to prescribe; nurse midwives do not need to.
Mississippi(M)	NP	Noncontrolled drugs only	Yes	Protocols are required in order to prescribe. They must be on file with the BON.
Missouri	APN[10], CNM, CNP, CNS, CRNA	Noncontrolled substances only	Yes	Can prescribe noncontrolled substances as a delegated medical act through collaborative agreement *or* protocols and the requirements are jointly determined by BON and BHA through rules.

---

[4]Bill signed by Louisiana legislature to provide limited prescriptive authority in collaborative practice, May 1995.

[5]Under new law, new NP must practice under supervision before he or she is allowed to practice independently. Also, the NP retains a copy of the collaborative agreement.

[6]Prescriptive authority for NPs only, not for nurse psychotherapists.

[7]Psychiatric clinical nurse specialist.

[8]In Massachusetts all prescription medications not classified by the federal government as II–V are categorized as Schedule VI.

[9]Michigan considering legislation on starter dosages.

[10]Under new law, new APN must practice under supervision before he/she is allowed to practice independently. Also, the new APN retains a copy of the collaborative agreement.

(continued)

TABLE 23-1. *(cont.)*

State	Type of Practitioner	Drug Schedules Under Which Practitioner Has Authority to Prescribe	Is Practice Agreement Collaboration, or Protocol Required to Prescribe?	Remarks
Montana*	NP Nurse Specialist to include: CNM and some CNS	II–V	No	No protocol required for prescribing. Schedule II limited to a 72-hour supply.
Nebraska	NP, CNS	III–V	Yes	This entire issue is in a state of flux. A legal opinion has been issued that states, because authority to prescribe is granted through the practice agreement by protocol, therefore DEA numbers cannot be issued. A final decision will be made soon.
Nevada*	APN, CNS[11]	Noncontrolled substances	Yes	Must also apply to Board of Pharmacy. No controlled substances drugs may be listed in protocol. APNs can only administer and dispense scheduled II–V drugs.
New Hampshire*	NP	II	No	Prescribing only allowed from state formulary for controlled and noncontrolled substances. No protocol required for prescribing.
New Jersey	NP, CNS+	Noncontrolled drugs	Yes	Medication protocols are required to prescribe. No practice protocols are required.
New Mexico*	NP, CNS+	II–V	No	Each NP must work under individual MD with formulary certified by the BON.
New York*	NP, CNM	II–V	Yes	Collaborative relationship, with written practice agreements and protocols.

[11]If certified as advanced practice nurses.

TABLE 23-1. *(cont.)*				
North Carolina*	NP	II–V	Yes	NPs and CNMs have authority to prescribe drugs including controlled substances according to site-specific protocols. NPs and CNMs may also be approved by the NCBOP to compound and dispense drugs.
North Dakota*	NP, CNS+, CNM	II–V	Yes	Scope of practice statement is required, to cover collaboration.
	CNS, NP	Noncontrolled drugs	Yes	Per formulary under supervision.
Ohio*[12]	CNM, CNS, NP	Noncontrolled drugs, site restrictions	Yes	Demonstration project only: Per formulary under supervision.
Oklahoma	CNM, CNS, CNP	III–V	Yes	CNSs, CNPs, and CRNAs may prescribe from an exclusionary formulary within scope of practice, with physician supervision.
	CRNA, CRNS	II–V and legend drugs	Yes	CRNAs may prescribe from an inclusionary formulary within scope of practice with physician supervision. CRNAs may order, select, obtain, and administer legend drugs, Schedule II–V CDS, devices, and medical gases only when engaged in the preanesthetic preparation and evaluation; anesthesia induction, maintenance, and emergence, and post-anesthesia care, and only the perioperative or peri-obstetrical period, and under the supervision of a MD, DO, or dentist licensed in Oklahoma.

[12]Ohio has a pilot program for prescriptive authority, which is conducted at three sites: University of Cincinnati, Wright State University, and Case Western Reserve University. The pilot programs were extended until the year 2010. Also, the biennial budget bill includes language to allow nurses in the pilot program to "personally supply" patients with five of the most commonly prescribed medications. Prior to this APNs were the only prescribers in Ohio prohibited from dispensing.

(continued)

TABLE 23-1. *(cont.)*

State	Type of Practitioner	Drug Schedules Under Which Practitioner Has Authority to Prescribe	Is Practice Agreement Collaboration, or Protocol Required to Prescribe?	Remarks
Oregon*	NP	III–V	No	Pursuant to formulary determined by the Board of Nursing. No protocol required for practice.
Pennsylvania*	CNM, CRNA, NP	Cannot prescribe without physician's signature	Yes[13]	
Rhode Island*	NP, CNS+	Cannot prescribe scheduled drugs	Yes	Although NPs cannot apply for their own DEA number, this may change. Formulary is now required; NP must be in collaboration with MD[14].
	CNM	III–V	Yes	Certified nurse midwives are permitted to apply for their own DEA number.
South Carolina*	NP, CNS	V	Yes	Listing of drugs in the MD-approved SBON-approved protocol.
South Dakota	NP	III–IV	Yes	The BON Rules and Regulations state that although the NP may apply for an independent DEA number, the NP is not permitted to use it. The NP must be authorized by the primary physician to prescribe and must use a code consisting of the supervisory physician's DEA number and the suffix of the first four numbers of the RN's license number. The order must be reviewed and countersigned by supervisory physician at least weekly and may not be refilled without consent of supervisory physician.

[13]Although statutory authorization exists, joint rules not completed by Board of Nursing and Board of Medicine.

[14]State presently considering legislation to authorize CNS prescriptive authority.

TABLE 23-1. *(cont.)*				
Tennessee	NP, CNS, CNM, CRNA	Noncontrolled drugs	Yes	Upon receipt of a BON Certificate of Fitness to prescribe, nurses in advanced practice may write and sign prescriptions and/or issue drugs.
Texas	APNs (NPs, CNSs, CNMs, CRNAs)	Dangerous/ Legend Drugs (Noncontrolled Substances)	Yes	APNs (NPs, CNSs, CNMs, & CRNAs) may prescribe under physician delegation using protocols, standing orders, or other orders. Protocols need not take cookbook approach and should be defined "to promote exercise of professional judgment of APN." BON and BOM have defined broadly as "legal authorization to initiate medical aspects of patient care." Prescriptive authority is site-based but most practice sites are covered.
Utah	APRN	III–V, PA	Yes	Utah requires collaboration with a physician. Prescriptive practice collaboration is spelled out in a consultation referral plan, signed by the collaborating physician.
Vermont*	NP, CNS, CNM, CRNA	II–V	Yes	Must prescribe under collaborative guidelines, which do not necessarily spell out formulary. The focus is on scope of practice, referral, consultation, and quality. The BON reviews the agreements.
Virginia	NP[15], CNS+	II–V, VI	Yes	A practice agreement is required to prescribe; however, Schedule VI are prescribed per formulary.
Virgin Islands	CNS, NP	Noncontrolled drugs	Yes	Independent prescriptive authority.
Washington*	NP	V	No	
West Virginia*(M)	NP, CNW	III–V	Yes	Collaboration agreement is required to prescribe, and must include written guidelines or protocols for prescriptive authority.

---

[15]With the exception of CRNA.

(continued)

TABLE 23-1. *(cont.)*

State	Type of Practitioner	Drug Schedules Under Which Practitioner Has Authority to Prescribe	Is Practice Agreement Collaboration, or Protocol Required to Prescribe?	Remarks
Wisconsin*(M)	NP, CNM, CRNA, CNS	II–V	No	Independent prescriptive authority: however nurses must facilitate collaboration. Limitations on Schedule II drugs nurses can prescribe.
Wyoming*	NP, CNS	III–V and Legend Drugs	Yes	The BON is seeking permission from the DEA for nurses who have prescriptive authority to apply for their own independent DEA registration number. NPs must have a plan of referral to work with a physician as needed.
Guam	NP	None	Yes	Collaboration is required.

G:\wyc\CHARTS\prescrip\dea

©Data compiled by Winifred Y. Carson, ANA Nurse Practice Counsel

M = minimum mandatory malpractice insurance for nurses who have prescriptive authority.

CONCLUSION

There are many exciting new opportunities for nurses within the rapidly changing health care field today. The roles of advanced practice nursing continue to expand, but with this growth come new and challenging legal ramifications. Clinical research and technology will continue to provide new techniques that will save lives and improve care in ways undreamed of today, but along with these improvements will come the need for advanced skills and knowledge. With the oversupply of physicians, the decrease in hospital beds, and fewer traditional hospital nursing jobs, may come restrictions on practice for those in independent or advanced nursing roles. In order to provide the highest quality nursing care, the advanced practice nurse must keep abreast of developments within the legal world as well as the medical world.

REFERENCES

American Nurses Association. (1996). Scope and standards of advanced practice nursing. Kansas City: American Nurses Association.

Blouin, A. S., & Brent, N. J. (1996). Collide or collaborate? Changing reimbursement and legal challenges facing advanced nurse practitioners and physicians. Journal of Nursing Administration, 26, 10–12.

Chally, P. S., & Yorker, B. C. (1989). Legal parameters for expanded roles in nursing. Journal of Neuroscience Nursing, 21, 258–260.

Edmunds, M. W. (1992). Council's pursuit of national standardization for advanced practice nursing meets with resistance. Nurse Practitioner, 17, 81–83.

Fennell, K. S. (1991). Prescriptive authority for nurse-midwives. Nursing Clinics of North America, 26, 511–521.

Guido, G. W. (1988). Legal issues in nursing. Norwalk, CT: Appleton & Lange.

Henry, P. F. (1992). Analysis of standardized procedures and protocols: A legal viewpoint. Nurse Practitioner Forum, 3, 122–123.

Hogue, E. E. (1993). Managing your risk of liability. Pediatric Nursing, 19, 366-368.

Inglis, A. D., & Kjervik, D. K. (1993). Empowerment of advanced practice nurses: Regulation reform needed to increase access to care. Journal of Law, Medicine and Ethics, 21, 193–205.

Jenkins, S. M. (1994). The myth of vicarious liability. Journal of Nurse-Midwifery, 39, 98–106.

Kraus, N. (1990). Practicing nurse-midwifery in the medical-legal climate. Journal of Nurse-Midwifery, 35, 307–314.

Loeb, S. (Ed.). (1992). Nurses handbook of law & ethics. Springhouse, PA: Springhouse Corp.

McBeth, A., Koerner, J., & Ethridge, P. (1993). Advanced licensure/mandatory credentialing: A nurse executive point of view. Nursing Management, 24, 45–47.

Moon, B. J. (1990). Prescriptive authority and nurse-midwives. Journal of Nurse-Midwifery, 35, 50–52.

Person, L. J. (1996). Annual update of how each state stands on legislative issues affecting advanced nursing practice. Nurse Practitioner, 21, 10–70.

Reinert, B. R., & Buck, E. A. (1989). Issues in liability insurance and the nursing consultant. Clinical Nurse Specialist, 3, 42–45.

Report of the Texas Medical Association Special Committee on the Texas Physicians Workforce. (Oct. 23, 1996).

Rowe, B. B. (1989). Expanding the nurse's role to diagnosis and treatment: Understanding the legal significance. AAOHN Journal, 37, 198–199.

Sharp, N. (1994). Recognizing APNs: It's now or never. Nursing Management, 25, 14–16.

Smith, S. A. (1993). Obtaining hospital privileges for the advanced practice nurse. Journal of Pediatric Health Care, 7, 292–293.

Smrcina, C. (1993). Licensure of advanced practice nursing: What's our position? Orthopaedic Nursing, 12, 9–13.

Survillo, A. I., & Levine, A. T. (1993). Strategies to limit CNS malpractice liability exposure. Clinical Nurse Specialist, 7, 215–220.

Williams, D. R. (1994). Credentialing Certified Nurse-Midwives. Journal of Nurse-Midwifery, 39, 258–264.

Yorker, B. C. (1989). Scope of Practice: Case Law. AAOHN Journal, 37, 80–81.

CASE CITATIONS

Bellegie v. Board of Nurse Examiners, 685 S. W.2d 431 (1985).

Chalmers-Francis v. Nelson, 6 Cal. 2d 402 (1936).

Commonwealth v. Porn, 196 Mass. 326, 82 N. E. 31 (1907).

Cooper v. National Motor Bearing Co., 136 Cal. App. 2d 229, 288 P.2d 581 (1955).

Corcoran v. United Heathcare, Inc. 91-3322 (U. S. Ct. App. 1992).

Fein v. Permanente Medical Group, 38 Cal. 3d 137 (1985).

Hernicz v. Fla. Dept. of Professional Regulation, 390 So. 2d 194 (Dist. Ct. App. 1980).

Kyslinger v. United States, 406 F. Supp. 800 (W. D. Pa. 1975).

Leigh v. Board of Registration in Nursing, 395 Mass. 670, 481 N.E.2d 1347 (1985).

Lunsford v. Board of Nurse Examiners, 648 S.W.2d 391 (Tex. Civ. App. Austin 1983).

Olson v. Bolstad, 161 Minn. 419, 201 N.W. 918 (1925).

O'Neill v. Montefiore Hospital, 202 N.Y.S. 2d 436, 11 A. D. 2d 132 (1960).

Sermchief v. Gonzales, 660 S.W.2d 683 (Mo. 1983).

Stablin v. Hilton Hotels Corp., 484 F.2d 580 (7th Cir. 1973).

Toth v. Community Hospital at Glen Cove, 239 N.E.2d 368 (N. Y. 1968).

Tuma v. Board of Nursing, 100 Idaho 74, 593 P. 2d 711 (1979).

Whitney v. Day, 100 Mich. App. 707, 300 N.W.2d 380 (Ct. App. 1980).

Wickline v. State of California, 192 Cal. app. 3d 1630, 228 Cal. Rptr. 661 (1986).

Wilson v. Blue Cross of Southern California, 222 Cal. App. 3d 660, 271 Cal. Rptr. 876 (1990).

CHAPTER 24

Computer Technology: Legal and Practice Issues

Cathy Beffa

You are a nurse working in a labor and delivery unit in a hospital. One of your patients happens to be the ex-wife of an emergency room physician in the hospital. Your patient has AIDS. You want to "protect" the other patients and staff so you access the physician's confidential medical file and find that he is HIV-positive. Is this appropriate use of computer information? Have you incurred any liability on your part and on behalf of the hospital? Was there a "need to know" this information, and what actions should you and the hospital take?

This is just one example of the many computer issues in health care today. In this example, the nurse did not have a "need to know" the HIV status of her OB patient's ex-husband who was a hospital physician. Without a "need to know" or "business purpose," accessing the physician's medical record would result in a legal breach of confidentiality by the nurse. The hospital would be liable for breach of confidentiality on the part of its nurse-employee.

A similar situation occurred in *Estate Of William Behringer, M.D. v. The Medical Center At Princeton* (1991). In this case, a physician was admitted to the hospital where he was on staff as a plastic surgeon. His admitting diagnosis was *pneumocystis carinii* pneumonia (PCP) and he was diagnosed as

HIV-positive during the same admission. The hospital was ultimately found liable for breach of confidentiality for failing to take reasonable precautions regarding its health care worker's (the doctor on its staff) medical record to prevent his AIDS-related diagnosis from becoming a matter of public knowledge. Furthering the invasion of the surgeon's right to confidentiality, upon delivering the diagnosis of AIDS at the bedside of the plastic surgeon, the treating physician, who was also a personal friend and colleague of the patient, stated that he had told his wife, who was also a personal friend, about the diagnosis. Privacy issues become even more blurred when coworkers are also friends.

Although technological advances increase the efficacy of health care delivery and reduce costs, the advances must be balanced against the patient's rights of privacy and confidentiality. A dilemma results in the slow development of protective laws and professional and organizational practice standards regarding privacy and confidentiality issues. The use of computers in the health care setting expands the nurse's professional and ethical role to include patient advocacy both at the bedside while delivering care and "at the keyboard" when transmitting and overseeing the use of confidential computer information.

THE LEGAL BASIS: PRIVACY AND CONFIDENTIALITY

Privacy includes the right of individuals to control disclosure of their personal medical information. Confidentiality includes the understanding that medical information will only be disclosed to an authorized user.

The legal right to privacy is a constitutional right, and is derived from the Fourteenth Amendment of the United States Constitution, which establishes the right of an individual to make autonomous decisions regarding his or her own medical care (*Roe v. Wade,* 1973). This landmark Supreme Court decision regarding a woman's right to an abortion clarified that an implied constitutional right to privacy exists within the explicit right to personal liberty.

Confidentiality is a right derived by statute. A statute is a state law, and all states have confidentiality statutes. These statutes attach legal rights and status to certain relationships including the relationship of doctor and patient, and lawyer and client (Feutz-Harter, 1993). Health maintenance organizations and other health care institutions are considered statutory entities and are obligated to maintain patient confidentiality. All employees, regardless of their position within the HMO, are under the umbrella of the confidentiality statute in their particular jurisdiction, and are bound by law to maintain patient confidentiality.

Nurses who have authorized access to patient information are under a professional obligation to avoid improperly disclosing that information. An ethical obligation also exists to be sensitive to certain types of patient information, which if released irresponsibly could damage an individual's employment status, reputation, and family relationships. Examples of the more sensitive types of health care information include mental health information; substance abuse information; HIV and AIDS information; and information regarding abortion, contraception, and sexually transmitted diseases. Numerous examples of the "potential for harm" pertaining to improper disclosure of HIV or AIDS information were cited in *Doe v. Barrington* (1990). Examples of a hysterical public reaction to AIDS included removal of a teacher with AIDS from teaching duties, refusal to rent an apartment to male homosexuals for fear of AIDS, and firebombing the home of hemophiliac children who tested positive for HIV.

Breaches of confidentiality can occur through improper use of computer information and by fax and answering machines, when private patient information is accessed, transmitted, or recorded.

THE AUTOMATED MEDICAL RECORD

Protecting the confidentiality of the written medical record is a simple and controlled process. A policy governing release of medical information and restricting access to the medical record area provides greater assurance of privacy and confidentiality than is afforded to individuals in this age of computer use, where information is literally at one's fingertips. Ironically, federal laws protect the privacy of video rental information, but no such protection is provided to ensure patient privacy regarding information found in medical records (*Washington Post,* 1996). Information systems are commonplace in many health care institutions, many with fully automated or computerized medical records, or large parts of the medical record on line. Nurses must be aware of the implications of computer use when it comes to the electronic use and disclosure of confidential information. The health care institution must enhance and support this awareness through appropriate policies, training regarding confidentiality, and adequate information systems and technology as a means to prevent electronic breaches of confidentiality and privacy. As *Behringer* demonstrates, more is required than simply instructing employees that medical records are confidential where charts are fully accessible to virtually all personnel.

COMPUTER SAFEGUARDS

Safeguards employed by an organization for computer use are only as good as the integrity of the employees who use them and to the degree the institution will oversee and safeguard the use of private computer information. Applicable computer safeguards include

- the use of individual access codes for computer use,
- policies covering the overall information system use,
- training regarding confidentiality and computer use, and
- frequent monitoring of access to information for a "need to know" purpose.

Access numbers for computer use allow an organization to control and monitor those who use the system and the appropriateness of that use. The number can be encrypted upon system entry and used as a check method later. This requires the cooperation of employees regarding the confidentiality and sole use of their individual access codes. Disciplinary measures should be implemented for improper code use, improper access of certain types of information, and certainly for improper disclosure of confidential information. Even an employee acting outside the scope of his or her employment would not preclude hospital liability for breach of confidentiality where the hospital has not taken reasonable measures to safeguard patient confidentiality (*Berbhringer,* 1991).

A policy governing confidential use of computer information is mandatory in health care organizations today. The use of computers makes it more difficult to protect patient privacy and confidentiality even though it offers better communication of patient information. A confidentiality policy governing computer use and information should include a requirement for the use of an individual access code, a provision requiring any outside vendor to sign and uphold the organization's confidentiality policy, provisions governing the use of modems that would allow outside or Internet access to the organization's network, and provisions related to access allowed only for "legitimate business purposes" as well as disciplinary action for "casual browsing" of files.

Training is an essential component of any organizational policy. Communication regarding confidentiality and computer use must be ongoing. An organizational policy is no defense to liability for breach of confidentiality or invasion of privacy if it has not been communicated

to the employees and implemented on a timely basis. Presentation to all new employees during new employee orientation assures that information regarding access codes and overall confidentiality measures and policies is adequately communicated.

However, some courts have gone so far as to say that an employer's policy need not be explicit if the employee "knew or should have known" that his or her actions would constitute a breach of confidentiality and that person's actions showed an intent to disregard a standard of behavior the employer had a right to expect (*Darlene Tehven v. Job Service North Dakota, 1992*). Tehven involved an employee of the medical records department who knew that she was not supposed to access her husband's medical records but did so anyway.

Organizations must make it a practice to monitor the appropriateness of employee computer use based on a "need to know" or "business purpose" rule. At Boston's Beth Israel Hospital, a "tag" is attached to any patient's information that has a greater risk of being looked at by another employee (Safran, 1995). If someone attempts to access this information, he or she is met with a broadcast message regarding confidentiality as a reminder that accessing the information may be communicated to the patient or the patient's physician. This is just one method used to curtail "browsing" of private information.

A critical legal responsibility of all health care organizations, which are said to "own" the medical record regardless of whether the records are written or computerized, is to maintain and preserve the medical record. The medical record is the property of the institution, which is the custodian of that medical record (Reed, 1996). As such, the institution is required to maintain that record for a certain period of time determined by the particular state or jurisdiction, which includes maintaining the privacy and confidentiality of the record at all times.

Nursing Practice Safeguards for Computer Use

Because it is usually the nurse who will enter important patient information into the computer, one commonsense reminder is to check the accuracy of that information to be entered. Once the information is computerized, there is less chance that an error will be discovered that could harm patient care or damage the patient at a later date. Electronic or computer error detection is more likely in other industries such as banking, where a mistake on an account can be detected immediately and corrected. Entering a mistaken diagnosis or test result on a medical record, such as HIV-positive, can have lasting repercussions and cause irreparable harm to the patient. Although some states allow patients access to their own medical record information, few patients know everything that has been recorded about them, which minimizes the chance to catch a serious error before it has been disseminated.

Nurses must be cognizant of the use of monitors. A nurse who will be steps away from the workstation for any time should check to be sure there is no private patient information that could be viewed by someone walking by the screen. Screen savers are recommended for this purpose, but prudent practice requires the nurse to sign off if away from the area for any substantial length of time.

Fax machines can also be a source of a breach of confidentiality. Fax machines are often located in public, high-traffic areas in health care settings. If faxing highly sensitive patient information (such as HIV status or test results, or substance abuse patient information), the nurse should make provisions for someone specific to be on the receiving end of the fax. Highly sensitive patient information should never be in public view. The same is true of answering machines. Private patient information should not be recorded on an answering machine or voice mail unless the patient expressly consents to receive information in this manner. Clearly, information contained in the medical record and that maintained on a health care computer network is private patient information, and must be treated with strict confidentiality. In most cases, that means that a signed patient consent is required for release of any of that confidential information. The limits of the consent should be documented in the medical record.

PUBLIC VERSUS PRIVATE INFORMATION

Standard III of the Joint Commission on Accreditation of Hospitals states: "Medical records shall be confidential, secure, current, authenticated, legible, and complete" (Accreditation Manual For Hospitals, 1996). A hospital that does not meet this requirement risks losing JCAHO accreditation. The commission is presently focusing on health care computer networks, and intends to provide a comprehensive evaluation of those systems.

Public information is information that is accessible through a public forum. The individual seeking public information usually has a "right to know" the information. The overall classification of the information is not deemed sensitive or harmful to an individual's privacy.

An example of the public "right to know" is found in the Freedom of Information Act, a broad act that allows individuals access to government agency information (The Freedom of Information Act, 5 U.S.C. §552), but does not allow for access to private individual records.

In 1993, an interesting situation occurred that illustrated the conflict between the public's right to know versus the protection of the private interests regarding when to release information. The situation involved Vince Foster, the White House counsel who allegedly committed suicide in the fall of 1993 while a member of the White House staff. An investigation ensued and information from his medical and personnel file at the White House was sought via the Freedom of Information Act. The information was not provided because neither medical nor personnel information could be released without the individual's signed consent (or in this case, the surviving family's consent) (*Washington Post,* 1993).

What then is the classification of a hospital or health care organization's computer information as it pertains to release of that information? First of all, the patient medical records and general business information "belong" to the organization, both in written and computerized form. These records are classified as "business assets" and the organization bears the responsibility of safeguarding the privacy and confidentiality of the patient medical record. The staff must uphold that responsibility and safeguard the confidentiality of the organization's "corporate assets," which include the medical records and any other data or information that is maintained or stored in the computer system. Both types of information must be accessed and released for appropriate business purposes only. This responsibility may be part of an internal policy, which might be discussed in a new employee orientation where new employees would then sign a confidentiality statement. In this age of technology where the use of computers is far ahead of legal protections when it comes to confidentiality or privacy, it is critical that institutions have sound policies that are well implemented and understood by all staff.

LEGISLATION: MEDICAL RECORDS ON THE INTERNET

The conflict surrounding the privacy of computerized medical records is evidenced by health care legislation involving the portability of health care insurance for individuals transferring or leaving jobs. This legislation is formally titled "The Health Insurance Portability and Accountability Act (Pub. L. 104-191) but is more often referred to as the "Kennedy-Kassebaum" bill after its cosponsors, Senators Nancy Landon Kassebaum (R-KS) and Edward Kennedy (D-MA). The bill was passed by Congress and signed into law by President Clinton in the summer of 1996, and has opened some hot debate on individual privacy and confidentiality due to the portability aspect of the bill. What does this mean for privacy and confidentiality?

In order to facilitate the "portability" feature of the bill, there are provisions for the development of a health information network and requirements that certain data be stored and transmitted electronically. The "Administrative Simplifications" portion of the bill contains computer regulations requirements for the network, which will be put in place for the transfer and storage of data that include private and confidential patient information (Sections 251 and 252 of Subtitle F of Title II of the House Bill).

Physicians and health care organizations will be required to have systems in place for the transfer and storage of this patient data, or to use data clearinghouses that will administer this aspect of the bill for them. Associated with this feature of the bill are requirements that have been promulgated by the Secretary of Health and Human Services regarding privacy and confidentiality safeguards.

The main issue becomes a balancing act between privacy and confidentiality versus access. Within 42 months of the enactment of the bill, there must be regulations in place designed to protect patient privacy and confidentiality associated with the electronic transfer and storage of confidential information. There are also privacy issues that deal with the storage and printing of this information.

Other organizations provide a variety of suggestions for maintaining principles of data integrity, confidentiality, and availability. The Electronic Privacy Information Center (EPIC) calls for security and controls that include

- medical records in storage or transit to be encrypted,
- audit trails that track every access to a patient's file, and
- access limited to a relevant function for each user.

In the absence of relevant state and federal computer privacy regulations, organizations and individuals must exert due diligence to safeguard patient privacy and confidentiality when it comes to the use of computer information.

ETHICAL RESPONSIBILITIES

Just as there exists the "letter and the spirit of the law" so too are there statutes and written organizational policies regarding confidentiality and the tone and manner in which they are upheld or maintained. The "spirit" of privacy and confidentiality for patients lies in each individual's ethical responsibility and accountability.

A question nurses should consider when determining whether they are upholding their ethical responsibility when it comes to privacy and confidentiality is how would they respond if they saw someone release confidential information inappropriately. Inappropriately includes through conversation, showing something on the screen to someone who did not have a business purpose for knowing it, and talking about a co-worker's test results or medical condition when there was no medical or business reason to be accessing that information or discussing it. The ethical response would be to intervene on the spot, or report it to the appropriate supervisor. Too many times the excuse of "not wanting to get involved" or "it's none of my business— I'm not the supervisor" causes nurses to overlook these breaches of confidentiality. The appropriate ethical and accountable response makes these issues everyone's responsibility. This is especially true regarding the fast advancing technological and computer information age about which security experts agree that it may be another two to three years before adequate privacy safeguards are in place when it comes to computer use, storage, and transfer of private patient information.

COMPUTER PRIVACY GUIDELINES FOR NURSES

The American Nurses' Association Code for Nurses states: "The nurse safeguards the client's right to privacy by judiciously protecting information of a confidential nature." This code provision predated the surge of technology in health care settings, and state boards of nursing now turn their attention to technological safeguards for patient information in health care settings.

The 1995 Delegate Assembly of the National Council of State Boards commissioned a Telecommunications Issues Task Force, which was charged with the duty to "study telecommunications practice across jurisdictional lines." Furthermore, the task force defined telenursing as "the practice of nursing over distance using telecommunications technology." Computers, e-mail, and faxes were among the types of technology more commonly used in the practice of telenursing. Examples of the practice of nursing using technology include obtaining test results,

patient education, teleconferencing, telephone triage across state lines, and electronic charting.

A hospital nurse who has authorized access to patients' medical charts is under a professional obligation not to disclose that information inappropriately. There is no technological mechanism to ensure that the nurse will not reveal any of the sensitive patient information. Lack of awareness regarding privacy and confidentiality is one of the main reasons for breaches of patient confidentiality. Increasing awareness of the basic tenets of private information, sensitizing nurses to types of private information, which when disclosed can cause irreparable harm, and enforcing penalties for breaches of confidentiality will often have positive and far-reaching results.

Guidelines for preventing breach of confidentiality can be used when using computers for charting, storing information, printing it, or otherwise transmitting the data. First, patient information should be consistent with the written medical record. Any patient information that is computerized is private and confidential including nurses' notes, lab and other test results, doctor's progress notes, and any consultations. It is the responsibility of the hospital or health care organization to implement meaningful restrictions on access to medical records (*Behringer,* 1991). Even demographic information is confidential and should not be accessed or disclosed without a business purpose, including name, address, and phone numbers of both staff and patients.

Without any national standards in place, actual workplace examples become instructive. Certain types of confidentiality situations arise in health care settings that illustrate the correct response to ensure patient and employee privacy. Examples include employer/employee issues, family members seeking patient information, employee confidentiality, clinical information in nonclinical settings, and third-party disclosure situations.

Employer/Employee Information

A staff nurse calls in sick one day and the supervisor wants more information about the illness. Can the supervisor access additional information about the sick employee in the computer if it's available? No, the information should not be obtained without the employee's consent. If an employee had a problem with chronic absenteeism, the supervisor would have a right to certain additional information to substantiate the illness and the employee's ability to work, but the information would still have to be obtained using proper channels.

Family Members Seeking Family Information

A man calls seeking information about his pregnant wife and wants appointment information related to her visit that day. The information is available on your computer, yet the nurse cannot answer his questions. Husbands and wives have strict confidentiality when it comes to individual medical record information including appointment histories. Policies typically include information regarding husband/wife situations when it comes to access of medical record information and include such measures as absolute restriction of that information on the part of either spouse. In a situation where that policy requirement was violated, a wife not only lost her longstanding job, but was also denied unemployment compensation benefits related to the breach of confidentiality (*Tehven,* 1992).

Specific health care issues give adolescents adult status regarding confidentiality Those issues include

- sexually transmitted disease information, pregnancy-related issues, including contraception and birth control;
- HIV;
- mental health concerns; and
- substance abuse.

(Maryland Code Annotated, Health-General §§20-101, -102, and -104). The rationale for this statutory protection is to encourage adolescents to seek treatment for such conditions. If they are not forced to tell an authority figure (such as a parent), they are more likely to seek treatment. In all other situations where the adolescent is under the age of majority (age 18 in most jurisdictions) parental consent is required to treat.

Confidentiality issues related to minors can be distinguished from consent-to-treat issues for minors. For example, an adolescent is being followed for pregnancy, which is one of the confidentiality exceptions. The information regarding her pregnancy can not be released without her consent. During her pregnancy, she needs surgery for an appendicitis. Consent must be obtained from a parent or guardian for the surgery.

Employee Information

One of your fellow nurses is having her birthday next month, but no one knows exactly what day. Is it appropriate to check her birth date in the computer if your nurse supervisor authorizes the search? No. Demographic staff information is confidential, including birth dates, telephone numbers, and addresses, unless the employee chooses to share that information. Accessing demographic information is a breach of confidentiality on the part of the staff person and the supervisor.

Clinical Information in a Non-Clinical Setting

You are working in the billing office of a large HMO. You receive a phone call from a man wanting to know the nature of his wife's office visit. (He just received the bill and she will be paying it.) The wife was seen for a positive pregnancy test, and has decided to terminate the pregnancy. Can you give him this information for billing purposes? No. Financial concerns are not a reason to breach patient confidentiality. Also, the husband–wife confidentiality principle prohibits disclosure of this information.

Third Party Disclosure

You are a nurse in a busy obstetric office practice. You get a phone call from someone you don't know who identifies himself as a doctor. This "doctor" says he is treating one of your patients (patients are sent to outside referrals for some conditions), and he says he is in a hurry. He is demanding at the outset. You're new and want to do a good job. He wants to know whether or not the patient has ever had an abortion. Can you give the "doctor" this information? No. First of all, a "red flag" should arise when information about abortion is being requested. Abortion information is in the more sensitive category of medical information, which if disclosed inappropriately can cause harm to an individual. Courts have classified abortion information as protected both as "vital record" information and "medical record" information and have denied access for confidentiality reasons even when requested under the Freedom of Information Act (*Arkansas Department of Health v. Westark Christian Action Council*, 910 S.W.2d, 322 Ark. 440.

Confidential patient information should never be given over the phone unless the identity of the caller is known and can be verified. Even if this were an outside consultant, a release of information signed by the patient should be in the medical record in order for you to release confidential information. In cases where you have personal knowledge of ongoing treatment and you are able to verify the identity of the caller, it could be appropriate to disclose this information.

These kinds of confidentiality questions, which arise in our health care environment today—and which may be even more complicated and confusing when it comes to computer use, storage, and transmittal of private patient data—mandate the nurse to have knowledge and awareness of an institution's internal computer confidentiality policy, as the first step toward avoiding breaches of confidentiality. However, knowledge alone is not enough. A level of sensitivity is also critical when making decisions about privacy and disclosure of patient information. Even if the information is not considered highly sensitive to most people, if it is a part of the medical record and stored or maintained in a computer database, it is confidential information. The patient has a right to disclose personal, confidential information. It is the responsibility of the nurse to maintain patient confidentiality.

Confidentiality Guidelines

Basic guidelines for easy reference are set forth in Display 24-1. When in doubt, the nurse should err on the side of caution and not disclose what might be protected information. There have been cases where well-meaning staff in the interest of "helping" someone, or making the person "feel better" about something they may have seen or heard about a patient, provide confidential patient information; as a result, patient confidentiality is breached. In family or social situations, nurses have been known to let their guard down and breach patient confidentiality.

CONCLUSION

As Congress moves forward to enact computer privacy regulations with other federal legislation on the horizon related to computer privacy, the basic principles regarding patient privacy issues and confidentiality remain the same. Patient privacy and confidentiality will only be safe to the extent that each individual health care provider remains professional and accountable.

REFERENCES

Feutz, Sheryl A. (1993). <u>Nursing and the Law</u> (5th ed.). Professional Education Systems.

Freedom of Information Act, 5 U.S.C.S.552.

Health Insurance Portability and Accountability Act, Pub. L. 104-191, (Sections 251 and 252 of Subtitle F of Title II of the House Bill.

DISPLAY 24-1

Confidentiality Guidelines

In general, do not discuss patient information with

- one patient about another patient
- relatives and friends of the patient
- visitors in any setting
- the news media
- fellow workers, except for a work situation
- your own relatives and friends in family and social settings

Joint Commission on Accreditation of Healthcare Organizations. (1996). <u>1996 Accreditation Manual for Hospitals.</u> Oakbrook Terrace, IL: Author.

Maryland Code Annotated, Health-General §20-101, -102, and -104.

Reed, Kimberly. (1996, November 4). Managing the security of computerized records. <u>Nurs Spectr, 6</u>(23), 5.

Safran, C., Rind, D., Citroen, M., Bakkar, A. R., Slack, W. V., & Bleich, H., L. Protection of confidentiality in the computer-based patient record. <u>MD Comput,</u> 12, 187–192.

Schwartz, John. (1996, August 4). Health insurance reform bill may undermine privacy of patients' records. <u>The Washington Post,</u> p. A23.

CASE CITATIONS

Arkansas Department of Health v. Westark Christian Action Council, 910 S.W.2d 199 (1995).

Darlene Tehven v Job Service North Dakota, 488 N.W. 2d 48 (1992).

Doe v. Barrington, 729 F. Supp. 384, n.

Estate of William Behringer, MD v. The Medical Center at Princeton, 592 A.2d 1251 (1991).

Roe v. Wade, 410 U.S. 113 (1973).

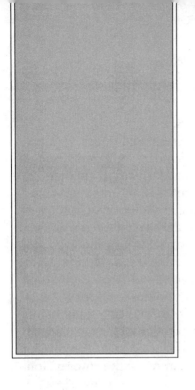

Glossary

Affidavit A written statement made or taken under oath before an officer of the court or a notary public or other person authorized to act.

Allegation In pleading, an assertion of fact.

Answer The pleading on the part of the defendant in response to the plaintiff's complaint.

Arbitration The conducting of a trial in front of one or more arbitrators (usually malpractice attorneys or retired judges) who act in place of the judge and jury, and who decide the case.

Attest To affirm as true; to sign one's name as a witness to the execution of the document; to bear witness to.

Bailiff A court attendant, usually a Sheriff's deputy, who maintains order in the courtroom.

Breach of Contract The failure to perform the terms of a contract as agreed without legal justification.

Case Law Decisions by the courts.

Cause of Action The particular facts that give rise to a right of action or legal right to sue.

Civil That branch of law that pertains to suits outside of criminal practice, pertaining to rights and duties of persons in contract, tort, and so on.

Common Law The system of jurisprudence that originated in England and was later applied to the United States. It is law based on judicial precedent.

Comparative Negligence The proportional sharing between plaintiff and defendant of compensation for injuries, based on the relative negligence of the two; the reduction of damages is made according to the relative negligence of each party.

Defendant The person against whom the suit is brought.

Deponent A witness; one who gives information, concerning some fact or facts known to him, under oath in a deposition. Any witness can be deposed, even if not a party to the lawsuit.

Deposition A method of pretrial discovery that consists of a statement of a witness under oath taken in question-and-answer form as it would be in court, with opportunity given to the adversary to be present and to cross-examine the witness.

Discovery Modern pretrial procedure by which one party gains vital information concerning the case held by the adverse party, including depositions and interrogatories.

Doctrine of Foreseeability Individual is liable for all natural and proximate consequences of any negligent acts to another individual to whom a duty is owed.

Due Care That degree of care or concern that would or should be exercised by an ordinary person in the same situation.

Evidence All means by which any alleged matter of fact is established or disproved.

327

Evidence includes the testimony of witnesses, introduction of records, documents, exhibits, and so on.

Expert Witness One who possesses special knowledge, skills, and experience in a specific area, and whose testimony as to his or her opinion is admissible as evidence.

Hearsay Rule Evidence of a statement that is made other than by a witness while testifying at a hearing or at a trial offered to prove the truth of the matter asserted. This evidence is inadmissible, unless one of the many exceptions to this rule apply. One important exception to this rule is statements made by a patient to a health care provider for the purpose of obtaining medical care. These statements are admissible.

Immunity Protection from being sued.

Impeachment The discrediting of a witness's testimony; the possible grounds include lack of knowledge or capacity, bias, or adverse interest.

Informed Consent Apprising a patient of the nature and risks and acceptable alternatives concerning the health care procedure or treatment proposed.

Interrogatories A method of pretrial discovery in which written questions are proposed by one party and served on the adversary party; written replies must be made under oath. Interrogatories can only be served to the parties named in the action.

Judgment A determination of the rights of the parties; a decision given by the court at the end of the proceedings.

Jurist A legal scholar; one versed in law; also used to refer to a judge.

Juror Person sworn as a member of a jury; also a person selected for jury duty but not yet chosen for a case.

Legal Permitted or authorized by law.

Liability An obligation one has incurred or might incur through any act or failure to act, responsibility for conduct falling below a certain standard, which is the cause of the plaintiff's injury.

Litigation A trial in court to determine legal issues and the rights and duties between parties.

Malpractice Professional misconduct, improper discharge of professional duties, or a failure to meet the standard of care by a professional that results in harm to another.

Negligence Failure to act as an ordinary prudent person; conduct contrary to that of a reasonable person under specific circumstances.

Party Any plaintiff or defendant involved in a given case.

Plaintiff The person who brings a civil suit seeking damages or other legal relief.

Privileged Communication Statements made to one in a position of trust, usually an attorney, physician, or spouse. Because of the confidential nature of the information, the law may protect it from being revealed, even in court, under certain circumstances.

Proximate Cause Legal concept of cause and effect; that which produces an event, and without which the injury would not have occurred.

Reasonable Care That degree of skill and knowledge customarily used by a competent health practitioner of similar education and experience in treating and caring for patients.

Records Written official documentation of what has happened to a particular patient during a specific period of time. An agency's business record.

Respondeat Superior "Let the master answer." The employer is responsible for the legal consequences of the acts of the employee while acting within the scope of his or her employment.

Standard of Care The conduct that a prudent nurse with similar education, training, and experience would undertake in similar circumstances; the standard to which the defendant's conduct is compared to ascertain negligence.

Statute of Limitations A legal limit on the time one has to file a suit in civil matters, usually measured from the time the wrong was or should have been discovered.

Subpoena A court order compelling the appearance of a witness at a judicial proceeding.

Tort A legal or civil wrong committed by one person against the person or property of another.

INDEX

Page numbers followed by d refer to displays; those followed by t refer to tables.

A